IAPSM's

Textbook of

Vaccinology

IAPSM's
Textbook of
Vaccinology

Editor-in-Chief

Annarao Kulkarni MBBS MD DPH DHA
Professor
Department of Community Medicine
Sri Madhusudan Sai Institute of Medical Sciences and Research
Karnataka, India

Editor

Krupal J Joshi MBBS MD PGDHHM FCMA FIMSA MNAMS
Associate Dean (Research) (I/C)
Associate Professor
Department of Community and Family Medicine
All India Institute of Medical Sciences
Rajkot, Gujarat, India

Associate Editors

Pentapati Siva Santosh Kumar MBBS MD FFM
Medical Officer – E (Assistant Professor)
Department of Preventive Oncology
Tata Memorial Centre
Varanasi, Uttar Pradesh, India

Anwita Khaitan MBBS MD
Assistant Professor
Department of Community and Family Medicine
All India Institute of Medical Sciences-CAPFIMS
New Delhi, India

Forewords

AM Kadri
Purushottam Giri

JAYPEE

JAYPEE BROTHERS MEDICAL PUBLISHERS
The Health Sciences Publisher
New Delhi | London

Jaypee Brothers Medical Publishers (P) Ltd

Headquarters
EMCA House
23/23-B, Ansari Road, Daryaganj
New Delhi 110 002, India
Landline: +91-11-23272143, +91-11-23272703
+91-11-23282021, +91-11-23245672
E-mail: jaypee@jaypeebrothers.com

Corporate Office
Jaypee Brothers Medical Publishers (P) Ltd.
4838/24, Ansari Road, Daryaganj
New Delhi 110 002, India
Phone: +91-11-43574357
Fax: +91-11-43574314
E-mail: jaypee@jaypeebrothers.com

Overseas Office
JP Medical Ltd.
83, Victoria Street, London
SW1H 0HW (UK)
Phone: +44-20 3170 8910
Fax: +44(0)20 3008 6180
E-mail: info@jpmedpub.com

Website: www.jaypeebrothers.com
Website: www.jaypeedigital.com

Inquiries for bulk sales may be solicited at: jaypee@jaypeebrothers.com

IAPSM's Textbook of Vaccinology / Annarao Kulkarni
First Edition: **2025**
ISBN: 978-93-6616-539-4
Printed at: Samrat Offset Pvt. Ltd.

Dedicated to

The tireless efforts of the vaccinators of our country—they are our guardian angels, making each life they touch less ordinary.

Contributors

Abhishek Kumar MBBS MD DNB MNAMS
Associate Professor
Community Medicine
Manipal Tata Medical College
Jamshedpur, Jharkhand
Manipal Academy of Higher Education
Manipal, Karnataka, India

Abhishek Padhi MBBS MD PDCC
Assistant Professor
Department of Microbiology
All India Institute of Medical Sciences
Rajkot, Gujarat, India

Achal Shetty MBBS MD MSc(Psychology)
Associate Professor
Department of Community Medicine
Father Muller Medical College
Mangaluru, Karnataka, India

Akanksha Gupta MBBS MD
Assistant Professor
Department of Microbiology
Dr Ram Manohar Lohia Institute of Medical Sciences
Lucknow, Uttar Pradesh, India

Animesh Jain MBBS MD DFH PGDBEME
Professor
Department of Community Medicine
Kasturba Medical College Mangalore
Manipal Academy of Higher Education
Manipal, Karnataka, India

Anit Kujur MBBS MD
Assistant Professor
Department of Community Medicine
Rajendra Institute of Medical Sciences
Ranchi, Jharkhand, India

Ankit Sheth MBBS MD PGDHMA
Medical Scientist 'E'
Head (Health Sciences Division)
ICMR – National Institute of Occupational Health
Ahmedabad, Gujarat, India

Annarao Kulkarni MBBS MD DPH DHA
Professor
Department of Community Medicine
Sri Madhusudan Sai Institute of Medical Sciences and Research
Karnataka, India

Anuj Bhatnagar MD DNB MBA PGDHHM PGDMLE MNAMS FIPHA MAHA DIT
Head
Public Health
Tata Steel Foundation
Jamshedpur, Jharkhand, India

Anwita Khaitan MBBS MD
Assistant Professor
Department of Community and Family Medicine
All India Institute of Medical Sciences-CAPFIMS
New Delhi, India

Aritrik Das MBBS MD
Senior Resident
Department of Community Medicine and School of Public Health
Postgraduate Institute of Medical Education and Research (PGIMER)
Chandigarh, India

Ashwini Agarwal MBBS MD PhD
Dean (Research)
Professor and Head
Department of Microbiology
All India Institute of Medical Sciences
Rajkot, Gujarat, India

Athulya V Ajith MBBS MD
Senior Resident
Department of Community Medicine and School of Public Health
Postgraduate Institute of Medical Education and Research (PGIMER)
Chandigarh, India

Bhautik Modi MBBS MD PGDHHM FIMSA MNAMS
Assistant Professor
Department of Community and Family Medicine
All India Institute of Medical Sciences
Rajkot, Gujarat, India

Hayfa Rajhi PhD
Assistant Professor
Department of Microbiology
University Hospital of Gabes, Tunisia

Harish Rangareddy MBBS MD
Assistant Professor
Department of Biochemistry
Haveri Institute of Medical Sciences
Karnataka, India

Jessica Fryer MBChB
Clinical Research Physician Meditrial
KwaZulu-Natal, South Africa

Jyotsna Agarwal MBBS MD
Professor and Head
Department of Microbiology
Dr Ram Manohar Lohia Institute of Medical Sciences
Lucknow, Uttar Pradesh, India

Krupal J Joshi MBBS MD PGDHHM FCMA FIMSA MNAMS
Associate Dean (Research) (I/C)
Associate Professor
Department of Community and Family Medicine
All India Institute of Medical Sciences
Rajkot, Gujarat, India

Madhu Gupta MBBS MD PhD
Professor
Department of Community Medicine
and School of Public Health
Postgraduate Institute of Medical
Education and Research (PGIMER)
Chandigarh, India

Mandar P Baviskar MBBS MD
Professor
Department of Community Medicine
Dr Balasaheb Vikhe Patil Rural
Medical College
Pravara Institute of Medical Sciences
Ahmednagar, Maharashtra, India

Manish Kumar Singh MD ACME
PGDHHM FIAPSM FIPHA FIMSA FIMAAMS
MAMS
Professor (JG)
Department of Community Medicine
Dr Ram Manohar Lohia Institute of
Medical Sciences
Lucknow, Uttar Pradesh, India

Neelima Tirkey MBBS MD
Lead, Public Health
Tata Steel Foundation
Jaipur, Rajasthan, India

Pankaj B Shah MBBS MD PhD
Associate Dean Research
Professor
Department of Community Medicine
SRMC and RI, SRIHER
Chennai, Tamil Nadu, India

Pentapati Siva Santosh Kumar
MBBS MD FFM
Medical Officer – E (Assistant
Professor)
Department of Preventive Oncology
Tata Memorial Centre
Varanasi, Uttar Pradesh, India

Praggya Mishra MBBS MS
Assistant Professor
Department of Ophthalmology
All India Institute of Medical Sciences
Rajkot, Gujarat, India

Radha A MBBS MD
Assistant Professor
Department of Pharmacology
Sri Madhusudan Sai Institute of
Medical Sciences and Research
Chikkaballapur, Karnataka, India

Rajvir Bhalwar MBBS MD PhD
PDF(Clinical Epid) PGDHM PGDMLE FAMS
FIPHA
Dean and Principal
Professor
Department of Community Medicine
Dr Balasaheb Vikhe Patil Rural
Medical College
Pravara Institute of Medical Sciences
Ahmednagar, Maharashtra, India

Smiti Narain MBBS MD
Senior Resident
Department of Community Medicine
Rajendra Institute of Medical Sciences
Ranchi, Jharkhand, India

Swati Shikha MD DNB MNAMS
Assistant Professor
Department of Community Medicine
Manipal Tata Medical College
Jamshedpur, Jharkhand, India

Vani Jayaraman MBBS MD
Professor and Head
Department of Pharmacology
Sri Madhusudan Sai Institute of
Medical Sciences and Research
Chikkaballapur, Maharashtra, India

Venkateshappa Chikkanarayanappa PhD
Professor
Department of Biochemistry
Sri Madhusudan Sai Institute of
Medical Sciences and Research,
Chikkaballapur, Maharashtra, India

Acknowledgments

Krishna M Jasani MBBS MD
Senior Resident
Department of Community and Family Medicine
All India Institute of Medical Sciences
Rajkot, Gujarat, India

Mohammed Shoyaib Khazi MBBS MD
Senior Resident
Department of Community and Family Medicine
All India Institute of Medical Sciences
Mangalagiri, Andhra Pradesh, India

Foreword

Vaccines have played a pivotal role in shaping global health, significantly reducing the burden of infectious diseases and preventing millions of deaths. The field of vaccinology continues to evolve, integrating cutting-edge scientific advancements with public health strategies to develop more effective and accessible immunization programs.

The *"IAPSM's Textbook of Vaccinology"* is designed as a comprehensive resource for students, researchers, educators, and healthcare professionals, providing in-depth knowledge on the principles and applications of vaccines. This book covers essential topics such as immune mechanisms, vaccine efficacy, technological innovations, and policy implications to offer a holistic perspective on vaccinology.

Through a structured approach, this book explores the core concepts of immunization, beginning with the foundational aspects of the immune response and progressing to specialized topics such as molecular insights, mucosal immunity, and vaccine efficacy evaluation. Advanced topics, including mRNA vaccines, therapeutic vaccines, and regulatory frameworks, provide insights into the latest breakthroughs in vaccine research and development.

This book serves as an invaluable guide for students seeking to build a strong foundation in vaccinology and for faculty members aiming to enrich their teaching methodologies with current scientific and clinical advancements. By addressing both theoretical and practical aspects, this book bridges the gap between research and real-world applications, fostering a deeper understanding of immunization practices.

We extend our sincere appreciation to all contributors who have enriched this book with their expertise. We hope that readers will find this resource useful in their academic and professional endeavors, contributing to the global efforts in disease prevention and public health enhancement.

AM Kadri
Executive Director
State Health System Resource Centre
Gujarat, India
President, IAPSM 2023–2024

Foreword

The purpose of this book is to provide a well-structured and detailed exploration of vaccinology, encompassing fundamental concepts, scientific advancements, and practical applications. It aims to bridge the gap between theoretical knowledge and real-world implementation, ensuring that readers gain a holistic understanding of vaccines and their role in disease prevention and control. Vaccination stands as one of the most significant achievements in the history of medicine, profoundly impacting global health by preventing infectious diseases and saving millions of lives. The "IAPSM's *Textbook of Vaccinology"* is designed to serve as a comprehensive guide for students, researchers, and healthcare professionals, providing an in-depth understanding of the science, technology, and public health aspects of vaccination.

This book is structured into 16 meticulously curated chapters, covering fundamental and advanced topics in vaccinology. It begins with the *Role of Vaccination in Public Health*, emphasizing the impact of immunization programs on disease control and eradication. The foundational principles of the immune response to vaccination are explored in *Foundations of Immune Response*, followed by *Molecular Insights into Immune Activation* and *Significance of Mucosal Immunity in Vaccination*, which delve into the intricate mechanisms of immune protection.

The book further examines the *Broad Spectrum Effects of Vaccines*, highlighting their benefits beyond direct disease prevention. *Evaluating Immunity: Laboratory Techniques and Innovations* provides insights into modern methodologies used to assess vaccine efficacy. Strategies to enhance vaccine effectiveness are discussed in *Enhancing Vaccine Efficacy: The Role of Adjuvant* and *Approaches to Determining Vaccine Efficacy*, offering valuable perspectives for vaccine development and implementation.

This book is the result of extensive collaboration among experts in immunology, public health, and vaccine research. We extend our gratitude to the contributing authors for their invaluable insights and dedication. We hope this textbook will serve as an essential resource, fostering a deeper understanding of vaccines and their pivotal role in global health.

Purushottam Giri
Secretary General
IAPSM (2022–2025)

Preface

Vaccination stands as one of the greatest triumphs of modern medicine, transforming global public health by preventing infectious diseases and saving millions of lives. The rapid evolution of vaccine science—marked by breakthroughs in mRNA technology, novel immunization strategies, and enhanced delivery systems—continues to shape our response to emerging and re-emerging health threats.

The "*IAPSM's Textbook of Vaccinology*" is a testament to the critical role of immunization in safeguarding health across populations. This book provides a comprehensive and structured approach to understanding vaccinology, bridging foundational immunological principles with real-world applications. It meticulously covers the mechanisms of immune response, vaccine development and evaluation, policy considerations, and implementation strategies. Additionally, it highlights the importance of targeted vaccination programs for special populations and explores the regulatory landscape, particularly in the Indian context.

Authored by esteemed experts in public health and vaccinology, this textbook serves as an essential resource for students, researchers, and healthcare professionals dedicated to advancing immunization programs. Its blend of scientific rigor and practical insights makes it an invaluable guide in the ongoing mission to control infectious diseases and improve public health outcomes.

I commend the editors and contributors for their diligent efforts in bringing forth this scholarly contribution, which will undoubtedly serve as a cornerstone for education, research, and policy development in vaccinology. I am confident that this textbook will not only enhance knowledge but also inspire professionals to strengthen vaccine delivery systems and ensure equitable access to immunization for all.

Annarao Kulkarni
President IAPSM (2024–2025)

Contents

CHAPTER 1

Role of Vaccination in Public Health

Animesh Jain

INTRODUCTION

Vaccination is the administration of a vaccine to stimulate the immune system to develop protection (immunity) against specific infectious diseases. Vaccines contain antigens derived from a pathogen, which may be in the form of live-attenuated, inactivated, or subunit components. Once vaccinated, the immune system "learns" to recognize and neutralize the pathogen if the individual is later exposed to the disease. This preemptive immunity prevents infection or significantly reduces the severity of the illness.

ROLE OF VACCINATION IN DISEASE PREVENTION

- *Individual immunity*: Vaccination protects individuals by equipping their immune systems to fight off specific pathogens before they can cause illness.
- *Community protection:* By reducing the number of susceptible individuals in a population, vaccination can help prevent the spread of infectious diseases, leading to *herd immunity*. This effect is crucial for protecting vulnerable individuals who cannot be vaccinated, such as those with compromised immune systems.
- *Global disease control:* Vaccination programs are instrumental in the control, elimination, and eradication of infectious diseases on a global scale.

EVOLUTION OF VACCINATION: FROM EARLY BEGINNINGS TO PUBLIC HEALTH CORNERSTONE

The practice of vaccination has evolved significantly since its inception.

- *Early beginnings:* The concept of inoculation, or variolation, was practiced in Asia and Africa centuries before modern vaccination. This involved exposing individuals to a small amount of a disease-causing agent, such as smallpox, to induce immunity.

  The breakthrough came in 1796 when Edward Jenner, an English physician, developed the first successful vaccine. He used material from cowpox lesions to protect individuals against smallpox, a deadly and widespread disease at the time. This discovery laid the foundation for modern vaccinology.
- *Scientific advances:* In the 19th and 20th centuries, scientific advances, led by pioneers such as Louis Pasteur and Robert Koch, contributed to the development of vaccines for diseases such as rabies, diphtheria, and tuberculosis.

  The introduction of vaccines for tetanus, pertussis (whooping cough), and polio in the mid-20th century further cemented vaccination's role in public health. The development of inactivated (Salk) and live-attenuated (Sabin) polio vaccines in particular played a pivotal role in efforts to eradicate poliomyelitis globally.

  The creation of combination vaccines, such as the DTP vaccine (diphtheria, tetanus, and pertussis), simplified immunization schedules and expanded the reach of vaccination programs.
- *Modern vaccination and global health:*
  - In the latter half of the 20th century, vaccination emerged as a global public health priority with the *expanded program on immunization (EPI)*, established by the World Health Organization (WHO) in 1974. This program aimed to ensure universal access to routine childhood vaccines and reduce the burden of preventable diseases.
  - Vaccination has eradicated smallpox (certified by the WHO in 1980) and brought the world close to eradicating polio. Ongoing global immunization programs continue to target diseases such as measles, rubella, and neonatal tetanus, reducing morbidity and mortality worldwide.

- *21st century innovations:*
    - The 21st century has seen remarkable innovation in vaccine technology, with the development of new platforms such as *mRNA vaccines* [e.g., coronavirus disease 2019 (COVID-19) vaccines], *recombinant protein vaccines,* and *vector-based vaccines.* These innovations enable rapid responses to emerging infectious diseases and improve the efficacy and safety of vaccines.
    - The global effort to develop and deploy COVID-19 vaccines has underscored the critical role vaccination plays in controlling pandemics and safeguarding global health.

CRITICAL ROLE OF VACCINATION IN PUBLIC HEALTH

- *Reducing disease burden*: Vaccination has dramatically reduced the global burden of many infectious diseases. For example, the widespread use of measles, mumps, and rubella (MMR) vaccines has reduced deaths from these diseases by millions. Immunization also prevents severe complications such as congenital rubella syndrome and encephalitis associated with measles.
- *Preventing outbreaks*: Vaccination breaks chains of transmission, preventing outbreaks, and containing the spread of diseases. For instance, routine immunization programs have been instrumental in controlling outbreaks of diseases such as polio, diphtheria, and pertussis. Vaccination campaigns have been essential in curbing outbreaks of emerging diseases, such as the Ebola virus in West Africa and cholera in humanitarian crises.
- *Global health security*: Vaccination is a cornerstone of *global health security,* helping to protect populations from infectious disease threats, including pandemics. By building immunity within communities, vaccines act as a first line of defense against the rapid spread of new and reemerging pathogens. The COVID-19 pandemic has highlighted the importance of robust immunization programs in both preventing health crises and reducing their impact.

Thus vaccination has evolved from early inoculation practices to a sophisticated, scientifically driven approach that underpins public health. It is a powerful tool for preventing infectious diseases, reducing the global disease burden, and strengthening health security worldwide. As a result, vaccination remains central to the goals of public health and global efforts to eliminate or eradicate infectious diseases.

HISTORICAL MILESTONES IN VACCINATION

Smallpox Eradication

Smallpox, a highly contagious and deadly disease, was one of the greatest scourges in human history. The development of the smallpox vaccine by Edward Jenner in 1796 marked a pivotal moment in the history of public health. Jenner demonstrated that inoculation with material from cowpox could protect individuals from smallpox, laying the foundation for modern vaccination.

In the 20th century, smallpox was responsible for millions of deaths annually. The WHO launched an intensive global campaign in 1967 aimed at eradicating smallpox through mass vaccination, surveillance, and containment strategies. By vaccinating large populations and closely monitoring outbreaks, the disease was successfully contained. In 1980, smallpox was declared eradicated, making it the first disease in history to be eliminated by human effort.

The smallpox eradication program had a profound impact on global health policies:

- It demonstrated the effectiveness of coordinated, global vaccination efforts
- It set the framework for future eradication programs and introduced surveillance as a key component of disease control
- The success of smallpox eradication inspired the development of the EPI, which aimed to provide universal access to vaccines for other infectious diseases.

Polio Eradication

Poliomyelitis (polio) was once a feared disease, causing paralysis and death worldwide, particularly in children. The development of the inactivated polio vaccine (IPV) by Jonas Salk in 1955, followed by the oral polio vaccine (OPV) by Albert Sabin in the 1960s, significantly reduced polio incidence. These vaccines became the backbone of polio prevention efforts.

In 1988, the WHO, in collaboration with other global health organizations, launched the Global Polio Eradication Initiative (GPEI) with the goal of eradicating polio worldwide. The GPEI implemented mass vaccination campaigns, targeted high-risk areas, and employed innovative strategies like "National Immunization Days (NIDs)" to reach millions of children.

The polio eradication program has had a lasting impact on global health:

- It showcased the importance of sustained political commitment and community engagement in vaccination campaigns.

- Lessons learned from polio eradication, such as the need for robust surveillance and rapid response to outbreaks, have informed broader vaccination strategies.
- The program strengthened health infrastructure in many countries, laying the groundwork for other vaccination initiatives, including efforts to combat measles, tetanus, and other diseases.

SHAPING GLOBAL HEALTH POLICIES AND VACCINATION STRATEGIES

The successes of smallpox and polio eradication have shaped modern public health in several keyways:

- *Comprehensive vaccination programs:* Both eradication efforts demonstrated that vaccines could not only reduce disease burden but eliminate diseases entirely. This has led to the development of comprehensive vaccination strategies under programs like the EPI, which provides routine immunization for diseases such as DPT.
- *Global health collaboration:* The coordinated, international response required to eradicate smallpox and control polio has highlighted the importance of global partnerships among organizations such as WHO, UNICEF, and GAVI, as well as national governments. This collaborative approach continues to guide responses to emerging infectious diseases.
- *Surveillance and response:* Both programs emphasized the critical role of disease surveillance, enabling early detection and rapid response to outbreaks. This principle is now central to global health strategies, particularly in combating diseases such as measles, cholera, and Ebola.

Impact of Vaccination on Public Health

- Reduction in morbidity and mortality
- Herd immunity
- Prevention of epidemics and pandemics

VACCINATION STRATEGIES IN PUBLIC HEALTH

As already established in earlier sections, vaccination programs are central to the prevention and control of infectious diseases worldwide. To achieve broad coverage and reach diverse populations, public health strategies include routine immunization programs, mass vaccination campaigns, and targeted vaccination efforts for high-risk populations. These approaches work synergistically to ensure that vaccines are accessible and effective in reducing disease burden across different contexts.

Routine Immunization Programs

Routine immunization programs provide regular, scheduled vaccines as part of public health infrastructure, particularly focusing on infants, children, and pregnant women. These programs are designed to deliver vaccines systematically and ensure long-term protection against a range of infectious diseases.

- *Expanded program on immunization:* Established by the *WHO* in 1974, the EPI aims to make vaccines accessible to all children, especially in low- and middle-income countries. It includes vaccines for diseases such as measles, diphtheria, tetanus, pertussis, and tuberculosis.
- *National immunization schedules:* Each country implements its own immunization schedule based on disease prevalence and health priorities. For example, India's *Universal Immunization Program (UIP)* provides vaccines for diseases such as polio, hepatitis B, *Haemophilus influenzae* type B (Hib), and rotavirus. These schedules ensure that vaccines are administered at specific ages for optimal efficacy and coverage.

Impact on Public Health

- Routine immunization has drastically reduced child mortality, with diseases such as diphtheria, measles, and tetanus being controlled in many parts of the world.
- It ensures widespread, sustained coverage that reduces the overall transmission of infectious diseases, contributing to *herd immunity*.

Mass Vaccination Campaigns

Mass vaccination campaigns are designed to rapidly immunize large segments of a population in a short period, typically in response to outbreaks, emergencies, or efforts to eliminate specific diseases. These campaigns are crucial for preventing epidemics and controlling outbreaks.

- *Polio National Immunization Days:* As part of the *GPEI*, many countries have organized NIDs, during which millions of children receive the OPV. These campaigns have been instrumental in driving polio to the brink of eradication.
- *Measles and rubella campaigns:* Measles mass vaccination campaigns have played a significant role in reducing measles-related mortality globally. In many countries, targeted campaigns aim to close immunity gaps in areas with low routine immunization coverage or during outbreaks.
- *Oral cholera vaccine (OCV) in outbreak settings:* During cholera outbreaks, mass vaccination campaigns using OCCs are deployed to rapidly protect at-risk

populations, particularly in regions experiencing humanitarian crises, such as in Yemen and Haiti.

Impact on Public Health

- Mass campaigns enable rapid control of infectious disease outbreaks, minimizing the spread and reducing mortality.
- They can be used to eliminate diseases at a national or regional level, as seen with smallpox and ongoing efforts against polio and measles.
- They are especially effective when high population immunity is needed quickly in a short timeframe, like during an outbreak or a humanitarian crisis.

Targeted Vaccination for High-risk Populations

Targeted vaccination strategies focus on immunizing specific populations that are at higher risk of contracting or spreading infectious diseases. These groups may include healthcare workers, people with chronic conditions, pregnant women, travelers, and populations living in epidemic-prone regions.

- *Healthcare workers:* Vaccination of healthcare workers is essential to prevent the transmission of diseases such as hepatitis B, influenza, and more recently, COVID-19. In many countries, hepatitis B vaccination is mandatory for healthcare professionals due to their increased risk of exposure to bloodborne infections.
- *Human papillomavirus (HPV) vaccine for adolescents*: Targeted HPV vaccination programs are designed to protect adolescents, particularly young girls, from HPV infection, which can lead to cervical cancer. Many countries have adopted school-based HPV vaccination programs to increase coverage.
- *Influenza vaccination for vulnerable groups*: Annual influenza vaccination is recommended for vulnerable groups, including the elderly, people with chronic diseases, and pregnant women. This approach reduces severe complications and hospitalizations associated with seasonal flu.
- *Epidemic-prone regions:* In regions prone to specific epidemics, targeted vaccination programs are implemented to prevent disease outbreaks. For example, *meningococcal vaccination* is targeted at populations living in Africa's "meningitis belt," where recurrent outbreaks of meningococcal disease are common.

Impact on Public Health

- Targeted vaccination reduces the incidence of disease in high-risk groups, thereby protecting both these groups and the broader community.
- It prevents healthcare-associated infections and ensures that critical populations (e.g., healthcare workers and pregnant women) are protected from severe disease outcomes.
- By focusing on vulnerable groups, targeted vaccinations contribute to reducing health disparities and enhancing public health resilience, especially in epidemic-prone regions.

CHALLENGES AND CONTROVERSIES IN VACCINATION

While vaccination is a critical tool in preventing infectious diseases and promoting public health, it faces several challenges and controversies that affect its implementation and success. These issues include vaccine hesitancy, access and equity concerns, and ethical and legal considerations.

Vaccine Hesitancy

Vaccine hesitancy, defined as the delay in acceptance or refusal of vaccines despite availability, is a growing concern worldwide. The WHO listed it among the top ten global health threats in 2019. Vaccine hesitancy arises from various factors, including misinformation, mistrust in health authorities, and concerns about vaccine safety.

- *Misinformation and myths:* Social media and misinformation campaigns have fueled public fears, such as unfounded claims linking vaccines to autism (particularly the MMR vaccine). These fears erode trust in vaccines, leading to lower coverage and outbreaks of vaccine-preventable diseases like measles.
- *Religious and cultural beliefs*: In some communities, cultural or religious beliefs play a significant role in vaccine refusal. For instance, certain groups have resisted polio vaccines due to misconceptions or distrust of health campaigns, particularly in areas of political instability.

Impact: Vaccine hesitancy can lead to dangerous drops in herd immunity, resulting in outbreaks of preventable diseases. Addressing hesitancy requires effective communication, community engagement, and efforts to rebuild trust in vaccines and public health systems.

Access and Equity Issues

Global inequities in access to vaccines remain a significant challenge. Disparities in vaccine distribution, affordability, and availability create barriers to achieving universal immunization.

- *Geographical barriers*: In low- and middle-income countries, particularly in rural and remote areas, infrastructure challenges—such as lack of transportation, cold chain facilities, and healthcare personnel—hinder vaccine delivery. This issue became especially evident during the COVID-19 pandemic, where wealthier countries secured vaccines early while poorer nations struggled to access them.

- *Economic inequities:* High vaccine costs can limit access, especially in low-resource settings where governments may lack funding to provide free or affordable vaccines. Initiatives such as *GAVI, the Vaccine Alliance*, and *COVAX* work to address these disparities by ensuring low-income countries receive vaccines at reduced or no cost.
- *Marginalized populations*: Vulnerable groups, including refugees, migrants, and people living in conflict zones, often have limited access to vaccines due to political and logistical barriers.

Impact: Inequities in vaccine access lead to uneven coverage rates, leaving some populations vulnerable to outbreaks. Ensuring equitable access is crucial to achieving global health security and protecting all populations from preventable diseases.

Ethical and Legal Considerations

Vaccination efforts often involve ethical and legal challenges, especially in balancing individual rights with the need to protect public health.

- *Mandatory vaccination*: Some governments implement mandatory vaccination policies for certain diseases (e.g., school-entry requirements for measles, mumps, rubella vaccines). These policies aim to achieve high coverage rates, but they also raise ethical debates about individual autonomy, religious freedom, and informed consent. Legal challenges sometimes arise when individuals or groups oppose mandatory vaccination based on personal beliefs.
- *Informed consent and vaccine trials:* In research settings, ethical considerations regarding informed consent are critical, particularly when conducting vaccine trials in vulnerable populations. Ensuring that participants understand the risks and benefits of the trial, as well as their right to withdraw, is a fundamental ethical requirement.
- *Global vaccine allocation*: During global health crises, such as the COVID-19 pandemic, ethical concerns about vaccine nationalism (where wealthy countries prioritize their own populations) emerged. The fair allocation of vaccines, especially to low-income nations, is a major ethical issue, underscoring the need for global solidarity and cooperation.

Impact: Ethical and legal challenges can slow down vaccination efforts or lead to public resistance. Clear communication, transparent policies, and respect for human rights are essential to address these issues and maintain public trust in vaccination programs.

FUTURE DIRECTIONS IN VACCINATION AND PUBLIC HEALTH

The future of vaccination is looks promising with significant advances in technology, strengthened global collaboration, and an expanded role in global health security.

Advances in Vaccine Technology

Recent innovations, such as *mRNA vaccines* (used for COVID-19), *viral vector vaccines*, and *recombinant protein vaccines*, are revolutionizing the field. These platforms enable faster vaccine development and higher efficacy. Advances in *nanotechnology*, *personalized vaccines*, and *therapeutic vaccines* targeting cancers and chronic diseases are also on the horizon, expanding the scope of vaccinology beyond infectious diseases.

Global Collaboration for Development and Distribution

The COVID-19 pandemic highlighted the importance of global cooperation in vaccine development and distribution. Initiatives such as *COVAX*, *GAVI*, and partnerships between governments, industry, and academia are critical to ensuring equitable access to vaccines, particularly in low-resource settings. Enhanced global collaboration is key to responding swiftly to future health emergencies.

Role of Vaccination in Global Health Security

Vaccination remains central to *global health security*, preventing not only routine diseases but also emerging infectious threats. By building immunity in populations, vaccines help mitigate the spread of pandemics, reduce health disparities, and strengthen global resilience against outbreaks, making them an essential tool in safeguarding public health on a global scale.

The future of vaccination promises more rapid, personalized, and equitable solutions to health challenges, with ongoing innovations and collaboration driving improvements in public health and global security.

Vaccination remains one of the most effective public health interventions, significantly reducing the burden of infectious diseases, preventing outbreaks, and saving millions of lives. This chapter highlighted the historical milestones of smallpox eradication and polio control, which have shaped global health policies and inspired modern immunization strategies. The various vaccination approaches—including routine immunization, mass campaigns, and targeted efforts—demonstrate the versatility and necessity of vaccines in different contexts.

Despite challenges such as vaccine hesitancy, inequitable access, and ethical considerations, vaccination continues to be a cornerstone of public health. Advances in vaccine technology and global collaboration have enhanced the development, distribution, and efficacy of vaccines, paving the way for future breakthroughs. Ultimately, vaccination plays a vital role in ensuring global health security, protecting populations from preventable diseases, and fostering a healthier, more resilient world.

RESEARCH METHODOLOGIES FOR VACCINE STUDIES (BRIEF OUTLINE—WILL BE EXPANDED LATER)

Research methodologies in vaccine studies are essential for evaluating the safety, efficacy, and immunogenicity of vaccines before they are approved for public use. These methodologies ensure that vaccines provide protection against diseases with minimal risks and guide their development, testing, and implementation. Key approaches include: Preclinical studies, Clinical trials, etc. These are briefly outlined below.

Preclinical Studies

Preclinical research involves laboratory and animal studies to assess the initial safety and immune response of a vaccine candidate. These studies are crucial for identifying potential vaccines and evaluating their biological effects before they proceed to human trials.

Clinical Trials

Vaccine clinical trials follow a phased approach:

- *Phase I trials:* These are small-scale trials (20–100 participants) focusing on the safety of the vaccine and determining appropriate dosage.
- *Phase II trials:* Larger groups (hundreds of participants) are tested to assess the vaccine's immunogenicity and safety further.
- *Phase III trials:* Involving thousands of participants, these trials determine the vaccine's efficacy in preventing disease in diverse populations, while continuing to monitor safety.

Randomized controlled trials (RCTs) are the gold standard in vaccine research. They involve randomly assigning participants to either the vaccine group or a placebo/control group to minimize bias and ensure accurate results.

Post-marketing Surveillance (Phase IV)

Once a vaccine is licensed for public use, post-marketing surveillance monitors its long-term safety and effectiveness in broader populations. This is done through pharmacovigilance systems, passive reporting, and active surveillance to detect rare adverse effects and ensure continued vaccine safety.

Epidemiological Studies

Epidemiological methods are used to measure vaccine impact in real-world settings, including *cohort studies*, *case-control studies*, and *observational studies*. These help to assess the effectiveness of vaccines in reducing disease incidence, transmission, and severity across populations.

In conclusion, robust research methodologies in vaccine studies, from preclinical to post-marketing surveillance, are critical for developing safe and effective vaccines that protect public health.

RECENT DEVELOPMENTS

Recently we have also seen expedited vaccine research and introduction of the vaccine especially during the COVID pandemic.

The COVID-19 pandemic led to an unprecedented global effort to develop vaccines in record time. The use of innovative technologies, such as mRNA vaccines and viral vector vaccines, allowed scientists to accelerate vaccine development while maintaining safety and efficacy standards.

COVID-19 vaccine research demonstrated the potential of cutting-edge technologies and global cooperation in addressing pandemics.

HUMAN CHALLENGE TRIALS

One of the controversial and ethically debatable trial was the human challenge trial where healthy humans were administered the vaccine and then they were to be exposed to the virus to check for the efficacy of the virus.

Human challenge trials are a type of vaccine study where healthy volunteers are intentionally exposed to a pathogen after receiving a vaccine, to rapidly assess its efficacy. During the COVID-19 pandemic, human challenge trials were considered and initiated in some regions to accelerate vaccine research. While these trials can provide valuable data on immune responses and vaccine protection, they raise significant *ethical concerns* due to the deliberate exposure of participants to potentially harmful pathogens.

In the case of COVID-19, challenge trials offered a controlled way to study how well vaccines work and speed up their development, particularly as traditional trials can take longer to show results. These trials require rigorous ethical oversight, informed consent, and safety protocols to protect participants from severe outcomes, making them a debated but potentially valuable tool in vaccine research, particularly in pandemic situations.

CONCLUSION

Vaccination has been a cornerstone of public health, transforming disease prevention and control on a global scale. From its early beginnings with smallpox inoculation to modern advancements like mRNA vaccines, immunization has significantly reduced morbidity and mortality from infectious diseases. It plays a crucial role in individual protection, community immunity, and global health security. While challenges such as vaccine hesitancy, access inequities, and ethical concerns persist, continuous innovation and collaborative public health efforts ensure that vaccination remains a powerful tool in preventing disease outbreaks and safeguarding populations worldwide.

SUGGESTED READINGS

1. Plotkin SA, Orenstein WA, Offit PA. Vaccines. 7th ed. Philadelphia: Elsevier; 2018.
2. World Health Organization. Global Vaccine Action Plan 2011-2020 [Internet]. Geneva: WHO; 2013 [cited 2025 Mar 25]. Available from: https://www.who.int/publications/i/item/global-vaccine-action-plan-2011-2020.
3. Centers for Disease Control and Prevention. Epidemiology and prevention of vaccine-preventable diseases. 14th ed. Washington, DC: Public Health Foundation; 2021.
4. Gavi, The Vaccine Alliance. Immunization coverage [Internet]. 2024 [cited 2025 Feb 25]. Available from: https://www.gavi.org/programmes-impact/
5. Andre FE, Booy R, Bock HL, Clemens J, Datta SK, John TJ, et al. Vaccination greatly reduces disease, disability, death and inequity worldwide. Bull World Health Organ. 2008;86(2):140-6.
6. Roush SW, Murphy TV, Vaccine-Preventable Disease Table Working Group. Historical comparisons of morbidity and mortality for vaccine-preventable diseases in the United States. JAMA. 2007;298(18):2155-63.
7. Jenner E. An inquiry into the causes and effects of the variolae vaccinae. London: Sampson Low; 1798.
8. Salk J. Studies in human subjects on active immunization against poliomyelitis. J Am Med Assoc. 1953;151(13):1081-98.
9. Sabin AB. Oral poliovirus vaccine: history of its development and use and current challenge to eliminate poliomyelitis from the world. J Infect Dis. 1985;151(3):420-6.
10. Patel MK, Goodson JL, Alexander JP Jr, Kretsinger K, Sodha SV, Rota PA, et al. Progress toward regional measles elimination—worldwide, 2000-2020. MMWR Morb Mortal Wkly Rep. 2021;70(45):1563-9.
11. World Health Organization. The Immunization Agenda 2030: A Global Strategy to Leave No One Behind [Internet]. 2021 [cited 2025 Mar 25]. Available from: https://www.who.int/publications/i/item/IA2030
12. Koff WC, Berkley SF. A universal coronavirus vaccine. Science. 2021;371(6531):759-62.

CHAPTER

2

Foundation of Immune Response

Smiti Narain, Swati Shikha

INTRODUCTION

The immune response is a sophisticated and highly organized defense system that safeguards the human body against infections, toxins, and malignancies. It is classified into innate immunity and adaptive immunity. Innate immunity is the immediate defense, providing quick and nonspecific responses to pathogens by physical barriers (e.g., skin, mucosa), soluble mediators (e.g., complement proteins, cytokines), and cellular elements like macrophages, dendritic cells, neutrophils, natural killer (NK) cells, eosinophils, basophils, and mast cells. On the other hand, adaptive immunity offers specific and long-term protection via T and B lymphocytes. These cells produce antigen-specific responses, with T cells coordinating cellular immunity and B cells secreting antibodies. In contrast to innate immunity, adaptive immunity forms immunological memory, enabling more effective responses on subsequent exposure to the same pathogen. The innate and adaptive immune systems interact together in harmony, with the antigen-presenting cells (APCs) bridging the two by activating T cells. Understanding these immune processes is essential for developing vaccines, immunotherapies, and treatments for infectious and autoimmune diseases, making immunology the foundation of modern medicine.

HISTORY

The term "immunology" originates from the Latin words "immunitas" and "immunis," meaning exemption from service or duty. Thucydides first documented immunity in 430 BC, noting during the plague in Athens that those who recovered could care for the sick without getting ill again, recognizing the body's ability to "learn" from exposure. In the Middle Ages, "immunis" referred to the Church's exemption from civil control.[1-4] Silverstein mentions that in AD 39, the Roman poet Marcus Annaeus Lucanus described the Psylli tribe's resistance to snakebites. In the 14th century, Colle used "immunis" during a plague epidemic. The Chinese and Turks in the 15th century attempted to induce immunity through variolation to prevent smallpox. In 1718, Lady Mary Wortley Montagu observed this practice in Turkey and had it performed on her children. Edward Jenner, known as the "Father of Immunology," advanced this in 1798 by inoculating a boy with cowpox fluid, making him immune to smallpox and coining the term "vaccine," a practice that spread across Europe. Nearly 100 years later, Louis Pasteur furthered immunology by demonstrating that weakened pathogens could confer immunity. He vaccinated sheep against anthrax in 1881 and administered the first human rabies vaccine in 1885, saving Joseph Meister, who later worked at the Pasteur Institute.[1,5-9]

FEW KEY CONCEPTS

The immune system protects the body from infectious agents, their toxins, and the damage they cause through various effector cells and molecules. This defense relies on white blood cells/leukocytes, which mostly originate in the bone marrow. Some immune cells, like the microglia in the central nervous system (CNS), develop from the yolk sac or fetal liver during embryonic development and remain self-renewing throughout life. Immune cells, once mature, are found in peripheral tissues, circulate in the bloodstream, or move within the lymphatic system, which drains extracellular fluid and returns it to the bloodstream.

The immune system operates through two main types of immunity: (1) innate and (2) adaptive. Innate immunity is the body's initial, nonspecific response to pathogens, involving barriers such as skin and immune cells that provide immediate defense. Adaptive immunity is more specific and involves the creation of immunological memory, allowing for a more efficient and targeted response to pathogens upon subsequent exposures.[10,11]

Antibody: Molecules produced by B (bursa derived) cells/B lymphocytes, consisting of immunoglobulin heavy and light chains, forming the B cell receptor (BCR). They can exist on B cell surfaces or as secreted molecules in plasma and other fluids.

Antigens: Foreign or self-molecules recognized by adaptive and innate immune systems, triggering immune responses, T (thymus derived) cell activation, and/or B cell antibody production.

Antimicrobial peptides: Small peptides (<100 amino acids) produced by innate immune cells with anti-infectious agent activity.

Apoptosis: Programmed cell death involving death receptors [e.g., tumor necrosis factor (TNF) receptors], caspase activation, and DNA cleavage, contrasting with necrosis which induces inflammation.

B lymphocytes: Bone marrow-derived cells expressing surface immunoglobulin (BCR) and secreting specific antibodies.

B regulatory cells: Suppressive B cells releasing cytokines like interleukin-10 (IL-10) to inhibit inflammation.

CD classification: System for naming leukocyte surface molecules using clusters of differentiation (CD), established in 1982.
- *CD4 T cells*: T lymphocytes aiding B cells in antibody production.
- *CD8 T cells*: Cytotoxic T lymphocytes destroying tumor cells and infected cells.

Complement: A series of plasma enzymes and proteins that lyse pathogens or mark them for phagocytosis by neutrophils and monocytes/macrophages.

Costimulatory molecules: Molecules (e.g., B7-1, B7-2, and CD40) on antigen-presenting cells (APCs) that activate T cells when bound by ligands (e.g., CD28 and CD40 ligand).

Cytokines: Soluble proteins regulating immune cell growth and activation, mediating inflammatory and immune responses.

The normal immune system has three key properties:
1. A highly diverse repertoire of antigen receptors that enables recognition of a nearly infinite range of pathogens
2. Immune memory, to mount rapid recall immune responses
3. Immunologic tolerance, to avoid immune damage to normal self-tissues.[12-18]

TYPES OF IMMUNITY

Innate Immunity

Innate immune system is an ancient immune recognition system with germline-encoded pattern recognition receptors (PRRs) recognizing pathogens. The innate immune system uses genetically inherited proteins to detect pathogens. It relies on cells such as macrophages, dendritic cells (DCs), and natural killer (NK) lymphocytes to identify common molecular structures on pathogens called pathogen-associated molecular patterns (PAMPs). These PAMPs are recognized by PRRs on host cells, which trigger the immune response. Key components of innate immunity include various PRRs [such as toll-like receptors (TLRs)], antimicrobial peptides, immune cells (like neutrophils and eosinophils), complement proteins, and cytokines that help mediate and regulate the immune response. The system is designed to recognize harmful microbes but not the body's own cells or harmless foreign molecules. When pathogens are detected, macrophages and NK cells can directly kill them or work with DCs to initiate processes that slow the infection and activate the adaptive immune system **(Table 1)**.

Natural killer cells: Natural killer cells are a type of large granular lymphocyte that make up 5–15% of peripheral blood lymphocytes. They play a key role in innate immunity by killing cells that lack human leukocyte antigens (HLAs) class I molecules, such as virus-infected, malignant, or foreign cells. NK cells have surface receptors such as CD16 and CD56 and can proliferate in response to IL-2.

TABLE 1: Component of innate immune system.

Pattern recognition receptors (PRRs)	Toll-like receptors (TLRs), C-type lectin receptors (CLRs), retinoic acid-inducible gene (RIG)-1-like receptors (RLRs), and NOD-like receptors (NLRs)
Antimicrobial peptides	α-defensins, β-defensins, cathelin, protegrin, granulysin, histatin, secretory leukoprotease inhibitor, and probiotics
Cells	Macrophages, dendritic cells, NK cells, NK-T cells, neutrophils, eosinophils, mast cells, basophils, and epithelial cells
Complement components	Classic and alternative complement pathway, and proteins that bind complement components
Cytokines	Autocrine, paracrine, endocrine cytokines that mediate host defense and inflammation, as well as recruit, direct, and regulate adaptive immune responses

They mediate antibody-dependent cellular cytotoxicity (ADCC), where they bind to antibody-coated target cells and induce cell lysis. NK cell activity is not restricted by major histocompatibility complex (MHC), allowing them to provide crucial immune surveillance. They balance inhibitory and activating signals to target harmful cells and can also recognize lipid antigens through NK T cells, contributing to the defense against certain bacteria.

Pattern recognition receptors: They are genetically encoded receptors on innate immune cells that detect pathogen-associated molecular patterns (PAMPs) on pathogens and damage-associated molecular patterns (DAMPs) on damaged cells. Major PRRs include transmembrane proteins such as TLRs and C-type lectin receptors (CLRs), as well as cytoplasmic proteins like retinoic acid-inducible gene (RIG)-1-like receptors (RLRs) and NOD-like receptors (NLRs). RLRs and NLRs are soluble proteins inside cells that monitor the cell's cytoplasm for internal pathogens.

T lymphocytes: Thymus-derived cells mediating adaptive cellular immune responses, including T helper, T regulatory, and cytotoxic T cell functions.

T cell receptor (TCR) for antigen: Surface molecule complex rearranging during T cell development, recognizing peptide fragments bound to MHC class I or II molecules on APCs, leading to effector functions.

Mannose-binding lectin (MBL) and other collectins (C-type lectin domains) as well as two other protein families—(1) the pentraxins (such as C-reactive protein and serum amyloid P) and (2) macrophage scavenger receptors—all have the property of opsonizing (coating) bacteria for phagocytosis by macrophages and can also activate the complement cascade to lyse bacteria.

Integrins are cell-surface adhesion molecules that affect attachment between cells and the extracellular matrix and mediate signal transduction that reflects the chemical composition of the cell environment. For example, integrins signal after cells bind bacterial lipopolysaccharide (LPS) and activate phagocytic cells to ingest pathogens.

Monocytes arise from bone marrow precursors, circulating for 1–3 days before migrating into tissues, where they become macrophages or proliferate in situ. Tissue macrophages are found in lymph nodes, spleen, bone marrow, connective tissues, serous cavities, skin, lungs (alveolar macrophages), liver (Kupffer cells), bone (osteoclasts), CNS (microglia), and synovium. As a first line of defense in innate immunity, monocytes-macrophages ingest and destroy microorganisms using toxic products such as hydrogen peroxide (H_2O_2) and nitric oxide (NO).

They produce inflammatory mediators (e.g., prostaglandins, leukotrienes, platelet-activating factor, cytokines such as IL-1, TNF-α, IL-6, IL-12, and chemokines) to attract neutrophils to infection sites. While DCs are the most potent APCs, monocytes-macrophages also present antigens and mediate innate immune functions, destroying antibody-coated bacteria, tumor cells, or normal hematopoietic cells in autoimmune cytopenias. They undergo apoptosis when ingesting bacteria or viruses, and DCs then phagocytose these apoptotic macrophages, "cross-presenting" antigens to T cells.

Activated macrophages can eliminate tumor cells without antibodies, mainly through cytokines (TNF-α and IL-1). They express specific surface receptors, including the LPS receptor CD14, and receptors for the Fc region of IgG, activated complement components, and various cytokines.

Dendritic cells: These include myeloid and plasmacytoid subsets. Myeloid DCs can become macrophages or tissue-specific DCs, while plasmacytoid DCs are inefficient APCs but produce type I interferon (IFN) (e.g., IFN-α) in response to viral infections. DC maturation is regulated by cell contact and soluble factors, attracting immune effectors through chemokine secretion. Upon encountering bacterial products, viral proteins, or danger signals, DCs activate via TLRs, releasing cytokines and chemokines to stimulate innate immunity and recruit adaptive immune cells.

Plasmacytoid DCs produce IFN-α, activating NK cells and T cells. Both DC types produce chemokines to attract T and B cells, polymorphonuclear cells, and regulatory T cells. TLR engagement on DCs upregulates MHC class II, CD80, and CD86, enhancing antigen presentation and cytokine production. DCs bridge innate and adaptive immunity and modulate immune responses through TLRs and other PRRs, determining the type and quality of adaptive immune responses.

Neutrophils, Eosinophils, and Basophils

Granulocytes enhance innate immune responses but can cause tissue damage if unchecked, as seen in neutrophil- and eosinophil-mediated vasculitis. They are derived from bone marrow stem cells, with each type originating from different progenitor cells.

Neutrophils express receptors for immunoglobulin G (IgG) (CD16a) and complement components (C3b and CD35). When interacting with opsonized bacteria, they release granules containing enzymes (myeloperoxidase, lysozyme, and elastase) and generate microbicidal superoxide radicals (O^{2-}), leading to tissue damage.

Eosinophils target parasites, regulated by IL-4 from T helper cells. Their granules contain cytotoxic proteins (major basic protein and eosinophil cationic protein) that damage tissues, contributing to hypereosinophilic syndromes. They also contain anti-inflammatory enzymes (histaminase and arylsulfatase) that downregulate inflammation.

Basophils and mast cells are cytokine reservoirs, responding to bacteria and viruses through TLRs and mediating immunity via antibodies. Basophils express IgE receptors (FcεRII and CD23). Cross-linking of IgE releases histamine and other mediators, causing allergic responses. They also have receptors for complement components (C3a and C5a), affecting mediator release and contributing to pathogen defense and allergies.[12-18]

Complement System

The complement system is a key component of innate immunity, consisting of plasma enzymes and regulatory proteins that work in a cascade to destroy harmful cells. There are four main pathways in the complement system:

1. *Classic pathway*: Activated when antibodies bind to antigens, triggering the complement protein C1q.
2. *MBL pathway*: Activated by microbes with mannose groups on their surfaces, using proteins called mannose-binding lectin-associated serine proteases (MASPs) to initiate the process.
3. *Alternative pathway*: Activated directly by microbes or tumor cells, starting with the complement protein C3.
4. *Terminal pathway*: All pathways converge here, leading to the formation of the membrane attack complex (MAC) that can lyse, or break apart, target cells.

The enzymes involved in the complement system are serine proteases. In the classic pathway, the immune complex binds to C1q, linking innate and adaptive immunity. The alternative pathway does not require antibodies and is activated by direct binding of C3 to pathogens or tumor cells. In diseases such as IgA nephropathy, IgA activates the alternative pathway, causing kidney damage. Both the classic and alternative pathways lead to the activation of C3, which is crucial for tagging pathogens for destruction (opsonization) and aiding phagocytosis.

Mannose-binding lectin-associated serine proteases (MASPs) are essential enzymes in the complement system, a key component of innate immunity. Among them, MASP-2 plays a pivotal role in activating complement proteins C4 and C2, which are crucial for initiating the lectin pathway. In contrast, MASP-1 and MASP-3 contribute to the activation of both the lectin and alternative complement pathways, enhancing the immune system's ability to recognize and eliminate pathogens.

Complement activation is essential for fighting infections, clearing microbes or damaged cells, enhancing inflammation, and lysing pathogens or opsonized cells through the MAC.[19,20]

Cytokines

Cytokines are essential soluble proteins produced by various cells, playing a critical role in both innate and adaptive immune responses. They regulate immune cell growth, development, and activation, and mediate inflammation. Cytokines can act on the same cell (autocrine), nearby cells (paracrine), or distant cells (endocrine). They belong to three main families: (1) hematopoietin, (2) TNF/IL-1/PDGF/TGF-β, and (3) chemokines, which regulate cell movement. Cytokines influence gene activation, leading to cellular growth, differentiation, and effector functions. T cells, e.g., secrete different cytokines for various immune responses: Th1 for cell-mediated, Th2 for humoral, and Th17 for defense against bacteria and fungi. Cytokine receptors are categorized into five families, and their signaling involves the Janus kinase (JAK) pathway, which activates gene expression. In innate immunity, cytokines are crucial for coordinating the body's immediate response to pathogens, promoting inflammation, and activating immune cells to fight infections.

There are *multiple connections between the innate and adaptive immune systems*; these include (1) a plasma protein, LPS-binding protein, that binds and transfers LPS to the macrophage LPS receptor, CD14; (2) a human family of proteins called TLR proteins, some of which are associated with CD14, bind LPS, and signal epithelial cells, DCs, and macrophages to produce cytokines and upregulate cell-surface molecules that signal the initiation of adaptive immune responses and three families of intracellular microbial sensors called NLRs and RLRs.[1-3]

Adaptive Immunity

Adaptive immunity features antigen-specific responses to foreign antigens or pathogens and includes immunologic memory, allowing faster and stronger responses upon reexposure. It comprises cellular and humoral branches: T lymphocytes mediate cellular immunity and B lymphocytes mediate humoral immunity. Both cell types originate from a common stem cell.

Bone marrow is the primary maturation site for B cells, monocytes-macrophages, DCs, and granulocytes, containing pluripotent stem cells that can differentiate into all hematopoietic cells. T cell precursors arise from these stem cells and mature in the thymus. Mature T and B lymphocytes, monocytes, and DCs circulate and home to peripheral lymphoid organs (lymph nodes and spleen), mucosal surface-associated lymphoid tissues (gut, genitourinary, and respiratory tracts), skin, and mucous

TABLE 2: Innate versus adaptive immunity.

Characteristics	Innate immunity	Adaptive immunity
Presence	Immunity already present in the body	Created in response to exposure to a foreign substance
Cells involved	Dendritic leukocyte, natural killer cells, mast cell, granulocytes/macrophages, basophils, etc.	Killer CD8+ T cells. Helper CD4+ T cells, B cells, antigen-presenting cells, etc.
Molecules involved	Cytokine, complement cells, interferon, acute phase reactants	Antibodies, cytokines
Order of defense	First line of defense of immune system	Action against pathogens that are able to evade or overcome innate immune defense
Specificity	Nonspecific	Specific
Response	Rapid	Slow (1–2 weeks)
Potency	Limited and lower potency	High potency
Memory	No memory	Long-term memory
Types of immune response	Inflammation, complement mediated killing, phagocytosis	Antibodies generation, microbe destruction by T helper cells and cytotoxic cells
Subsequent exposure	Immune response remains same on repeated exposure	Immune response gets stronger with repeated exposure
Allergic reaction	None	Immediate and delayed hypersensitivity

membranes, ready for activation by foreign antigens. **Table 2** explains the differences between innate and adaptive immunity.

Cell-mediated Adaptive Immunity

T cells: Effector T cells are produced in the thymus early in life and maintained by continuous thymic production and expansion into memory T cells. The thymus exports about 2% of thymocytes daily, decreasing by around 3% each year over four decades. Mature T lymphocytes comprise a significant portion of peripheral blood lymphocytes, thoracic duct lymphocytes, lymph node cells, and spleen lymphoid cells. T cells are crucial for cell-mediated immunity: CD8+ cytotoxic T cells destroy virus-infected or foreign cells, while CD4+ T cells support the development of CD8+ T cells and B cells. Memory T cells, including effector memory cells in nonlymphoid organs and central memory T cells in lymphoid organs, respond rapidly to infections. T cell precursors from bone marrow migrate to the thymus, where they differentiate into TCR-αβ or TCR-γδ cells. These cells recognize antigen peptides presented by MHC molecules on APCs and undergo selection to ensure they do not attack self-antigens. TCRs, along with CD3 subunits, are essential for T cell activation, and the process of gene recombination in the thymus creates diverse TCRs, enabling the immune system to recognize a wide array of antigens.

B cells: B cells make up a smaller percentage of peripheral blood lymphocytes but are crucial for producing antibodies and presenting antigens. They express surface immunoglobulins (Igs) as BCRs for antigens, allowing them to recognize and respond to whole, unprocessed antigens. B cells also have receptors for IgG and complement components, which enhance their ability to produce antibodies and present antigens. B cells develop from bone marrow precursors, undergoing antigen-independent maturation in primary lymphoid organs and antigen-dependent maturation in secondary lymphoid organs. Upon encountering an antigen, B cells can become memory B cells, switch Ig classes, and form plasma cells that secrete antibodies. The process of somatic hypermutation and gene rearrangement creates diverse and high-affinity antibodies. Cytokines such as IL-4 and transforming growth factor-beta (TGF-β) drive Ig class switching, while others such as IL-1, IL-2, IL-4, IL-5, IL-6 promote B cell proliferation and differentiation. This complex interaction between T and B cells ensures a robust and adaptive immune response, tailored to effectively combat a wide range of pathogens.

Humoral Mediators of Adaptive Immunity: Immunoglobulins

Immunoglobulins are antibodies produced by B cells, mediating the humoral immune response. They bind to antigens to neutralize or eliminate toxins, microbes, and other foreign substances. Each Ig molecule consists of two heavy and two light chains. The isotype (G, M, A, D,

E) is determined by the heavy chain type, with IgG and IgA further divided into subclasses.

Immunoglobulins have variable (V) and constant (C) regions. Light chains have one V and one C unit, while heavy chains have one V and three or four C units. The C regions perform biological functions, such as complement activation and binding to Fc receptors on various immune cells. The V regions form the antigen-binding (Fab) region, with hypervariable regions for antigen specificity.

IgG: Comprises 75–85% of serum Igs, with four subclasses. IgG is important in secondary antibody responses and can bind Fc receptors and activate complement. Deficiencies in IgG subclasses can lead to increased susceptibility to infections.

IgM: A pentamer that appears first in immune responses and is important in primary antibody responses and as an antigen receptor on B cells. It is significant in autoimmune diseases, such as rheumatoid arthritis.

IgA: Makes up 7–15% of serum Igs and is predominant in secretions (e.g., tears and saliva). Secretory IgA (sIgA) prevents viral binding in respiratory and gastrointestinal tracts.

IgD: Found in low serum quantities and acts as an antigen receptor on naïve B cells.

IgE: Present in very low serum concentrations, it binds to mast cells and basophils, playing a major role in allergic responses by releasing mediators upon antigen cross-linking.

Immunoglobulins are crucial for immune defense, mediating antigen recognition, complement activation, and interactions with immune cells to protect against pathogens and regulate immune responses.[21-25]

CELLULAR INTERACTIONS IN REGULATION OF NORMAL IMMUNE RESPONSES

In normal immune responses, T and B lymphocytes play crucial roles in eliminating antigens. T cells and B cells go through stages of activation, proliferation, differentiation, and performing their specific functions. CD4+ helper T cells, including subsets such as Th1, Th2, Th17, Th9, and Tfh cells, secrete different cytokines to support immune functions. Th1 cells help in intracellular killing and support cytotoxic T cells, while Th2 cells regulate antibody production and limit Th1 responses. Th17 cells are involved in defense against bacteria and fungi, and Th9 cells play roles in atopic diseases and anti-tumor immunity. Tfh cells assist B cells in producing high-affinity antibodies. T cell responses are influenced by PAMPs, TLRs, DCs, and cytokines. Regulatory T cells (Tregs) maintain tolerance to self-antigens and control the immune response's magnitude. B cells require T cell help for producing high-affinity antibodies through processes such as antigen processing, binding of the TCR complex and CD40 ligand, antibody isotype switching, and affinity maturation. Naive B cells express IgD and IgM and need T cell cytokines for gene recombination and isotype switching, with CD40 ligand being crucial for B cell responsiveness.[26-28]

VACCINATION AND IMMUNIZATION

Vaccination and immunization are often used interchangeably, but they are distinct. Vaccination refers specifically to the administration of a vaccine, while immunization is the process of inducing or providing immunity, which can be either active or passive. Vaccination does not always result in immunization.

MECHANISMS OF IMMUNE RESPONSE

Vaccines stimulate the immune system by introducing antigens, which are either weakened or inactivated parts of pathogens. This exposure allows the immune system to recognize these antigens as foreign invaders, leading to the initiation of an immune response. When a vaccine is administered, specialized immune cells, B-lymphocytes (B-cells), and T-lymphocytes (T-cells), become activated. B-cells produce antibodies that specifically target the antigens present in the vaccine, while T-cells play a crucial role in identifying and destroying infected cells. This process generates two essential components of the immune response: (1) active immunity and (2) immunological memory. The active immune response involves the production of antibodies and cytokines that help to eliminate the foreign invaders. Furthermore, some of the B-cells and T-cells differentiate into memory cells, which persist long after the vaccination has occurred. These memory cells enhance the immune system''s ability to recognize and fight off the actual pathogen more efficiently during subsequent exposures. This rapid recall response is vital in preventing illness since it allows the immune system to react quickly before the pathogen can replicate to harmful levels. While the immune response triggered by vaccination usually takes time to build, it prepares the body for future infections, significantly reducing the risk of severe disease.

Immunosuppressive Effects and Monoclonal Antibodies

In addition to providing immediate protection, passive immunization can have immunosuppressive effects,

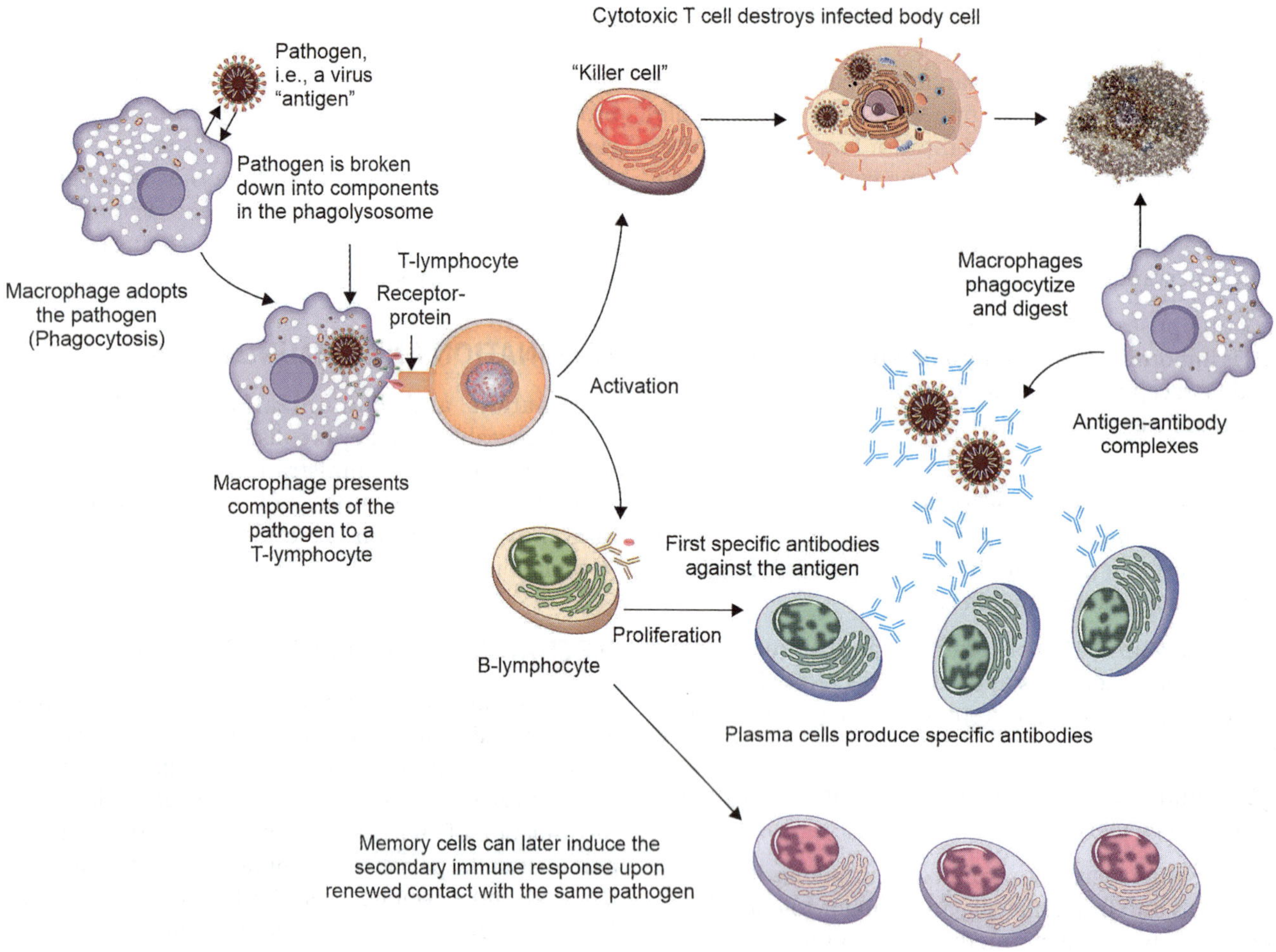

FIG. 1: Primary immune response steps.

Source: Pickett S. Understanding immunological memory [Internet]. Washington, DC: American Society for Microbiology; 2023 May 15 [cited 2025 Mar 28]. Available from: https://asm.org/articles/2023/may/understanding-immunological-memory

useful in conditions like hemolytic disease of the newborn. Monoclonal antibodies, derived from a single clone of B cells, offer targeted therapies for cancer and autoimmune diseases. These antibodies are engineered to reduce immunogenicity and improve therapeutic efficacy.

The immune response to vaccination involves activating the body's immune system to recognize and combat pathogens. This process has two main phases: (1) primary and (2) secondary immune responses.

1. *Primary immune response*: Upon first exposure to an antigen, B and T lymphocytes are activated, leading to the production of specific antibodies. This initial immune response peaks around 14 days after exposure. During this phase, memory cells are also created, which help the body respond more quickly to future encounters with the same antigen. When a vaccine is given, there is a delay of several days before the immune system's response is detectable. Circulating antibodies typically appear within 7–10 days. The response starts with the production of low-affinity IgM antibodies, followed by the later appearance of high-affinity IgG antibodies. CD4+ T-helper cells help switch the production from IgM to IgG for certain antigens. Some individuals may not respond to vaccines due to the absence of necessary MHC determinants, resulting in primary vaccine failure **(Fig. 1)**.
2. *Secondary immune response*: Upon subsequent exposure to the same antigen, the immune system mounts a rapid and stronger response due to memory cells. This secondary response occurs within 2–3 days and is more robust than the initial response. While the primary immune response mainly produces IgM antibodies, the secondary response generates higher-affinity IgG antibodies, providing better protection. This quick reaction, occurring within 4–5 days, is due to the immunologic memory formed during the first exposure and involves the proliferation of IgG-producing B cells and effector T cells **(Fig. 2)**.

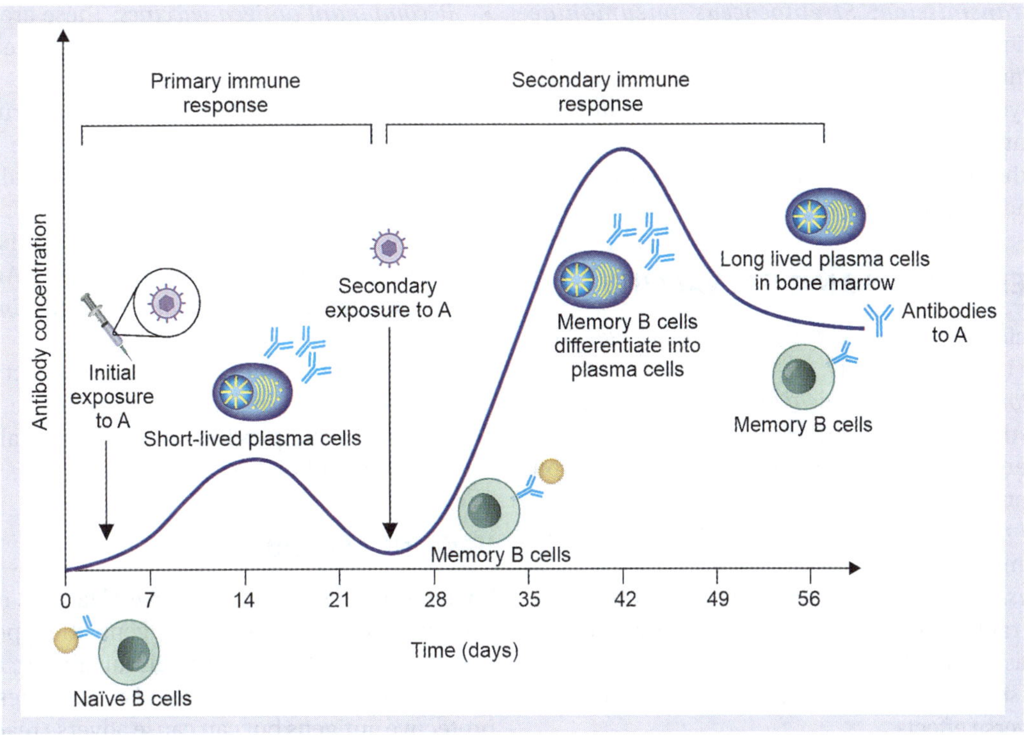

FIG. 2: Primary versus secondary immune response.

Source: Landsteiner K. The Specificity of Serological Reactions. Cambridge: Harvard University Press; 1947.

Hypersensitivity reactions: Vaccination can cause hypersensitivity reactions. Example: Killed measles vaccine previously caused atypical measles syndrome inducing humoral and cell-mediated immune system.

Mucosal immunity: Some pathogens induce secretory IgA at mucosal sites, blocking initial infection steps. Effective for organisms confined to mucosal surfaces or those that invade across mucosa.

Measurement of immune response: Typically gauged by specific antibody concentrations in serum. While seroconversion is a reliable indicator, it does not always correlate with protection. The development of circulating antibodies after immunization often correlates directly with clinical protection (e.g., against measles or rubella).[29-32]

HERD IMMUNITY AND VACCINATION

Herd immunity refers to a form of indirect protection from infectious diseases that occurs when a significant portion of a population becomes immune, either through vaccination or previous infections. When a large number of individuals in a community are immune to a particular pathogen, the spread of disease is hindered, ultimately protecting those who are not immune or cannot be vaccinated due to medical reasons, such as allergies or compromised immune systems. This principle is grounded in the idea that the more people who are immune to a disease, the less likely it is for the pathogen to find hosts to infect, thus reducing the overall transmission rates.

Vaccination plays a crucial role in achieving herd immunity, as it allows for a higher proportion of the population to gain immunity without the need for natural infection, which can carry significant health risks and complications. The threshold for achieving herd immunity varies depending on the disease; for instance, highly contagious diseases like measles require around 95% of the population to be immune to prevent outbreaks, whereas less contagious diseases might require lower percentages.

Notably, herd immunity does not eliminate the disease entirely but lowers the chances of an outbreak, providing safety for vulnerable groups within the population. It is important to maintain high vaccination rates to uphold herd immunity, as reduced immunization coverage can result in resurgence of diseases once thought to be under control. Public health policies emphasizing vaccination campaigns and community awareness play a vital role in achieving and sustaining herd immunity, thereby contributing to the overall health and well-being of society.

Examples:

- *High transmission*: Measles and varicella require higher vaccine coverage for herd immunity.

- *Lower transmission*: *Streptococcus pneumoniae* requires lower coverage.

Herd immunity can cease disease transmission, as seen with poliomyelitis and measles. However, interruptions in immunization programs or refusal to vaccinate (e.g., pertussis in the UK and Japan) can lead to the loss of herd immunity and large outbreaks.[33-36]

CHARACTERISTICS OF AN IDEAL VACCINE

An ideal vaccine should possess several key characteristics to effectively induce immunity:

- *Generation of immunological memory*: The vaccine should stimulate the formation of memory B and T cells, ensuring rapid and robust responses upon subsequent exposures to the pathogen.
- *Lifelong immunity*: Ideally, a single dose should confer lifelong immunity.
- *Noninvasive administration*: Vaccines should be administrable through noninvasive methods such as oral or nasal delivery.
- *Minimal side effects*: The vaccine should have minimal or no adverse effects.
- *Broad immune activation*: It should stimulate both humoral (antibody-mediated) and cell-mediated immunity.
- *Stability and cost-effectiveness*: The vaccine should be inexpensive, easily manufactured, and stable under various environmental conditions.[37-41]

TYPES OF VACCINES

Vaccines can be categorized based on their composition and preparation methods:

- *Live attenuated vaccines*: These contain live pathogens that have been weakened so they cannot cause disease in healthy individuals. Examples include the BCG vaccine for tuberculosis and the MMR vaccine for measles, mumps, and rubella.
- *Inactivated vaccines*: These contain killed pathogens that cannot replicate but can still induce an immune response. Examples include the Salk polio vaccine and the hepatitis A vaccine.
- *Toxoid vaccines*: These contain inactivated toxins produced by the pathogen, used to induce immunity against the toxin rather than the pathogen itself. Examples include the diphtheria and tetanus vaccines.
- *Polysaccharide vaccines*: These use long chains of sugar molecules that make up the surface capsule of certain bacteria. Examples include the vaccines for pneumococcal pneumonia and meningococcal meningitis.
- *Recombinant antigen vaccines*: These are made using recombinant DNA technology to produce antigens. An example is the hepatitis B vaccine.
- *Viral vector vaccines*: These use a virus to deliver pathogen genes into cells to provoke an immune response. An example in clinical trials is an HIV vaccine using a canarypox virus vector.
- *Bacterial vector vaccines*: These use bacteria as a delivery system for pathogen antigens. An example is an attenuated strain of *Salmonella typhimurium* used as a vector for a cholera vaccine.
- *DNA vaccines*: These involve the direct injection of DNA encoding an antigen to produce an immune response. Examples include experimental vaccines for rabies and influenza.[1,42,43]

VACCINE EFFICACY

Vaccine efficacy depends on several factors, including the presence of cross-reactive antigens, the type of vaccine, genetic variability, route of administration, age, and the use of adjuvants. Whole-organism vaccines contain all protective antigens but can cause adverse reactions due to nonprotective components. The route of administration, such as oral, intranasal, or intramuscular, influences the type and speed of the immune response. Age affects vaccine response, with young infants and the elderly often requiring adjustments in dosage. Adjuvants, like aluminum salts, enhance the immune response by converting soluble antigens into particulate form and prolonging antigen release. Polysaccharide vaccines elicit T cell-independent responses, which are not boosted by repeated doses, but conjugating them to proteins makes them T cell-dependent, allowing for memory and stronger secondary responses. Vaccine-induced antibody levels may decline over time, but revaccination or exposure can quickly restore protection through a rapid IgG response. Detectable antibodies postvaccination do not always guarantee clinical protection, as a minimum antibody level is required for certain diseases, like tetanus.[38,40]

ACTIVE, PASSIVE, AND ADOPTIVE IMMUNITY

Active Immunity

Mechanism: Activation of humoral and cell-mediated responses by exposure to an antigen.

Examples: Natural infection and vaccination

Advantages: Long-term protection due to immunologic memory

Limitations: Delay in response initiation

Passive Immunity

Mechanism: Transfer of preformed antibodies

Examples: Maternal antibodies, immune serum globulin, and antitoxins

Advantages: Immediate protection

Limitations: Temporary immunity, no memory cells generated

Adoptive Immunity

Mechanism: Transfer of immune cells

Examples: Tumor-infiltrating lymphocytes, hematopoietic stem cell transplantation

Advantages: Potential for long-term protection

Limitations: Risk of rejection, high cost.[44-47]

BIOLOGIC IMPEDIMENTS IN VACCINE DEVELOPMENT

Technical Challenges

- *Influenza virus*: Characterized by antigenic drift, requiring new vaccines for emerging strains.
- *Pneumococcal vaccines*: Many serotypes circulate, each requiring specific immunity. The current vaccine includes 23 polysaccharides but has limitations due to poorly immunogenic serotypes.

Strategy for Vaccine Development

- *Animal studies*: Identify protective antigens
- *Presentation to immune system*: Determine effective presentation methods
- *Human safety and immunogenicity*: Small-scale trials across various ages
- *Large-scale trials*: Evaluate safety and efficacy in target populations

Phases: After successful animal studies and small human trials (phases 1 and 2), large clinical trials (1,000–10,000 participants) are conducted. Postlicensing monitoring is crucial to identify rare adverse effects.

Development and cost: Cost and liability—high costs and uncertain success hinder vaccine development.

Production of Vaccines

- *Quality assurance*: Ensured by manufacturers and regulated by the Food and Drug Administration (FDA). Continuous monitoring post-licensure.
- *Good manufacturing practices (GMPs) standards*: Ensure safety, efficacy, sterility, and purity.
- *Production issues*: Decline in vaccine manufacturers may be due to high development costs and better profitability from other products.

Administration of Vaccines

- *Healthcare worker precautions*: Handwashing and safe disposal of needles to prevent disease spread.
- *Combining vaccines*: Avoid mixing vaccines unless approved.
- *Multiple injections*: Parental concerns addressed by combining vaccines and ensuring administration of all indicated vaccines at each visit.

Coverage and Access

- *High coverage rates*: Achieved through effective primary health care and public education.
- *Multiple-dose schedules*: Systematic attention needed to ensure completion.
- Effective vaccine development and administration depend on overcoming biological impediments, ensuring quality production, managing costs, and maintaining high coverage through education and systematic healthcare practices.[44-47]

CONCLUSION

Vaccines are a cornerstone of public health, providing protection against a wide range of infectious diseases. By understanding the mechanisms of the immune response and leveraging modern technologies, researchers continue to develop safer and more effective vaccines. The goal is to achieve long-lasting immunity with minimal side effects, enhancing both individual and community health.

REFERENCES

1. Owen JA, Punt J, Stranford SA, Jones PP, Kuby J. Kuby Immunology, 8th edition. New York: Macmillan Learning; 2019.
2. Khan FA. Elements of Immunology. Chennai: Pearson Education; 2021.
3. Murphy K, Weaver C. Janeway's immunobiology. New York: Garland Science; 2016.
4. Juan I. From the Old Immunitas to the Modern Immunity: Do We Need a New Name for the Immune System? Curr Immunol Rev. 2015;11:55-6.
5. Silverstein AM. History of immunology: cellular versus humoral immunity: determinants and consequences of an epic 19th-century battle. Cell Immunol. 1979;48(2):208-21.

6. Matzinger P. The evolution of the danger theory. Interview by Constable L. Expert Rev Clin Immunol. 2012;8(4):311-5.
7. Medawar PB. The immunology of transplantation: the Harvey lectures, 1956–1957. New York: Academic Press; 1958.
8. Burnet FM. The Clonal Selection Theory of Acquired Immunity. Cambridge: Cambridge University Press; 1959.
9. Descour L. Pasteur and his work. Trans. Wedd AF, Wedd BH. London: T. Fisher Unwin; 1922.
10. Landsteiner K. The Specificity of Serological Reactions. Cambridge: Harvard University Press; 1947.
11. Metchnikoff E. Immunity in Infectious Diseases. New York: Macmillan; 1905.
12. Haurowitz F. Immunochemistry. Annu Rev Biochem. 1960;29:395-420.
13. Williams MA, Bevan MJ. Effector and memory CTL differentiation. Annu Rev Immunol. 2007;25:171-92.
14. Billingham RE, Brent L, Medawar PB. Actively acquired tolerance of foreign cells in skin-graft transplantation. Nature. 1953;172:603-6.
15. Beutler B, Rietschel ET. Innate immune sensing and its roots: the story of endotoxin. Nat Rev Immunol. 2003;3(2):169-76.
16. Bowie AG, Unterholzner L. Viral evasion and subversion of pattern-recognition receptor signaling. Nat Rev Immunol. 2008;8(12): 911-22.
17. Brubaker SW, Bonham KS, Zanoni I, Kagan JC. Innate immune pattern recognition: a cell biological perspective. Annu Rev Immunol. 2015;33:257-90.
18. Gordon S. Phagocytosis: an immunobiologic process. Immunity. 2016;44(3):463-75.
19. Aleshin AE, Schraufstatter IU, Stamatoyannopoulos G, Skokos EA, Torrance S, Bolen JB, et al. Structure of complement C6 suggests a mechanism for initiation and unidirectional, sequential assembly of the membrane attack complex (MAC). J Biol Chem. 2012;287(13):10210-22.
20. Alexander JJ, Anderson AJ, Barnum SR, Stevens B, Tenner AJ. The complement cascade: Yin-Yang in neuroinflammation--neuro-protection and -degeneration. J Neurochem. 2008;107(5): 1169-87.
21. Übelhart R, Werner M, Jumaa H. Assembly and function of the precursor B-cell receptor. Curr Top Microbiol Immunol. 2016;393:3-20.
22. Mescher MF, Curtsinger JM, Agarwal P, Casey KA, Gerner M, Hammerbeck CD, et al. Molecular basis for checkpoints in the CD8+ T cell response: tolerance versus activation. Semin Immunol. 2007;19(3):153-61.
23. Caton AJ, Cozzo C, Larkin J. CD4+CD25+ regulatory T cell selection. Ann N Y Acad Sci. 2004;1029:101-14.
24. Kisielow P, Blüthmann H, Staerz UD, Steinmetz M, von Boehmer H. Tolerance in T-cell receptor transgenic mice involves deletion of nonmature CD4+8+ thymocytes. Nature. 1988;333(6175):742-6.
25. Hogquist KA, Jameson SC, Bevan MJ. Strong agonist ligands for the T cell receptor do not mediate positive selection of functional CD8+ T cells. Immunity. 1995;3(1):79-92.
26. Lemaitre B. The road to Toll. Nat Rev Immunol. 2004;4(7):521-7.
27. Gross CP, Sepkowitz KA. The myth of the medical breakthrough: smallpox, vaccination, and Jenner reconsidered. Int J Infect Dis. 1998;3(1):54-60.
28. Romani L. Immunity to fungal infections. Nat Rev Immunol. 2011;11(4):275-88.
29. Coffman RL, Sher A, Seder RA. Vaccine adjuvants: putting innate immunity to work. Immunity. 2010;33(4):492-503.
30. Bloom BR (Ed). Tuberculosis: pathogenesis, protection and control. Washington: ASM Press; 1994.
31. Liu MA. DNA vaccines: an historical perspective and view to the future. Immunol Rev. 2011;239(1):62-84.
32. Anderson RM, May RM. Infectious diseases of humans: dynamics and control. Oxford: Oxford University Press; 1991.
33. Fine P, Eames K, Hiatt M. "Herd immunity": A rough guide. Clim Chang. 2011;105(3):1-12.
34. World Health Organization. (2023). Immunization coverage and herd immunity. [online] Available from https://www.who.int/immunization/coverage [Last accessed March, 2025].
35. Orenstein WA, Ahmed R. Simply put: vaccination saves lives. The importance of vaccines in the present context. Immunity. 2017;47(2):425-8.
36. Männikkö N. Etymologia: Variola and Vaccination. Emerg Infect Dis. 2011;17(4):680.
37. Rappuoli R, Mandl CW, Black S, De Gregorio E. Vaccines for the twenty-first century society. Nat Rev Immunol. 2011;11(12): 865-72.
38. Plotkin SA. Correlates of protection induced by vaccination. Clin Vaccine Immunol. 2010;17(7):1055-65.
39. O'Hagan DT, MacKichan ML, Singh M. Recent developments in adjuvants for vaccines against infectious diseases. Biomol Eng. 2001;18(3):69-85.
40. Cunningham AL, Garçon N, Leo O, Friedland LR, Strugnell R, Laupèze B, et al. Vaccine development: From concept to early clinical testing. Vaccine. 2016;34(52):6655-64.
41. Hotez PJ. Neglected parasitic infections and poverty in the United States. PLoS Negl Trop Dis. 2014;8(9):e3012.
42. Stevens DC, Miller LE. Clinical Immunology and Serology: A Laboratory Perspective, 5th edition. Philadelphia: F.A. Davis Company; 2017.
43. Mahalingam S, Peter J, Xu Z, Bordoloi D, Ho M, Kalyanaraman VS, et al. Landscape of humoral immune responses against SARS-CoV-2 in patients with COVID-19 disease and the value of antibody testing. Heliyon. 2021;7(4):e06836.
44. Schietinger A, Greenberg PD. Tolerance and exhaustion: defining mechanisms of T cell dysfunction. Trends Immunol. 2014;35(2): 51-60.
45. Restifo NP, Dudley ME, Rosenberg SA. Adoptive immunotherapy for cancer: harnessing the T cell response. Nat Rev Immunol. 2012;12(4):269-81.
46. Maloy K, Powrie F. Regulatory T cells in the control of immune pathology. Nat Immunol. 2001;2:816-22.
47. Gill S, June CH. Going viral: chimeric antigen receptor T-cell therapy for hematological malignancies. Immunol Rev. 2015;263(1):68-89.

CHAPTER 3

Molecular Insights into Immune Activation in Vaccine Response

Venkateshappa Chikkanarayanappa, Harish Rangareddy, Jessica Fryer, Achal Shetty, Hayfa Rajhi

INTRODUCTION

The human body has a defense mechanism comprised of immune cells present throughout the body that protects it from harmful microorganisms and substances, which are encountered frequently. The immune system is organized in such a way in the immune organs that allows regulated immune response which is immediate and magnified to kill the infective agents or halt the spread of infection. These defensive reactions involve two closely interrelated systems: (1) innate immunity and (2) adaptive immunity based on which the cells of the immune system have been classified into two general groups.[1] Innate immunity provides immediate, nonspecific defense against pathogens through phagocytosis and inflammation while adaptive immunity recognizes and targets specific antigens encountered during infection or vaccination. Innate immunity includes cells such as macrophages, neutrophils, dendritic cells (DCs), natural killer cells, and complement proteins. Adaptive immunity has T cells and B cells that are antigen-specific and have pathogen immune memory through specific memory cells.[1,2]

MOLECULAR BASIS OF VACCINE DESIGN

Evolution of Vaccines

The history of vaccines is a tale of scientific ingenuity and the relentless pursuit of public health. The journey began in the late 18th century with Edward Jenner's pioneering work on smallpox, where he observed that milkmaids who had contracted cowpox were immune to smallpox. Jenner's innovative approach led to the development of the first vaccine—a method that involved the deliberate exposure of individuals to cowpox to confer immunity against smallpox.[3] This marked the birth of vaccinology and laid the foundation for modern immunization strategies.

As the 19th and 20th centuries progressed, the field of vaccinology evolved significantly. Louis Pasteur's development of vaccines for rabies and anthrax introduced the concept of attenuated vaccines, where weakened forms of pathogens were used to stimulate immunity without causing the disease. The discovery of the polio vaccine by Jonas Salk in 1955 further showcased the potential of vaccines in eradicating diseases that had once caused widespread fear and devastation.[4]

Traditional vaccines, such as live-attenuated, inactivated, and subunit vaccines, have since been instrumental in controlling infectious diseases such as measles, mumps, rubella, and hepatitis. However, these traditional methods, while effective, have limitations, including the potential for adverse reactions, limited effectiveness in certain populations, and challenges in producing vaccines for complex or mutating pathogens. However, contemporary vaccine strategies have shifted toward more targeted approaches, including subunit, recombinant, and nucleic acid vaccines (DNA and mRNA).[4,5] These approaches focus on the expression of specific viral or bacterial antigens that are recognized by the immune system, thereby inducing protective immunity without the risk of infection. The molecular identification of pathogen-associated antigens, such as viral surface glycoproteins or bacterial toxins, has provided key targets for vaccine development.[5]

Molecular Revolution

Vaccines have revolutionized public health by preventing a range of infectious diseases, contributing to the control and elimination of pathogens worldwide. The molecular basis of vaccine design has evolved significantly with advances in immunology, molecular biology, and biotechnology. Modern vaccines aim to elicit a robust immune response, specifically targeting key molecules of pathogens that drive immunity without causing disease. At the core of vaccine development lies a deep understanding of the molecular interactions between pathogens and the host immune system.[6]

The advent of molecular biology in the late 20th century marked a paradigm shift in vaccine development. The ability to decode and manipulate genetic material revolutionized the way vaccines were conceptualized and produced. This molecular revolution brought about the era of recombinant DNA technology, where genes encoding specific antigens could be cloned and expressed in various systems to produce vaccines. This allowed for the development of safer and more targeted vaccines, such as the recombinant hepatitis B vaccine, which became the first vaccine to be produced using genetic engineering techniques.[4,5] The ability to manipulate genetic material for antigen production, coupled with innovative delivery systems like lipid nanoparticles (LNPs) and adjuvants, has transformed vaccine efficacy and safety profiles.[7] Furthermore, the growing understanding of immune responses at the molecular level, such as antigen presentation, T-cell activation, and B cell response, has further enhanced vaccine design to optimize both the quality and duration of immunity.[6]

Advances in genomics and proteomics have further expanded the horizons of vaccine design. With the complete sequencing of the human genome and the genomes of numerous pathogens, scientists gained unprecedented insights into the genetic underpinnings of immunity and disease. This wealth of genetic information has enabled the identification of novel vaccine targets, the prediction of immune responses, and the design of vaccines tailored to specific populations or even individuals.[8]

Rise of Immunoinformatics

Immunoinformatics, a multidisciplinary field that integrates immunology and bioinformatics, has become an essential tool in modern vaccine design. By utilizing computational models and algorithms, researchers can predict which regions of a pathogen's proteome are most likely to trigger a robust immune response. These predictive models are particularly valuable for identifying peptide epitopes—short sequences of amino acids that are recognized by the immune system and can serve as the foundation for vaccine development.[9]

The combination of immunoinformatics with high-throughput screening technologies has facilitated the development of epitope-based vaccines, which focus on specific antigenic components of a pathogen rather than the entire organism. This approach offers several advantages, including a reduced risk of adverse reactions and the ability to design vaccines that target multiple strains of a pathogen or even different pathogens simultaneously. To manage the vast array of immunological data, immunoinformatics employs a variety of bioinformatics tools that span multiple domains, including the creation and management of databases, the definition of both structural and functional signatures, and the development of predictive algorithms.[10]

These strategies enable a deeper understanding of immune system function in both humans and animals and provide new opportunities for tackling complex diseases with unpredictable pathogenesis. The intricate nature of vertebrate immune systems, along with the diversity of pathogens and environmental antigens, requires the analysis of large datasets to unravel immune system mechanisms. Traditionally, the complexity of the immune system and pathogen virulence posed challenges for vaccine development. However, with the advent of computational vaccinology, vaccine research has become more efficient, precise, and tailored to specific needs.[11]

The application of immunoinformatics in disease research involves a comprehensive understanding of disease pathogenesis, immune system dynamics, and computational vaccinology. It also requires extensive database searches, sequence alignment, structural modeling, and motif analysis. These methods have proven invaluable in analyzing disease pathogenesis and identifying potential vaccine candidates, marking a significant advancement in the field of vaccine development.

Broadening the Scope: Vaccines Beyond Infectious Diseases

Traditionally, vaccines have been synonymous with the prevention of infectious diseases. However, the principles of immunology are not confined to pathogens alone. The concept of vaccination has expanded into the realms of oncology and autoimmune diseases, where the immune system plays a central role.

In the early stages of cancer, the immune system performs immunosurveillance, identifying and eliminating abnormal cells to prevent tumor formation. However, cancer cells employ various mechanisms to evade immune detection, allowing tumors to grow and progress. Immunotherapies, including immune checkpoint inhibitors (ICIs) and chimeric antigen receptor (CAR) T-cell therapy, have revolutionized cancer treatment by harnessing the immune system to fight cancer.[12] Despite these advancements, some patients may not respond to immunotherapy or may develop resistance, underscoring the need for further research into the immune-cancer interaction. Gaining a deeper understanding of these mechanisms will be key to developing new therapeutic strategies and identifying predictive biomarkers to improve patient outcomes. Cancer vaccines primarily function by stimulating both innate and adaptive immune responses to recognize, attack, and eliminate neoplastic cells. This section will explore the detailed mechanisms underlying their action.[13]

In autoimmune diseases, where the immune system erroneously attacks the body's own tissues, vaccine design presents a distinct challenge. The goal here is to induce immune tolerance rather than activation. By carefully modulating the immune response, it is possible to prevent or even reverse the progression of autoimmune disorders. Tolerogenic vaccines, which promote the development of antigen-specific regulatory T cells (Tregs), as well as induce anergy and apoptosis in autoreactive T cells, have shown success in animal models of autoimmune diseases.[14]

Various platforms for tolerogenic vaccines have been explored, including protein/peptide, nanoparticle, cell-based, and DNA/RNA vaccines. These approaches have been studied for their ability to enhance immunogenicity in preclinical and clinical research, particularly in multiple sclerosis (MS).[15]

Molecular Techniques in Immunology

The complexities of some pathogens, such as human immunodeficiency virus (HIV) and influenza, and the need for rapid vaccine development in response to emerging threats like coronavirus disease 2019 (COVID-19), have highlighted the need for more advanced and flexible vaccine design strategies. The integration of molecular biology into immunology has opened new avenues for vaccine development. Molecular techniques allow for the precise identification and manipulation of genes and proteins involved in the immune response, leading to the creation of vaccines that are safer, more effective, and quicker to develop than traditional methods.

One of the most significant breakthroughs in molecular vaccine design has been the advent of recombinant DNA technology. This technique involves inserting the gene encoding an antigen from a pathogen into a vector, such as a plasmid or virus, which is then introduced into a host cell. The host cell produces the antigen, which can then be purified and used as a vaccine. The recombinant hepatitis B vaccine, which was first approved in the 1980s, was the first vaccine to be produced using this technology, demonstrating the potential of molecular techniques to revolutionize vaccine design.[16]

Messenger RNA (mRNA) technology has emerged as a groundbreaking approach in vaccine development, gaining widespread attention during the COVID-19 pandemic. mRNA vaccines work by introducing synthetic mRNA sequences that encode viral antigens into host cells. These cells then use the mRNA to produce the corresponding antigens, which triggers an immune response.[17] This method offers several advantages, including rapid vaccine development, the ability to target multiple antigens simultaneously, and the potential for high efficacy. The success of mRNA vaccines against severe acute respiratory syndrome coronavirus 2 (SARS-CoV-2) has spurred interest in expanding this technology for the prevention of other infectious and noninfectious diseases.

The foundational development of mRNA vaccines dates back over three decades, initially explored for influenza. Early efforts focused on encapsulating mRNA coding for viral proteins in LNPs, a strategy that was later applied to the COVID-19 vaccines, particularly targeting the spike (S) protein of SARS-CoV-2. Recent studies, utilizing genetic and epidemiological data, have raised concerns about the theoretical fragmentation of mRNA into smaller RNA sequences. Such fragmentation could potentially interfere with essential biosynthetic processes, such as the production of β-globin, though further research is needed to clarify these risks.[18]

Key considerations regarding mRNA vaccines include: (1) the potential for mRNA fragmentation and its biological consequences and (2) the role of LNPs in the delivery and biodistribution of the mRNA. To address these challenges, it is crucial to refine LNP formulations to improve vaccine targeting and minimize adverse effects.[17] Additionally, personalizing vaccine administration, particularly for high-risk populations such as chronic disease patients, may help optimize efficacy and reduce potential side effects. Furthermore, adapting mRNA vaccines to target the least mutated viral proteins could enhance their effectiveness and longevity, ensuring a more reliable immune response.

Key Immunological Concepts: Antigens, Epitopes, and Adjuvants

To design effective vaccines, it is essential to understand several key immunological concepts: Antigens, epitopes, and adjuvants.

- *Antigens* are molecules, typically proteins or polysaccharides, that are recognized by the immune system as foreign. When an antigen is introduced into the body, it triggers an immune response, leading to the production of antibodies or the activation of immune cells that specifically target the antigen. In the context of vaccines, antigens are the components that stimulate immunity, and selecting the right antigen is crucial for the vaccine's effectiveness.[19]
- *Epitopes* are specific regions of an antigen that are recognized by immune receptors, such as antibodies

or T-cell receptors (TCRs). An antigen can have multiple epitopes, each of which can elicit a different immune response. In vaccine design, identifying and selecting the most immunogenic epitopes is a critical step in ensuring that the vaccine effectively stimulates the desired immune response. Techniques such as *epitope mapping* and *in silico epitope prediction* are used to identify these key regions of the antigen.[20]

- *Adjuvants* are substances that are added to vaccines to enhance the immune response to the antigen. They work by stimulating the immune system in various ways, such as by activating antigen-presenting cells (APCs) or promoting the release of cytokines. Common adjuvants include aluminum salts (alum), which have been used in vaccines for decades, and newer adjuvants such as MF59 and AS01, which are used in vaccines such as the influenza and malaria vaccines. The choice of adjuvant can significantly impact the effectiveness of a vaccine, particularly in populations with weaker immune responses, such as the elderly.[21]

Transition from Empirical to Rational Vaccine Design

Traditional vaccine development has often been an empirical process, involving the trial-and-error testing of various vaccine candidates in animal models and human trials.[22] While this approach has led to many successful vaccines, it is time-consuming, costly, and not always effective, particularly for complex diseases such as HIV, malaria, and cancer.

Molecular techniques are transforming vaccine design into a more rational process, where decisions are guided by a detailed understanding of the immune system and the pathogen. This rational approach involves:

- *Targeted antigen selection:* Using genomic and proteomic data to identify the most relevant antigens for a given pathogen, reducing the need for broad, less specific approaches.[22,23]
- *Epitope-based design:* Focusing on specific epitopes known to elicit strong and protective immune responses, rather than using entire pathogens or large portions of them.[22,23]
- *Personalized vaccines:* Leveraging genomic and immunological data from individual patients to create vaccines tailored to their specific immune profiles, particularly in the context of cancer and chronic diseases.[22,23]
- *Rapid response technologies:* Employing platforms like mRNA and viral vectors to quickly develop and deploy vaccines in response to emerging infectious diseases.[22,23]

Genomic Data in Identifying Vaccine Targets

Genomics, the study of an organism's complete set of DNA, has revolutionized many fields of medicine, particularly vaccine design. The ability to sequence entire genomes of pathogens and hosts has provided researchers with a detailed map of the genetic material involved in disease processes and immune responses. This information is invaluable in identifying potential vaccine targets—genes or proteins that play critical roles in pathogen survival or virulence and are likely to elicit a strong immune response.[22]

The identification of vaccine targets through genomics begins with *comparative genomics*, where the genomes of pathogenic strains are compared to nonpathogenic strains or closely related organisms. This comparison helps to identify genes that are unique to the pathogen or are highly conserved across different strains, making them ideal targets for vaccine development. For example, the success of the meningococcal B vaccine (4CMenB) was largely due to the identification of novel antigens through comparative genomics, which were not present in earlier vaccines.[22,24]

Another approach involves *reverse vaccinology*, a technique pioneered in the early 2000s. In reverse vaccinology, researchers start with the genome of the pathogen and use bioinformatics tools to predict which proteins are located on the surface of the pathogen and are likely to be recognized by the immune system. These predictions are then validated through laboratory experiments, leading to the identification of promising vaccine candidates.[25] This method bypasses the need for traditional antigen identification, which relied on cultivating the pathogen and testing various components—a time-consuming and often incomplete process.

Advances in High-throughput Sequencing Technologies

The ability to rapidly sequence DNA has been one of the key drivers behind the integration of genomics into vaccine design. High-throughput sequencing technologies, often referred to as next-generation sequencing (NGS), have dramatically reduced the time and cost associated with genome sequencing. These technologies can sequence entire genomes in a matter of days, providing a wealth of data that can be mined for vaccine development.[26]

Whole-genome sequencing (WGS) is one of the most comprehensive approaches, as it provides the complete DNA sequence of an organism. WGS allows researchers to identify all the genes present in a pathogen, including those involved in virulence, antibiotic resistance, and immune evasion.[27] This holistic view is particularly useful for pathogens with complex genomes or those that undergo frequent genetic changes, such as influenza and HIV.

Transcriptomics is another important tool, focusing on the RNA transcripts produced by a pathogen or host cell during infection. By analyzing which genes are actively expressed during different stages of infection, researchers can identify potential vaccine targets that are critical for pathogen survival or immune evasion. Transcriptomic data can also reveal how the host's immune system responds to infection, helping to identify which aspects of the immune response should be targeted or enhanced by a vaccine.[28]

Genomics-driven Vaccine Development

To illustrate the impact of genomics on vaccine development, let us explore a few examples where genomic data played a crucial role in designing effective vaccines.

- *Meningococcal B vaccine (4CMenB)*: Meningococcal disease, caused by *Neisseria meningitidis*, is a leading cause of bacterial meningitis and septicemia. While vaccines for several serogroups of *N. meningitidis* were available, developing a vaccine for serogroup B (MenB) proved challenging due to the poor immunogenicity of its polysaccharide capsule. The breakthrough came with the use of reverse vaccinology, where the genome of *N. meningitidis* was sequenced, and potential surface-exposed proteins were identified as vaccine candidates. These candidates were then tested in preclinical and clinical trials, leading to the development of the 4CMenB vaccine, which has significantly reduced the incidence of MenB disease.[24]
- *Influenza vaccines*: Influenza viruses undergo frequent genetic changes, leading to the emergence of new strains that can evade immunity from previous infections or vaccinations. Genomic surveillance of circulating influenza strains is essential for selecting the appropriate strains to include in the seasonal influenza vaccine. High-throughput sequencing has enabled the rapid identification of genetic changes in the hemagglutinin and neuraminidase proteins, which are the primary targets of influenza vaccines. This genomic data ensures that the vaccine components are updated annually to match the most prevalent strains, improving vaccine efficacy.[29]
- *COVID-19 mRNA vaccines*: The rapid development of COVID-19 vaccines, particularly the mRNA vaccines showcases the power of genomics in responding to emerging infectious diseases. Within weeks of the SARS-CoV-2 virus being identified, its genome was sequenced and made publicly available. Researchers quickly identified the spike (S) protein as the key antigen for vaccine development. The mRNA vaccines were designed to encode the S protein, prompting the body to produce the protein and generate an immune response.[17,18] The success of these vaccines, with their high efficacy and rapid deployment, demonstrates the potential of genomics-driven vaccine design in addressing global health emergencies.

Proteomics and Its Role in Immunology

Proteomics is the large-scale study of proteins, the workhorses of the cell that carry out a wide array of functions essential to life. In the context of immunology and vaccine development, proteomics provides critical insights into the structure, function, and interactions of proteins, particularly those involved in pathogen-host interactions and immune responses. By analyzing the proteome—the complete set of proteins expressed by an organism—researchers can identify and characterize the proteins that are most likely to serve as effective vaccine targets.[28]

While genomics focuses on the DNA blueprint, proteomics reveals how these genetic instructions are translated into the functional molecules that drive biological processes. This is particularly important in vaccine design, as the immune system often recognizes and responds to specific proteins (antigens) on the surface of pathogens. Proteomic techniques allow for the identification of these antigens, the mapping of epitopes (the specific regions of the antigen that are recognized by the immune system), and the characterization of the immune response they elicit.[8,22]

Techniques in Proteomics for Vaccine Design

Several proteomic techniques are crucial in identifying and characterizing proteins for vaccine development:

- *Mass spectrometry*: Mass spectrometry is one of the most powerful tools in proteomics. It allows for the precise identification and quantification of proteins within a complex mixture. In vaccine development, it is used to identify potential antigens by analyzing the protein composition of pathogens. The technique can also be used to map post-translational modifications, such as glycosylation or phosphorylation, which can affect how antigens are recognized by the immune system.[30]
- *Two-dimensional gel electrophoresis (2D-GE)*: This technique separates proteins based on their iso-electric point and molecular weight, allowing for

the resolution of thousands of proteins in a single experiment. 2D-GE is often used in combination with mass spectrometry to identify proteins that are differentially expressed during infection, which may represent potential vaccine targets.[30]

- *Western blotting*: A technique used to detect specific proteins in a sample, Western blotting is valuable for validating the presence of target proteins identified through mass spectrometry or 2D-GE. In vaccine research, it helps confirm the expression of antigens in pathogen samples or vaccine formulations.[30]
- *Protein microarrays*: Protein microarrays allow for the simultaneous analysis of thousands of proteins, making them a powerful tool for studying immune responses. In vaccine design, they are used to identify which proteins or epitopes are recognized by antibodies in sera from infected or vaccinated individuals, helping to pinpoint the most immunogenic components of a pathogen.[30]

Uncovering Peptide Epitopes for Vaccine Development

One of the key applications of proteomics in vaccine design is the identification of peptide epitopes—short sequences of amino acids within proteins that are recognized by immune cells. These epitopes are crucial for the development of subunit and epitope-based vaccines, which aim to induce immunity by targeting specific, highly immunogenic regions of a pathogen's proteome.

The process of epitope discovery involves several steps:

- *Epitope prediction*: Using computational tools, researchers can predict potential epitopes based on the amino acid sequence of a protein. These tools analyze factors such as the protein's secondary structure, binding affinities to major histocompatibility complex (MHC) molecules, and similarity to known epitopes.[31]
- *Experimental validation*: Predicted epitopes must be validated through laboratory experiments. This often involves synthesizing the peptide epitopes and testing their ability to bind to MHC molecules or be recognized by T cells or antibodies. Techniques such as enzyme-linked immunosorbent assays (ELISA), flow cytometry, and peptide-MHC tetramer staining are commonly used in this phase.[32]
- *Epitope mapping*: Once potential epitopes are identified, they are mapped to determine their precise location within the protein and their accessibility to the immune system. This mapping is essential for understanding how the epitope is presented on the pathogen's surface and how it interacts with immune receptors.[32,33]

The identification of peptide epitopes has been particularly useful in developing vaccines for viruses that undergo frequent mutations, such as influenza and HIV. By targeting conserved epitopes—regions of the viral proteome that remain unchanged across different strains—researchers can design vaccines that provide broader protection against diverse or rapidly evolving pathogens.

MOLECULAR MECHANISMS IN IMMUNE ACTIVATION

A profound comprehension of the intricate molecular mechanisms that adaptive immune response relies on the sequential activation of different types of immune cells, viz., APCs become activated when they encounter a pathogen and subsequently pathogen-derived peptides bind to MHC molecules on APCs and engage the TCR on T cells followed by activation of T cells and other mechanisms underlying immune activation is an imperative pursuit in vaccination for advancing vaccine efficacy, safety, and personalized approaches.

Antigen-presenting Cells: Gatekeepers of the Immune System

Antigen-presenting cells play a pivotal role in initiating the adaptive immune response. They are responsible for capturing, processing, and presenting antigens to T cells, thereby bridging the innate and adaptive immune systems.[1,2]

- *Types of APCs*: The main types of APCs include DCs, macrophages, and B cells. Each type has distinct functions and tissue distributions, contributing to the overall immune response.[1,2,33]
  - *Dendritic cells*: DCs are considered the most potent APCs and are key players in initiating immune responses. They capture antigens through endocytosis or phagocytosis, process them into peptides, and present these peptides on MHC molecules. DCs then migrate to lymph nodes where they interact with T cells.[34-36]
  - *Macrophages*: Macrophages are versatile immune cells that can act as APCs. They engulf and digest pathogens, present antigens to T cells, and produce cytokines that influence the immune response. Macrophages are particularly important in tissue surveillance and response to chronic infections.[1,2]
  - *B cells*: B cells can also function as APCs. They internalize antigens through specific receptors

(e.g., B cell receptors), process them, and present antigenic peptides to helper T cells. B cells are crucial for generating antigen-specific antibody responses.[1,2]

- *Antigen processing and presentation*: The process of antigen processing involves the breakdown of pathogen-derived proteins into peptides. These peptides are then loaded onto MHC molecules. There are two main classes of MHC molecules:
    - *MHC class I*: Presents peptides derived from endogenous proteins (e.g., those synthesized within the cell) to CD8+ cytotoxic T cells (CTLs). This pathway is crucial for detecting and eliminating infected or cancerous cells.[34-36]
    - *MHC class II*: Presents peptides derived from exogenous proteins (e.g., those taken up from the extracellular environment) to CD4+ helper T cells. This pathway is essential for coordinating immune responses and helping B cells to produce antibodies.[34-36]

T-cell Activation: From Naïve to Effector

The activation of T cells is a complex process that involves several key steps:

- *Antigen recognition*: Naïve T cells circulate through lymph nodes, where they encounter APCs presenting antigens on MHC molecules. The interaction between the TCR and the peptide-MHC complex is the first critical step in T-cell activation.[1,2]
- *Costimulation*: In addition to TCR signaling, T cells require additional signals from costimulatory molecules to become fully activated. Key costimulatory molecules include CD80/CD86 on APCs and CD28 on T cells. This second signal is crucial for ensuring a robust and regulated immune response.[34-36]
- *Activation and proliferation*: Once activated, T cells undergo clonal expansion, rapidly dividing to produce a large population of antigen-specific cells. This proliferation is driven by cytokines such as interleukin-2 (IL-2), which promote T-cell growth and differentiation.[34-36]
- *Differentiation*: Activated T cells differentiate into various subsets with distinct functions:
    - *CD4+ T helper cells*: These cells help orchestrate the immune response by releasing cytokines that influence the activity of other immune cells. They can differentiate into various subsets, including Th1, Th2, Th17, and Tregs, each with specific roles in immune regulation and pathogen defense.[34-36]
    - *CD8+ cytotoxic T cells*: These cells are specialized in killing infected or malignant cells. They recognize and destroy target cells presenting the antigen on MHC class I molecules.[34-36]

Understanding the Immune System's Response to Vaccines

The immune system's response to a vaccine is a highly orchestrated process involving various cells and molecules. The goal of vaccination is to prime the immune system to recognize and combat specific pathogens without causing disease. A vaccine's efficacy depends on its ability to stimulate both innate and adaptive immune responses effectively.

- *Innate immune response*: The first line of defense, the innate immune response, is triggered immediately upon vaccination. It involves the activation of APCs such as DCs and macrophages, which recognize pathogen-associated molecular patterns (PAMPs) on the vaccine antigens. Innate immunity is the body's first line of defense, mediated through the recognition of PAMPs by pattern recognition receptors (PRRs). Key PRRs include toll-like receptors (TLRs) and NOD-like receptors (NLRs), which trigger signaling cascades essential for immune activation. Upon recognition of PAMPs, TLRs activate the nuclear factor kappa B (NF-κB) pathway, leading to inflammatory cytokine production. Additionally, type I interferon (IFN) responses are activated through the detection of viral RNA by receptors like RIG-I, enhancing antiviral defenses. These cells process the antigens and present them to T cells, bridging the innate and adaptive immune responses.[34,35]
- *Adaptive immune response*: The adaptive immune response is more specific and involves the activation of T cells and B cells. T cells can differentiate into helper T cells (Th), which aid in activating other immune cells, or CTLs, which directly kill infected cells. B cells produce antibodies that neutralize pathogens or mark them for destruction by other immune cells. The formation of memory T and B cells is crucial, as they provide long-term protection by responding more rapidly and robustly upon subsequent exposures to the pathogen.[2,34]

The molecular mechanisms driving adaptive immunity are closely linked to the innate immune system, particularly through the activation of PRRs and the subsequent activation of APCs like DCs.

Bridging Innate and Adaptive Immune Defenses

A key event in the initiation of adaptive immunity following vaccination is the bridging of innate and adaptive responses, a process largely mediated by PRRs, especially TLRs on DCs. PRRs recognize conserved molecular patterns on pathogens, such as lipopolysaccharides (LPS) and viral RNA, which trigger innate immune responses. These receptors are instrumental in activating DCs, which then link innate immune signals to adaptive immunity by presenting antigens to T lymphocytes.[35]

Role of Dendritic Cells in Linking Innate and Adaptive Immunity

Dendritic cells are pivotal in the initiation of adaptive immune responses. Upon recognition of vaccine-derived antigens, DCs become activated and undergo several key processes that promote the transition from innate to adaptive immunity:

- *Antigen uptake and maturation*: After taking up the vaccine antigen via phagocytosis or endocytosis, DCs mature. This maturation process is regulated by PRR signaling, which includes the upregulation of costimulatory molecules (e.g., CD80, CD86, and CD40) and antigen-presenting molecules (e.g., MHC class II), necessary for effective T-cell activation.[36]
- *Migration to lymph nodes*: Activated DCs migrate from the site of infection or vaccination to regional lymph nodes, where they encounter T lymphocytes. This migration is directed by chemokines and changes in the expression of chemokine receptors, such as CCR7, which guide DCs to the lymphatic system.[36]
- *Antigen presentation*: In the lymph nodes, mature DCs present processed antigenic peptides via MHC molecules to naïve T cells. The interaction between the antigen presented by DCs and the TCR on T cells initiates T-cell activation, a cornerstone of adaptive immunity.[36]
- *Activation of T lymphocytes*: Once TCRs engage with the antigen-MHC complex, costimulatory signals provided by the upregulated costimulatory molecules (CD80, CD86, and CD40) are crucial for T cell activation. In addition, cytokine secretion by DCs during this interaction provides signals that drive T cell differentiation into specific subtypes, such as helper T cells (Th1, Th2, and Th17) or CTLs.[36]

Dendritic Cell Subsets and their Roles in Immune Activation

Dendritic cells are not a homogeneous population, and distinct subsets of DCs express different sets of TLRs and other PRRs, which contribute to the diversity of their functions. These subsets can be broadly classified into *conventional DCs (cDCs)* and *plasmacytoid DCs (pDCs)*, each playing unique roles in immune responses:[37]

- *Conventional DCs*: These cells are critical for activating T cells and initiating the adaptive immune response. They are equipped with a broad range of TLRs and are particularly important in recognizing bacterial and fungal pathogens. Their functions include antigen uptake, processing, and presentation to T cells, as well as the secretion of proinflammatory cytokines that promote T-cell activation and differentiation.[37,38]
- *Plasmacytoid DCs*: These cells are primarily involved in the early antiviral immune response due to their ability to recognize viral nucleic acids through TLR7 and TLR9. Upon activation, pDCs secrete large amounts of type I IFNs, which play a pivotal role in shaping the adaptive immune response, especially in the context of viral infections.[37,38]

The nonoverlapping expression of TLRs between these DC subsets and their selective tissue distribution is believed to underlie the diversity in their functions. This specificity allows DCs to fine-tune the immune response based on the pathogen type and the site of infection, ensuring that the adaptive immune system is appropriately activated.

Integration of Innate and Adaptive Responses

The activation of T lymphocytes by DCs initiates the adaptive immune response, leading to the generation of effector T cells that clear infections and the formation of memory T and B cells, providing long-term immunity. CD4+ T helper cells coordinate both cellular and humoral immunity, while CD8+ CTLs directly target and kill infected cells. Concurrently, B cells are activated through antigen presentation and T cell assistance, resulting in the production of antibodies that neutralize pathogens. The formation of memory cells ensures a quicker and more robust immune response upon future exposure to the same pathogen. The interaction between the innate immune system, particularly the activation of DCs via PRRs like TLRs, and the adaptive immune system facilitates a coordinated immune defense following vaccination, which not only enhances immediate responses but also provides the foundation for long-lasting protection. The effectiveness of a vaccine depends on this interplay, although different pathogens and vaccines may require tailored immune responses, with viral vaccines often needing robust cytotoxic T lymphocyte (CTL) responses, while bacterial vaccines may rely more on antibody production. Fine-tuning these immune mechanisms is crucial for optimizing vaccine efficacy.[34-36]

Strategies for Enhancing Immunogenicity

To ensure that vaccines elicit a strong and appropriate immune response, several strategies are employed to enhance their immunogenicity:

- *Adjuvants*: Adjuvants are substances added to vaccines to boost the immune response. They work by stimulating the innate immune system, increasing the recruitment and activation of APCs, and enhancing antigen presentation to T cells.[21] Common adjuvants include aluminum salts (alum), oil-in-water emulsions (e.g., MF59), and TLR agonists. The choice of adjuvant depends on the type of immune response desired. Many adjuvants function as ligands for PRRs, triggering an innate immune response. This receptor activation can then initiate signaling pathways that activate transcription factors, leading to the production of cytokines and chemokines. These molecules help to guide the immune response toward specific types, such as Th1 or Th2 responses, and regulate the recruitment of immune cells to the injection site. Additionally, inflammasome activation has been identified as a potential mechanism through which some adjuvants exert their effects. This activation results in the release of proinflammatory cytokines, such as IL-1β and IL-18. Some adjuvants can also enhance antigen presentation by MHC molecules. Notably, certain adjuvants may work through multiple pathways; for instance, alum has been proposed to influence antigen uptake, PRR signaling, inflammasome activation, and immune cell recruitment.[39]
- *Antigen engineering*: The structure and presentation of the antigen can significantly impact the immune response. Antigen engineering involves modifying the antigen to enhance its immunogenicity. This can include *glycosylation modifications* to mimic natural pathogen structures, the inclusion of *multimeric forms* of antigens to improve B cell receptor cross-linking, or the design of *chimeric antigens* that incorporate multiple epitopes from different strains of a pathogen.[40] For example, the respiratory syncytial virus (RSV) new vaccine, antigen based on the RSV fusion protein (RSV F), stabilized in its native prefusion conformation, has shown promise. This prefusion form is created by preventing hinge movements in the first refolding region and avoiding proteolytic exposure of the fusion peptide. This stable prefusion RSV F induces neutralizing antibodies in cotton rats and provides full protection against viral infection.[41]
- *Prime-boost strategies*: Prime-boost strategies involve administering multiple doses of a vaccine, with the first dose (prime) establishing an initial immune response and subsequent doses (boosts) enhancing and prolonging this response. This approach can increase the magnitude and duration of the immune response, particularly for vaccines that require strong T cell-mediated immunity.[42] For example, the malaria vaccine RTS,S uses a prime-boost regimen with a protein-based vaccine followed by a viral vector-based boost to enhance the immune response against the *Plasmodium* parasite.[43]
- *Route of administration*: The route by which a vaccine is administered can influence the type of immune response generated. Intramuscular and subcutaneous injections are common, but other routes, such as intranasal, oral, or intradermal, may be more effective for certain pathogens. For instance, the oral polio vaccine (OPV) is administered orally because it mimics the natural route of infection, leading to strong mucosal immunity in the gut, where poliovirus replicates.[44]

Molecular Pathways of Immune Activation

The molecular pathways involved in immune activation are intricate and involve a series of signaling events that lead to T-cell activation and effector function. Key pathways include:

T-cell receptor signaling pathway: The TCR signaling pathway is initiated when the TCR binds to the peptide-MHC complex. This interaction activates a cascade of intracellular signaling events involving protein tyrosine kinases (e.g., Lck and ZAP70), adaptor proteins (e.g., LAT and SLP-76), and downstream signaling molecules [e.g., mitogen-activated protein kinases (MAPKs) and NF-κB]. These signals lead to T-cell activation, cytokine production, and cell proliferation[45] as shown in **Flowchart 1**.

NF-κB pathway: The NF-κB pathway is a critical regulator of immune responses. NF-κB transcription factors are activated in response to various signals, including TCR signaling and costimulatory signals. NF-κB exerts its immune response through classical pathway and noncanonical pathway as shown in **Table 1**. NF-κB promotes the expression of genes involved in T-cell activation, survival, and inflammation.[46]

MAPK pathway: The MAPK pathway is involved in regulating cellular responses to growth factors, cytokines, and stress signals. MAPKs such as ERK, JNK, and p38 are activated by TCR signaling and contribute to T-cell proliferation, differentiation, and effector functions.[47]

Step 1: Pathogen targeting of MAPK pathways

- Many pathogens target host MAPK pathways to inhibit immune responses.

Step 2: MAPK pathways activation

- Key MAPK pathways involved:
  - p38 MAPK
  - JNK
  - ERK
- These pathways induce the production of immunomodulatory cytokines (e.g., TNF-α, IL-1, IL-10, and IL-12).

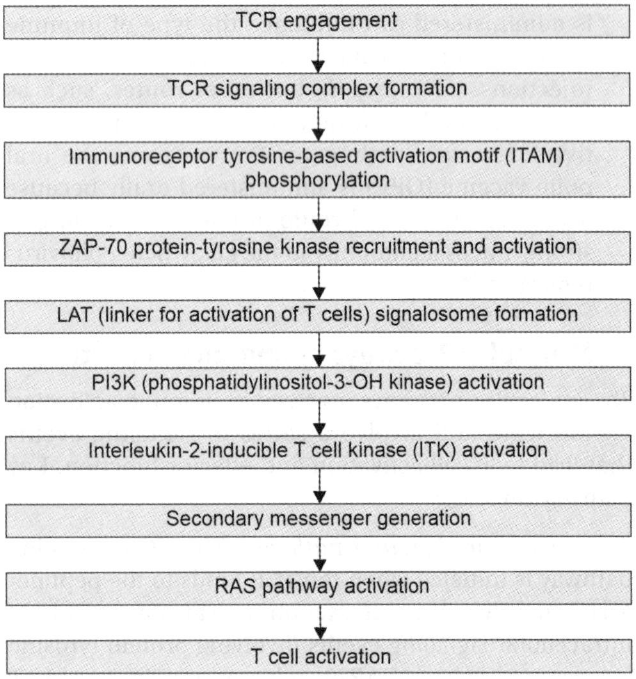

FLOWCHART 1: Steps in T cell receptor (TCR) signaling pathway.

Th1 response (intracellular pathogens):

Step 3: p38 MAPK and IL-12 production

- Activation of *p38 MAPK* regulates IL-12 production
- IL-12 promotes differentiation of *Th1 cells*

Step 4: Th1 cell action

- Th1 cells release proinflammatory cytokines *(IL-2, IFN-γ, and TNF-α/β)*
- These cytokines mediate killing of intracellular pathogens (e.g., *Leishmania species, Trypanosoma cruzi*)

Th2 response (extracellular pathogens):

Step 5: ERK1/2 and IL-10 production

- Activation of *ERK1/2* regulates IL-10 production
- IL-10 promotes differentiation of *Th2 cells*

Step 6: Th2 cell action

- Th2 cells release anti-inflammatory cytokines *(IL-4, IL-5, IL-9, and IL-13).*
- These cytokines mediate the humoral immune response and elimination of extracellular pathogens.

Step 7: Regulation of inflammation by IL-10

- IL-10 also acts as a *negative regulator of inflammation* to prevent tissue damage

MAPK1 plays a role in regulating inflammatory cytokine production (e.g., IL-1 and TNF-α). Vaccines targeting this pathway can enhance protective immune responses by promoting balanced cytokine profiles, aiding in the development of Th1 or Th2 immune responses depending on the desired outcome. Advanced computational tools like molecular docking and virtual screening facilitate the identification of peptide-based vaccines and compounds that interact optimally with

TABLE 1: Differences between classical and noncanonical pathway of NF-κB signaling.

Steps	Classical pathway	Noncanonical pathway
Triggering the pathway	Activated by proinflammatory cytokines (e.g., IL-1β, IL-18, and TNF-α) and PRR ligands (e.g., RIG-I and TLRs)	Activated by TNF superfamily members
Signal initiation	TAK1, or transforming growth factor β-activated kinase-1, activates IKK, or I-kappa B kinase complex	NF-κB-inducing kinase (NIK) activates IκB kinase α (IKKα) by phosphorylating it on serine residue 176 in the activation loop
Phosphorylation events	IKKβ phosphorylates IκBα at Ser32 and Ser36	IKKα phosphorylates p100 at Ser866 and Ser870
Protein degradation	Phosphorylated IκBα is ubiquitinated and degraded by the 26S proteasome	Phosphorylated p100 undergoes partial degradation to generate the p52 subunit
Release and translocation	RelA/p50 dimers are released and translocate to the nucleus	RelB/p52 dimers are generated and translocate to the nucleus
Gene activation	Regulates innate immunity	Regulates adaptive immunity

(IL-1β: interleukin-1beta; IL-18: interleukin-18; NF-κB: nuclear factor kappaB; TLRs: toll-like receptors; TNF-α: tumor necrosis factor-alpha)

MAPK1. These methods ensure high specificity and reduced risk of off-target effects.[48]

Modulating the Immune Response: Th1, Th2, and Beyond

The adaptive immune response can be broadly classified into different types based on the cytokine profiles and the immune cells involved:

- *Th1 response*: It is characterized by the production of interferon-gamma (IFN-γ) and the activation of CTLs, the Th1 response is critical for combating intracellular pathogens, such as viruses and certain bacteria. Vaccines designed to elicit a Th1 response often incorporate adjuvants that stimulate TLRs and promote the secretion of IFN-γ.[49]
- *Th2 response*: The Th2 response is associated with the production of cytokines such as IL-4, IL-5, and IL-13, which promote B cell activation and antibody production. This response is important for defending against extracellular pathogens, such as helminths and toxins.[50]
- *Th17 and Treg responses*: In addition to Th1 and Th2, other T helper cell subsets play important roles in immune regulation. Th17 cells, which produce IL-17, are involved in mucosal immunity and protection against fungi and some bacteria. Tregs help to maintain immune tolerance and prevent autoimmunity by suppressing excessive immune responses.[14,34-36] Fine-tuning the balance between these different T cell responses is crucial for developing vaccines that are not only effective but also safe, minimizing the risk of immune-mediated adverse effects.
- *Cross-presentation*: Cross-presentation refers to the process by which DCs present extracellular antigens on MHC class I molecules, leading to the activation of CTLs. This mechanism is particularly important for vaccines against viruses and tumors, where a strong CD8+ T cell response is needed. Enhancing cross-presentation through the use of specific adjuvants or antigen delivery systems can improve the efficacy of these vaccines.[51]

Long-term Immunity and Memory Formation

One of the ultimate goals of vaccination is to induce long-lasting immunity, providing protection against future exposures to the pathogen. The formation of memory T and B cells is central to this process:

- *Memory T cells*: After the initial immune response, some of the activated T cells differentiate into memory T cells, which persist long-term in the body. These cells can be quickly reactivated upon reexposure to the antigen, providing rapid and robust protection. Memory T cells can be broadly categorized into central memory T cells, which reside in lymphoid tissues and provide long-term protection, and effector memory T cells, which circulate in the blood and peripheral tissues and provide immediate protection.[52]
- *Memory B cells and long-lived plasma cells*: Similarly, some activated B cells become memory B cells, which can rapidly produce antibodies upon reexposure to the antigen. Additionally, long-lived plasma cells reside in the bone marrow and continuously secrete antibodies, providing sustained protection. The longevity of these cells and their ability to produce high-affinity antibodies are key factors in the duration of vaccine-induced immunity.[53]

To enhance long-term immunity, vaccine developers often focus on optimizing the initial priming and boosting phases, ensuring that memory cells are generated and maintained. The use of adjuvants, antigen design, and delivery methods that promote memory cell formation is critical in this regard.

Beyond Infectious Diseases

Traditionally, vaccines have been developed to protect against infectious diseases, leveraging the body's immune system to prevent or mitigate the effects of pathogens such as bacteria, viruses, and parasites. However, recent advances in molecular biology, immunology, and biotechnology are expanding the scope of vaccine design to include noninfectious conditions such as cancer, autoimmune diseases, allergies, and even neurological disorders.

These next-generation vaccines are not merely preventive; they are also therapeutic, aiming to treat existing diseases by modulating the immune system in targeted and innovative ways. This expansion marks a significant shift in the role of vaccines in medicine, transforming them from a tool solely for disease prevention to a powerful therapeutic strategy for a broad range of conditions.

Cancer Vaccines: Targeting Tumors with Precision

Cancer vaccines are designed to stimulate the immune system to recognize and attack cancer cells. Unlike traditional vaccines, which prevent disease, cancer vaccines are typically therapeutic, used to treat existing cancers or prevent their recurrence. The development of cancer vaccines is particularly challenging due to the complexity of cancer biology and the immune system's ability to distinguish between normal and malignant cells.

- *Tumor-associated antigens (TAAs) and neoantigens*: Cancer cells often express abnormal proteins known as TAAs or neoantigens that are not present on normal cells. TAAs are derived from proteins that are overexpressed or aberrantly expressed in cancer cells, while neoantigens arise from mutations unique to the tumor. The identification of TAAs and neoantigens through genomic and proteomic approaches is a critical step in designing cancer vaccines.[54] These antigens are used to train the immune system to recognize and eliminate cancer cells without harming normal tissues.
- *Types of cancer vaccines*: There are several types of cancer vaccines, each utilizing different strategies to elicit an antitumor immune response:
  - *Peptide-based vaccines*: These vaccines use short sequences of amino acids (peptides) from TAAs or neoantigens to stimulate T cells. The peptides are often combined with adjuvants or delivery systems that enhance their immunogenicity. Peptide vaccines are highly specific, but their effectiveness can be limited by the patient's human leukocyte antigen (HLA) type, which determines how well the peptides are presented to the immune system.[55]
  - *Dendritic cell vaccines*: Dendritic cells are potent APCs that play a key role in initiating the immune response. DC vaccines involve isolating DCs from a patient's blood, loading them with tumor antigens, and then reintroducing them into the patient. The loaded DCs present the antigens to T cells, stimulating a targeted immune response against the tumor. An example of this approach is Sipuleucel-T (Provenge), a DC vaccine approved for the treatment of metastatic prostate cancer.[56]
  - *Virus-like particles (VLPs)*: VLPs are noninfectious particles that mimic the structure of viruses but do not contain viral genetic material. They can be engineered to display TAAs on their surface, making them highly immunogenic. VLP-based cancer vaccines have shown promise in preclinical studies and are being explored for various cancers.[57]
  - *Oncolytic virus vaccines*: Oncolytic viruses are genetically modified viruses that selectively infect and kill cancer cells. These viruses can also be engineered to express TAAs, enhancing the antitumor immune response. Oncolytic virus vaccines have the dual benefit of directly destroying cancer cells and stimulating the immune system to recognize and attack tumors.[58]

Vaccines for Autoimmune Diseases: Restoring Immune Tolerance

Autoimmune diseases occur when the immune system mistakenly attacks the body's own tissues, leading to chronic inflammation and tissue damage. The goal of vaccines for autoimmune diseases is to restore immune tolerance, preventing the immune system from targeting self-antigens while preserving its ability to fight infections.

- *Multiple sclerosis vaccines*: As an autoimmune disease that targets the central nervous system, MS presents unique challenges for vaccine development. Experimental vaccines for MS aim to induce tolerance to myelin antigens or to modulate the immune response to reduce inflammation and prevent further damage to the nervous system. Despite the failure of a phase III clinical trial using a peptide vaccine to show significant clinical benefit, the tolerogenic approach remains under investigation in MS patients using several vaccine platforms.[59]
- Recently, Krienke et al. demonstrated the successful induction of immune tolerance in a mouse model of experimental autoimmune encephalomyelitis (EAE), induced by myelin oligodendrocyte glycoprotein (MOG35-55), using a noninflammatory mRNA-based vaccine. Notably, although double-stranded RNA is typically proinflammatory, its inflammatory properties were minimized by replacing uridine with 1-methylpseudouridine (m1Ψ). This modified mRNA vaccine, encoding MOG35-55, effectively prevented disease onset and progression in mice. It induced MOG35-55-specific FOXP3+ Treg cells and suppressed MOG35-55-specific Th1 and Th17 cells. Furthermore, the expression of inhibitory molecules such as PD1 and CTLA4 was upregulated on antigen-specific cells. The protective effects of the vaccine were negated when PD1 and CTLA4 checkpoint inhibitors were administered, highlighting the role of these immune checkpoints in regulating the tolerogenic response.[60]

Vaccines for Neurological Disorders: A New Frontier

Neurological disorders, including Alzheimer's disease, Parkinson's disease, and MS, represent a new frontier for vaccine development. These conditions often involve complex interactions between the immune system and the nervous system, leading to chronic inflammation, neurodegeneration, or autoimmune responses. Vaccines for neurological disorders aim to modulate these immune processes to prevent or slow disease progression.

- *Alzheimer's disease vaccines*: Alzheimer's disease is characterized by the accumulation of amyloid-β plaques and tau protein tangles in the brain, leading to neurodegeneration. Vaccine strategies for Alzheimer's focus on eliciting an immune response against these pathological proteins, either by targeting amyloid-β, tau, or both. Newer approaches are exploring ways to fine-tune the immune response to reduce inflammation while promoting the clearance of amyloid-β and tau.[48,61]
- *Parkinson's disease vaccines*: Parkinson's disease involves the loss of dopamine-producing neurons in the brain, leading to motor and cognitive symptoms. α-synuclein, a protein that aggregates in the brains of Parkinson's patients, is a key target for vaccine development. Vaccines targeting α-synuclein aim to stimulate the immune system to clear these aggregates and protect neurons from further damage.[62]

SYSTEMS VACCINOLOGY APPROACH

Systems vaccinology integrates omics technologies such as genomics, proteomics, and transcriptomics to study vaccine responses at a systems level, enabling the identification of molecular signatures that predict efficacy and guide personalized strategies. By analyzing genetic variations, protein biomarkers, and gene expression profiles, this approach provides insights into immune cell activation, cytokine patterns, and antibody production, facilitating the optimization of vaccine formulations and safety. Computational models further enhance the ability to predict individual and population-level outcomes, uncover novel targets, and refine vaccine design, advancing the development of effective and tailored immunization strategies.[22,25,28]

CHALLENGES IN VACCINATION AFFECTING THE IMMUNE RESPONSES

Vaccine development and vaccination face various challenges such as vaccine hesitancy, vaccine inequity, and vaccine-preventable disease outbreaks. The delicate nature of antigen structures, viz., thermosensitive vaccines is a factor that determines the vaccine potency laying the emphasis on the cold chain logistics to be maintained stringently.[63] Supply of the vaccines requiring low to ultra-low temperature storage to remote areas and low- and middle-income countries is a challenge.[64,65] Overcoming these challenges requires a comprehensive understanding of the factors underlying vaccine uptake and adherence.

Cold Chain Challenges: Maintaining Vaccine Potency

The effectiveness of many vaccines is highly sensitive to temperature. Proper cold chain management is crucial to ensure that vaccines remain potent from production to administration.

- *Thermosensitive vaccines*: Some vaccines, such as mRNA vaccines, require storage at very low temperatures (–70°C or lower). Maintaining these temperatures throughout the supply chain is challenging, particularly in remote or resource-limited settings.[66]
- *Logistical issues*:
  - *Transportation*: Ensuring that vaccines are transported under the required temperature conditions can be logistically complex and costly.[65]
  - *Storage infrastructure*: Providing adequate storage facilities with temperature control is essential for maintaining vaccine potency.[63]
- *Strategies to overcome cold chain challenges*:
  - *Innovative packaging*: Developing advanced packaging solutions, such as temperature-controlled containers and sensors, can help maintain vaccine stability.[63]
  - *Local solutions*: Investing in local cold chain infrastructure and exploring alternative storage technologies can improve vaccine delivery in challenging environments.[67]
  - *Training and capacity building*: Training healthcare workers and logisticians on cold chain management and best practices can help ensure that vaccines are stored and transported correctly.

FUTURE DIRECTIONS FOR LEVERAGING MOLECULAR INSIGHTS

The field of vaccine development stands on the brink of a new era, driven by advancements in molecular insights and technologies. Personalized vaccine strategies, informed by an individual's unique immune profile, hold the promise of significantly enhancing vaccine efficacy and safety. Understanding factors that influence vaccine response variability, such as age, genetics, and prior immune history, is crucial for developing these tailored approaches.

Personalized Vaccine Strategies

Personalized vaccines aim to optimize vaccine efficacy by tailoring formulations and delivery methods to the specific characteristics of an individual. This approach is informed by a comprehensive understanding of the individual's immune profile, including genetic, proteomic, and immunological factors. The use of omics technologies—spanning genomics, proteomics, and metabolomics—combined with measures of innate and adaptive immunity, as well as insights into host genetics, pathogen interactions, and the microbiome, provides a comprehensive framework for vaccine research. These datasets are analyzed through multilevel approaches, including unsupervised methods, individual parameter assessments, and pathway/network/module analyses integrating known biological functions. Computational and predictive modeling techniques, such as prediction analysis for microarrays, K-nearest neighbor, support vector machines, and generalized linear models, are then applied to predict immunogenicity and vaccine efficacy with precision.[68]

The integration of artificial intelligence (AI) into vaccine development marks a transformative milestone in modern biomedical research. AI-driven methodologies, particularly those utilizing machine learning (ML) and deep learning (DL) algorithms, offer robust frameworks for accelerating and optimizing vaccine design. These technologies leverage vast datasets, encompassing genomic sequences, protein structures, and immunological interactions, to predict antigenic epitopes, evaluate immunogenicity, and prioritize candidate antigens for experimental validation. By harnessing AI, researchers can also facilitate the rational design of immunogens and identify novel adjuvants with enhanced safety and efficacy profiles, contributing to the development of next-generation vaccines. AI's utility extends to epitope mapping, where predictive models analyze complex datasets to identify regions of antigens capable of eliciting strong immune responses. Moreover, AI algorithms streamline the identification and optimization of adjuvants by evaluating their potential to modulate immune responses effectively. Despite these advances, several challenges remain, including the heterogeneity of datasets, the interpretability of AI models, and the need for regulatory frameworks to ensure safe and ethical implementation.[69,70]

CONCLUSION

The future of vaccine development lies in leveraging molecular insights to create personalized vaccine strategies and apply systems-level approaches. By understanding and addressing factors that influence vaccine response variability, researchers can develop more effective and targeted vaccines. The integration of cutting-edge technologies will further enhance our ability to design and implement vaccines that meet the diverse needs of individuals and populations. As we advance toward a more personalized approach to vaccination, it is crucial to continue exploring new technologies, addressing challenges, and ensuring equitable access to the benefits of these innovations.

REFERENCES

1. InformedHealth.org [Internet]. Cologne, Germany: Institute for Quality and Efficiency in Health Care (IQWiG); 2006. In brief: The innate and adaptive immune systems.
2. Spiering MJ. Primer on the Immune System. Alcohol Res. 2015;37(2):171-5.
3. Riedel S. Edward Jenner and the history of smallpox and vaccination. Proc (Bayl Univ Med Cent). 2005;18(1):21-5.
4. Conti AA. Vaccination through time: from the first smallpox vaccine to current vaccination campaigns against the COVID-19 pandemic. Acta Biomed. 2021;92(S6):e2021453.
5. Vashishtha VM, Kumar P. The durability of vaccine-induced protection: an overview. Expert Rev Vaccines. 2024;23(1):389-408.
6. Tripathi T. Advances in vaccines: revolutionizing disease prevention. Sci Rep. 2023;13(1):11748.
7. Bezbaruah R, Chavda VP, Nongrang L, Alom S, Deka K, Kalita T, et al. Nanoparticle-Based Delivery Systems for Vaccines. Vaccines (Basel). 2022;10(11):1946.
8. Khan MA, Amin A, Farid A, Ullah A, Waris A, Shinwari K, et al. Recent Advances in Genomics-Based Approaches for the Development of Intracellular Bacterial Pathogen Vaccines. Pharmaceutics. 2022;15(1):152.
9. Hegde NR, Gauthami S, Sampath Kumar HM, Bayry J. The use of databases, data mining and immunoinformatics in vaccinology: where are we? Expert Opin Drug Discov. 2018;13(2):117-130.
10. Pritam M, Singh G, Swaroop S, Singh AK, Singh SP. Exploitation of reverse vaccinology and immunoinformatics as promising platform for genome-wide screening of new effective vaccine candidates against Plasmodium falciparum. BMC Bioinformatics. 2019;19(Suppl 13):468.
11. Michalik M, Djahanshiri B, Leo JC, Linke D. Reverse Vaccinology: The Pathway from Genomes and Epitope Predictions to Tailored Recombinant Vaccines. Methods Mol Biol. 2016;1403:87-106.
12. Chen DS, Mellman I. Elements of cancer immunity and the cancer-immune set point. Nature. 2017;541(7637):321-30.
13. Liu D, Che X, Wang X, Ma C, Wu G. Tumor Vaccines: Unleashing the Power of the Immune System to Fight Cancer. Pharmaceuticals (Basel). 2023;16(10):1384.
14. Jung SM, Kim WU. Targeted Immunotherapy for Autoimmune Disease. Immune Netw. 2022;22(1):e9.
15. Moorman CD, Sohn SJ, Phee H. Emerging Therapeutics for Immune Tolerance: Tolerogenic Vaccines, T cell Therapy, and IL-2 Therapy. Front Immunol. 2021;12:657768.

16. Nascimento IP, Leite LC. Recombinant vaccines and the development of new vaccine strategies. Braz J Med Biol Res. 2012;45(12):1102-11.
17. Demongeot J, Fougère C. mRNA COVID-19 Vaccines-Facts and Hypotheses on Fragmentation and Encapsulation. Vaccines (Basel). 2022;11(1):40.
18. Lan J, Ge J, Yu J, Shan S, Zhou H, Fan S, et al. Structure of the SARS-CoV-2 spike receptor-binding domain bound to the ACE2 receptor. Nature. 2020;581(7807):215-20.
19. Stewart J. Immunological principles: antigens and antigen recognition. In: Greenwood D, Barer M, Slack R, Irving W, (Eds). Medical Microbiology, 18th edition. Churchill Edinburgh: Livingstone; 2012. pp. 98-108.
20. Eng CLP, Tan TW, Tong JC. Immunoinformatics databases. In: Ranganathan S, Gribskov M, Nakai K, Schönbach C, (Eds). Encyclopedia of Bioinformatics and Computational Biology. Amsterdam; Academic Press; 2019. pp. 931-9.
21. Facciolà A, Visalli G, Laganà A, Di Pietro A. An Overview of Vaccine Adjuvants: Current Evidence and Future Perspectives. Vaccines (Basel). 2022;10(5):819.
22. Rinaudo CD, Telford JL, Rappuoli R, Seib KL. Vaccinology in the genome era. J Clin Invest. 2009;119(9):2515-25.
23. Okuyama R. mRNA and Adenoviral Vector Vaccine Platforms Utilized in COVID-19 Vaccines: Technologies, Ecosystem, and Future Directions. Vaccines (Basel). 2023;11(12):1737.
24. Bodini M, Brozzi A, Giuliani M, Nohynek H, Vainio A, Kuusi M, et al. Genomic Characterization of Invasive Meningococcal Serogroup B Isolates and Estimation of 4CMenB Vaccine Coverage in Finland. mSphere. 2020;5(5):e00376-20.
25. Rappuoli R. The application of reverse vaccinology, Novartis MenB vaccine developed by design. In: van Alphen L, van Ley P, van den Dobbelsteen G, editors. 16th International Pathogenic *Neisseria* Conference. Rotterdam, The Netherlands, 2008.
26. Croucher NJ, Harris SR, Fraser C, Quail MA, Burton J, van der Linden M, et al. Rapid pneumococcal evolution in response to clinical interventions. Science. 2011;331(6016):430-4.
27. Wizemann TM, Heinrichs JH, Adamou JE, Erwin AL, Kunsch C, Choi GH, et al. Use of a whole genome approach to identify vaccine molecules affording protection against *Streptococcus pneumoniae* infection. Infect Immun. 2001;69(3):1593-8.
28. Betts JC. Transcriptomics and proteomics: tools for the identification of novel drug targets and vaccine candidates for tuberculosis. IUBMB Life. 2002;53(4-5):239-42.
29. Lopez CE, Legge KL. Influenza A Virus Vaccination: Immunity, Protection, and Recent Advances Toward A Universal Vaccine. Vaccines (Basel). 2020;8(3):434.
30. Galassie AC, Link AJ. Proteomic contributions to our understanding of vaccine and immune responses. Proteomics Clin Appl. 2015;9(11-12):972-89.
31. Yurina V, Adianingsih OR. Predicting epitopes for vaccine development using bioinformatics tools. Ther Adv Vaccines Immunother. 2022;10:25151355221100218.
32. Sidney J, Peters B, Sette A. Epitope prediction and identification-adaptive T cell responses in humans. Semin Immunol. 2020;50:101418.
33. Mogensen TH. Pathogen recognition and inflammatory signaling in innate immune defenses. Clin Microbiol Rev. 2009;22(2):240-73.
34. Kawai T, Akira S. The role of pattern-recognition receptors in innate immunity: update on Toll-like receptors. Nat Immunol. 2010;11(5):373-84.
35. Iwasaki A, Medzhitov R. Control of adaptive immunity by the innate immune system. Nat Immunol. 2015;16(4):343-53.
36. Chen P, Liu X, Sun Y, Zhou P, Wang Y, Zhang Y. Dendritic cell targeted vaccines: Recent progresses and challenges. Hum Vaccin Immunother. 2016;12(3):612-22.
37. Gi M, Im W, Hong S. Dendritic cells as danger-recognizing biosensors. Sensors (Basel). 2009;9(9):6730-51.
38. Soto JA, Gálvez NMS, Andrade CA, Pacheco GA, Bohmwald K, Berrios RV, et al. The Role of Dendritic Cells During Infections Caused by Highly Prevalent Viruses. Front Immunol. 2020;11:1513.
39. Reed SG, Orr MT, Fox CB. Key roles of adjuvants in modern vaccines. Nat Med. 2013;19(12):1597-608.
40. Caradonna TM, Schmidt AG. Protein engineering strategies for rational immunogen design. NPJ Vaccines. 2021;6(1):154.
41. Krarup A, Truan D, Furmanova-Hollenstein P, Bogaert L, Bouchier P, Bisschop IJM, et al. A highly stable prefusion RSV F vaccine derived from structural analysis of the fusion mechanism. Nat Commun. 2015;6:8143.
42. Dale CJ, Thomson S, De Rose R, Ranasinghe C, Medveczky CJ, Pamungkas J, et al. Prime-boost strategies in DNA vaccines. Methods Mol Med. 2006;127:171-97.
43. Dunachie SJ, Hill AV. Prime-boost strategies for malaria vaccine development. J Exp Biol. 2003;206(Pt 21):3771-9.
44. Song Y, Mehl F, Zeichner SL. Vaccine Strategies to Elicit Mucosal Immunity. Vaccines (Basel). 2024;12(2):191.
45. Courtney AH, Lo WL, Weiss A. TCR Signaling: Mechanisms of Initiation and Propagation. Trends Biochem Sci. 2018;43(2): 108-23.
46. Struzik J, Szulc-Dąbrowska L. NF-κB as an Important Factor in Optimizing Poxvirus-Based Vaccines against Viral Infections. Pathogens. 2020;9(12):1001.
47. Soares-Silva M, Diniz FF, Gomes GN, Bahia D. The Mitogen-Activated Protein Kinase (MAPK) Pathway: Role in Immune Evasion by Trypanosomatids. Front Microbiol. 2016;7:183.
48. Arfat Y, Zafar I, Sehgal SA, Ayaz M, Sajid M, Khan JM, et al. In silico designing of multiepitope-based-peptide (MBP) vaccine against MAPK protein express for Alzheimer's disease in Zebrafish. Heliyon. 2023;9(11):e22204.
49. Huang L, Krieg AM, Eller N, Scott DE. Induction and regulation of Th1-inducing cytokines by bacterial DNA, lipopolysaccharide, and heat-inactivated bacteria. Infect Immun. 1999;67(12):6257-63.
50. Allen JE, Sutherland TE. Host protective roles of type 2 immunity: parasite killing and tissue repair, flip sides of the same coin. Semin Immunol. 2014;26(4):329-40.
51. Baljon JJ, Wilson JT. Bioinspired vaccines to enhance MHC class-I antigen cross-presentation. Curr Opin Immunol. 2022;77:102215.
52. Lauvau G, Soudja SM. Mechanisms of Memory T Cell Activation and Effective Immunity. Adv Exp Med Biol. 2015;850:73-80.
53. Ionescu L, Urschel S. Memory B Cells and Long-lived Plasma Cells. Transplantation. 2019;103(5):890-8.
54. Leko V, Rosenberg SA. Identifying and Targeting Human Tumor Antigens for T Cell-Based Immunotherapy of Solid Tumors. Cancer Cell. 2020;38(4):454-72.
55. Abd-Aziz N, Poh CL. Development of Peptide-Based Vaccines for Cancer. J Oncol. 2022;2022:9749363.
56. Gardner TA, Elzey BD, Hahn NM. Sipuleucel-T (Provenge) autologous vaccine approved for treatment of men with asymptomatic or minimally symptomatic castrate-resistant metastatic prostate cancer. Hum Vaccin Immunother. 2012;8(4): 534-9.
57. Ruzzi F, Semprini MS, Scalambra L, Palladini A, Angelicola S, Cappello C, et al. Virus-like Particle (VLP) Vaccines for Cancer Immunotherapy. Int J Mol Sci. 2023;24(16):12963.

58. Tian Y, Xie D, Yang L. Engineering strategies to enhance oncolytic viruses in cancer immunotherapy. Signal Transduct Target Ther. 2022;7(1):117.
59. Freedman MS, Bar-Or A, Oger J, Traboulsee A, Patry D, Young C, et al. A phase III study evaluating the efficacy and safety of MBP8298 in secondary progressive MS. Neurology. 2011;77:1551-60.
60. Krienke C, Kolb L, Diken E, Streuber M, Kirchhoff S, Bukur T, et al. A noninflammatory mRNA vaccine for treatment of experimental autoimmune encephalomyelitis. Science. 2021;371(6525):145-53.
61. Song C, Shi J, Zhang P, Zhang Y, Xu J, Zhao L, et al. Immunotherapy for Alzheimer's disease: targeting β-amyloid and beyond. Transl Neurodegener. 2022;11(1):18.
62. Romero-Ramos M, von Euler Chelpin M, Sanchez-Guajardo V. Vaccination strategies for Parkinson disease: induction of a swift attack or raising tolerance? Hum Vaccin Immunother. 2014;10(4):852-67.
63. Pambudi NA, Sarifudin A, Gandidi IM, Romadhon R. Vaccine cold chain management and cold storage technology to address the challenges of vaccination programs. Energy Reports. 2022;8:955-72.
64. Bajrovic I, Croyle MA. Challenges in vaccine transport: can we deliver without the cold chain? Expert Rev Vaccines. 2023; 22(1):933-6.
65. Dadari IK, Zgibor JC. How the use of vaccines outside the cold chain or in controlled temperature chain contributes to improving immunization coverage in low- and middle-income countries (LMICs): A scoping review of the literature. J Glob Health. 2021;11:04004.
66. Uddin MN, Roni MA. Challenges of Storage and Stability of mRNA-Based COVID-19 Vaccines. Vaccines (Basel). 2021;9(9):1033.
67. Lugelo A, Hampson K, Bigambo M, Kazwala R, Lankester F. Controlling human rabies: The development of an effective, inexpensive, and locally made passive cooling device for storing thermotolerant animal rabies vaccines. Trop Med Infect Dis. 2020;5(3):130.
68. Kennedy RB, Ovsyannikova IG, Lambert ND, Haralambieva IH, Poland GA. The personal touch: strategies toward personalized vaccines and predicting immune responses to them. Expert Rev Vaccines. 2014;13(5):657-69.
69. Olawade DB, Teke J, Fapohunda O, Weerasinghe K, Usman SO, Ige AO, et al. Leveraging artificial intelligence in vaccine development: A narrative review. J Microbiol Methods. 2024;224:106998.
70. Russo G, Reche P, Pennisi M, Pappalardo F. The combination of artificial intelligence and systems biology for intelligent vaccine design. Expert Opin Drug Discov. 2020;15(11):1267-81.

CHAPTER 4

Significance of Mucosal Immunity in Vaccination

Manish Kumar Singh, Akanksha Gupta, Jyotsna Agarwal

INTRODUCTION

Mucosal surfaces come in direct contact with air, food, water, and environment and thus are potential entry points for more than 90% of the pathogenic microorganisms, especially viruses. The mucosal surfaces provide the first line of host defenses against most infections at the point of entry and also prevent secondary transmission by decreasing shedding of pathogens from mucosal surfaces.[1-3] Till recently, immune protection was only supposed to be provided by hematopoietic immune cells (neutrophils, macrophages, and T and B lymphocytes). New evidences demonstrate that nonhematopoietic cells like the mucosal epithelial cells have a role to play in mounting immune responses.[2]

Mucosal defense mechanism includes the physical, biochemical, and immunological barriers. Microbial homeostasis is needed to maintain the gut barrier, and any alteration in it is associated with intestinal microbial dysbiosis and ultimately an abnormal gut mucosal barrier. Mucosal vaccines administered through the mucosal surfaces are expected to have the potential to protect the host at the initial site of contact with the pathogen itself and have been a point of interest for vaccine developers and researchers.[3]

MUCOSAL BARRIER: STRUCTURE AND FUNCTION

Structure

The gastrointestinal, respiratory and urogenital tracts, eye conjunctiva, inner ear, and ducts of exocrine glands are all covered by mucous membranes, also known as mucosa. Body's mucosa has a large surface area, around 200 times more than the skin surface, making it the body's largest protective barrier.[1]

Mucosa has three layers: Outermost epithelium, middle lamina propria, and innermost muscularis mucosae. In most organs, the mucosal barrier is just a single layer of epithelial cells. The mucosal barrier separates the internal milieu of the body from the external environment. It is a selectively permeable barrier which allows passage of water, nutrients, and electrolytes but prevents the passage of bacteria and their toxins.

Lamina propria is composed of connective tissue, nerves, blood, lymphatic vessels, and associated lymphoid tissues. Muscularis mucosa is the innermost layer of smooth muscle fibers. It is made up of two layers of smooth muscle cells, including inner circular layer and outer longitudinal layer.

Mucosae are classified into two types, i.e., type I and type II. Type I mucosa is present in the respiratory tract, most of the gastrointestinal tract (GIT), tonsils, and adenoids, while type II mucosa is found in the oral cavity and urogenital tract **(Figs. 1A and B)**.

Type I mucosa is lined by columnar epithelium with goblet cells that secrete mucus all over. The lamina propria has mucosa-associated lymphoid tissue (MALT), dendritic cells (DCs), and specialized microfold (M) cells that play a pivotal role in mucosal immunity. It also has a neonatal Fc receptor (FcRN) for transport of immunoglobulin G (IgG) and polymeric Ig receptor (pIgR) for transport of dimeric IgA.

Type II mucosa is lined by stratified squamous epithelium. Unlike type I, it does not have goblet cells and mucus is secreted by nearby glands. The pIgR receptor is also not present in type II mucosa and only FcRN is present; thus, IgG is the predominant antibody in these sites

Functions

Epithelium: Mucosal epithelium acts as a physical, biochemical, and immunological barrier between the body and external environment as it lines the external and internal structures of the body. Physical barriers consist of tight junctions among epithelial cells, cilia, and thick

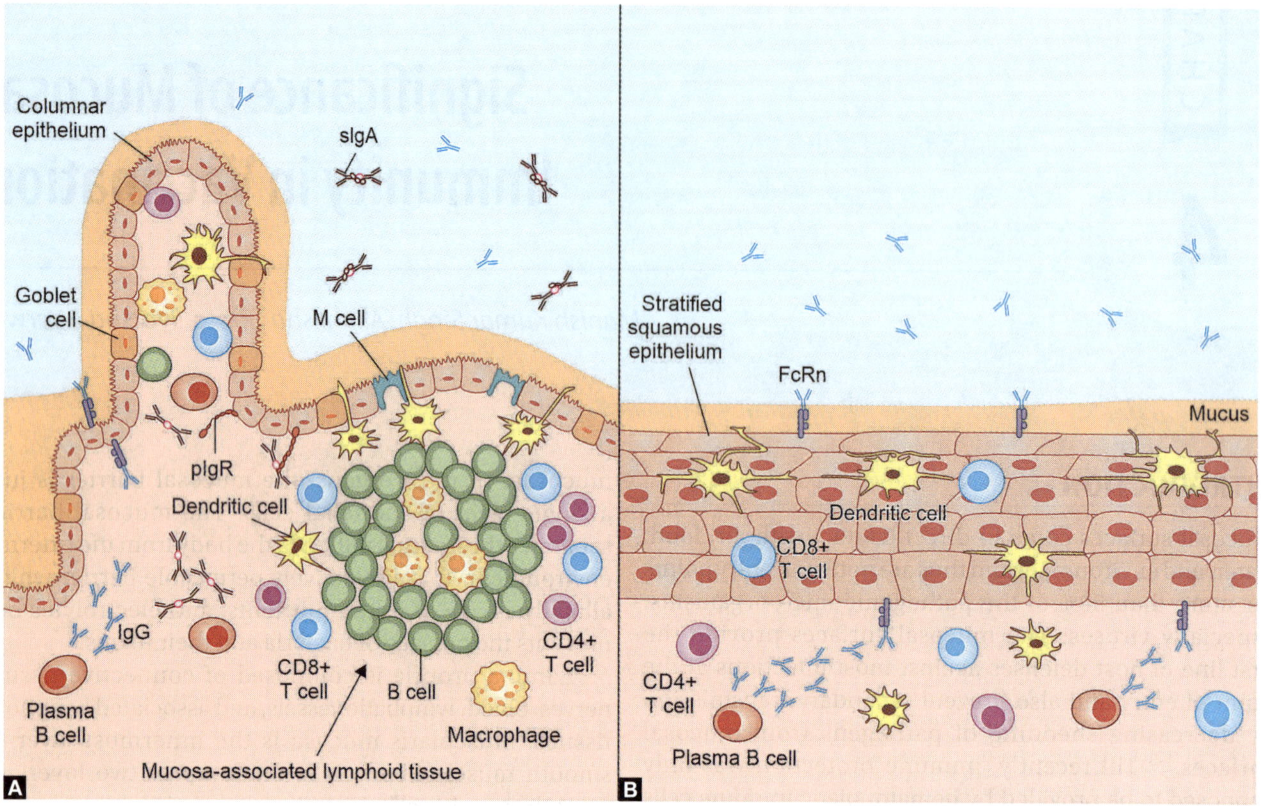

FIGS. 1A AND B: Difference in the structure of (A) Type I; and (B) Type II mucosa.
(pIgR: polymeric Ig receptor; sIgA: secretory IgA)
Source: Iwasaki A. Exploiting mucosal immunity for antiviral vaccines. Ann Rev Immunol. 2016;34:575-608.

layer of mucus which protects the body from irritants and toxins. Biochemical barrier is provided by microbiota producing antimicrobial peptides (AMPs) and differences in pH. Other functions of epithelial cells include secretion, absorption, sensation, protection, and transport depending upon the type of epithelium. Nonkeratinized epithelium mainly provides protection against mechanical stress and friction. Columnar epithelium is specialized for absorption and secretion.

The squamous epithelium which lines the lungs, blood vessels, and body cavities serves as a barrier against infection and injury. It also provides a nonspecific innate defense mechanism by secreting substances such as mucins, antimicrobial proteins, enzyme, secretory antibodies, and other components of the intraluminal mucosal environment.[1] Ciliated cells in the respiratory tract push the pathogens out of the airways by mucociliary clearance.

Lamina propria: It supplies blood to epithelium, provides structural role, and hosts the lymphoid tissue which plays an important role in the mucosal immune defense mechanism.

Muscularis mucosae: They help the mucosa to stretch and contract along with the organs.

MUCOSAL IMMUNITY: COMPONENT AND MECHANISM

The mucosal immune system (MIS) constitutes a network of innate immune components, immune cells, and antibodies that together mediate immune responses to pathogens.[2]

Common Mucosal Immune System

Common mucosal immune system (CMIS) is a highly integrated and regulated system. It is broadly classified as inductive sites and effector sites based on anatomical and functional properties. At inductive sites, antigen-specific B and T cells are initiated and harbor precursor cytotoxic lymphocytes (pCTLs), while in the effector sites, adaptive immune responses are mediated and activated CD8+ CTLs mediate their function.[4,5] Migration of immune cells from inductive to effector sites via the lymphatic system forms the cellular basis for immune responses in the GIT, upper respiratory tract, and urogenital tract.[6]

Intraepithelial lymphocytes (IEL) are important components of the mucosal epithelium which consists of various subsets of T cells to maintain normal homeostatis.[6]

Exposure of a foreign antigen to the mucosal surface can lead to either activation of humoral or cell-mediated immunity or to systemic anergy or mucosal tolerance[5] **(Fig. 2)**.

Inductive Sites

Organized secondary lymphoid tissues containing B-cell follicles, T-cell areas, and antigen-presenting cells (APCs) such as DCs in the URT and GIT which promotes sensing and sampling of antigens, antigen uptake, its processing and presentation for induction of the mucosal immune responses are known as mucosal inductive sites. Mucosal inductive sites comprise MALT, including the gut-associated lymphoid tissue (GALT) in the intestine, nasopharyngeal-associated lymphoid tissue (NALT), and lymphoid sites. Inductive sites are concentrated either in areas which are most likely to be the entry point of pathogens (e.g., NALT in tonsils, adenoids, etc.) or in areas with high microbial density (e.g., GALT in the lower intestinal tract) **(Box 1)**.

BOX 1 Distribution of inductive sites.

GALT (gut-associated lymphoid tissue):
- Peyer's patches (PP) (large clusters of lymphoid follicles in the mucosa of distal ileum, B-cell follicle is surrounded by interfollicular T cells)
- Mesenteric lymph nodes (MLN)
- Isolated lymphoid follicles (ILFs) throughout small intestine, colon, and rectum

NALT (nasopharyngeal-associated lymphoid tissue):
- Tonsils/adenoids
- Inducible bronchus-associated lymphoid tissue (iBALT)
- Cervical lymph nodes (CLNs)
- Hilar lymph nodes (HLNs)

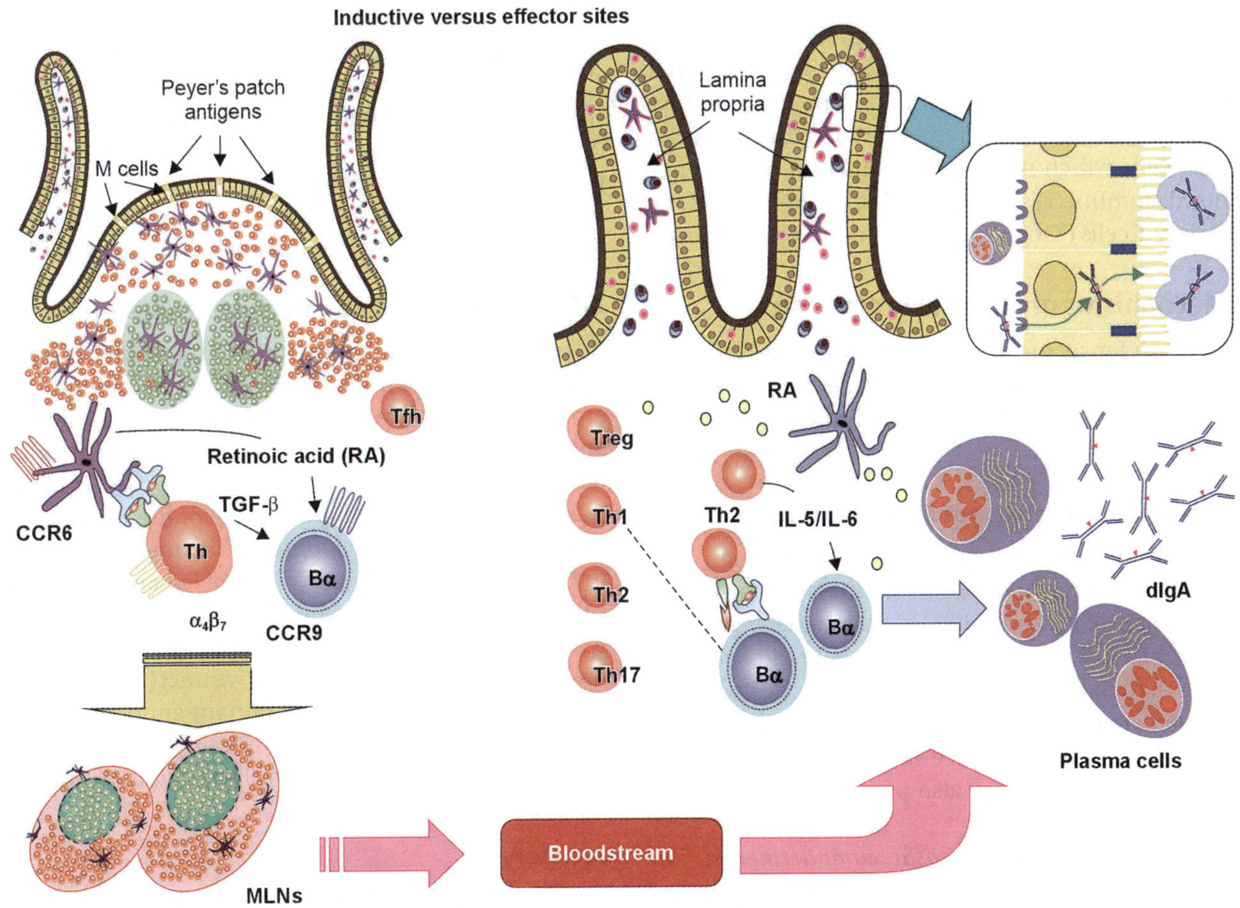

FIG. 2: Luminal antigens sampled by M cells or DCs activate antigen-specific B and T cells in MALT. Homing of lymphocytes via receptors helps in its movement to effector sites, where specific B cells differentiate into mucosal IgA-secreting plasma cells.

(DCs: dendritic cells; MALT: mucosa-associated lymphoid tissue)

Source: McGhee JR, Fujihashi K. Inside the mucosal immune system. PLoS Biol. 2012;10(9):e1001397.

Mucosa-associated lymphoid tissue has the basic structural features required for transportation, processing, and presentation of the antigens on one hand and clonal expansion and induction of the antigen-specific effector lymphocytes on the other hand. A single layer of cuboidal epithelial cells, known as follicle-associated epithelium (FAE), separates the MALT from the luminal epithelium. A distinctive population of specialized epithelial cells (M cells) is present in the FAE which helps in sampling of antigens. M (microfold) cells are specialized for performing endocytosis and rapid transepithelial transport described later in "antigen sampling". M cells are present only in some areas; the rest of the FAE are enterocytes having apical microvilli with a coating of thick brush border glycocalyx.

Mucosa-associated lymphoid tissue consists of DCs, macrophages, innate lymphoid cells, intraepithelial T cells, regulatory T cells, IgA-secreting plasma cells, and source of memory B and T cells.[1]

Effector Sites

Effector sites comprise lamina propria regions in the mucosal barriers of upper respiratory, gastrointestinal, and reproductive tracts and also along secretory glandular tissues. These contain different types of antigen-specific effector cells which make up the mucosal cellular and humoral immune responses, including helper T cells, regulatory T cells (Treg), and IgA-producing plasma cells.

Mechanisms of Mucosal Protection

Mucosal defense mechanism includes the physical, biochemical, and immunological barriers. Immunological defense components are innate and adaptive immune responses.

Innate Immune Response at Mucosal Surfaces

Innate immune mechanisms include the following:

- *Antimicrobial peptides (AMPs)*: These are produced by immune cells and epithelial cells in the presence of microbial invasion, and they possess broad-spectrum antimicrobial activity against infections. AMPs provide immediate protection against the invading pathogen, even before the adaptive immunity can mount a specific response. They also promote recruitment of immune cells.
- *Microbiome of the mucosal compartments*: The microbiome (microbiota) of the mucosal compartment interacts with the mucosal immune system (MIS) by various mechanisms. It stimulates the production of AMPs and regulates the development and function of immune cells, T cells, and B cells within lymphoid tissues of MIS. In some compartments, the microbiota alters the environment making it hostile for the pathogens to invade; e.g., in the female genital tract, *Lactobacilli* maintain a low pH in vagina which is unfavorable for most of the invading pathogens.[1]
- Innate immune cells including macrophages, DCs (most important mucosal APC), and natural killer (NK) cells, which not only promote phagocytosis and removal of pathogen but can also act as APCs and thus trigger adaptive immune responses.
- Cytokines like interferons and chemokines to co-ordinate with the adaptive immune responses.[7] Epithelial cells can also sense dangerous pathogen components through pathogen recognition receptors (PRRs) like toll-like receptors (TLRs) and send signals to DCs and macrophages to in turn activate innate and adaptive immune responses.[1,8]

Till recently, immunological memory was supposed to be limited only to the adaptive immune system and not innate immunity. Recent evidences suggest that after infection or vaccination, some innate cells like NK cells or myeloid cells can show long-term nonspecific heterologous immunity during second stimulation. This increased innate immune response is termed "trained innate immunity" (TII). This latest development in the knowledge of innate immunity serves as an important potential of protection against *Mycobacterium tuberculosis* infection using the respiratory mucosal route of tuberculosis (TB) vaccination in the early stage of TB.[1]

Adaptive Immune Response at Mucosal Surfaces

Adaptive immunity comprises nonencapsulated lymphoid follicles known as mucosal-associated lymphoid tissue embedded in the mucosa and submucosa, localized antibody, and tissue resident memory T and B cells. It has two arms: Humoral and cellular mucosal immunity (CMI). An important characteristic of the humoral arm of adaptive immune response at the mucosal surface is the local production and secretion of IgA antibody in high concentration by mucosal B cells. IgA is mostly found in type I mucosae (URT) while in type II mucosae [cornea, oral, esophageal, lower reproductive tract (LRT), or female genital tract] IgG is the predominant antibody isotype.[1] The cellular arm of adaptive immunity comprises tissue resident memory T and B cells (TRM and BRM) mucosal CTLs, and mucosal helper T cells.

Secretory IgA

IgA is the only antibody isotype which can resist degradation in the protease-rich environment of mucosal surface, because of dimerization and high degree of glycosylation during its synthesis in the plasma cells.[8] The highest concentration of IgA is present in the secretions associated with the mucosal surfaces. IgA can be expressed in mucosal surfaces in both monomeric and dimeric secretory IgA forms. More than 90% of the body's IgA is produced by GALT, the principal precursor source being Peyer's patches (PP). Secretory IgA (sIgA) is formed, while dimeric IgA is being transported across the epithelial cells to the lumen via polymeric immunoglobulin receptor (pIgR) (produced by the epithelial cells and located on the basal membrane side of epithelial cells). Glycosylated fragment derived from pIgR during this transport associates with dimeric IgA and constitutes the secretory component. This also provides protease resistance to sIgA. sIgA has numerous roles in mucosal immunity:

- *"Immune exclusion" of exogenous antigens*: sIgA entraps the normal commensal bacteria without affecting their growth, thus preventing them from invading the epithelium and mounting immune response. It also limits inflammatory responses at mucosal surfaces.[5]
- sIgA coats the pathogen and these are internalized by M cells via sIgA specific receptor into PP or exploit M cells for delivery of antigens to DCs, thus leading to immune response.
- *sIgA promotes the clearance of immune complexes*: Mucophilic nature of secretory component increases attachment of bacteria to mucous membrane and then these immune complexes can be cleared either by mucociliary action or by peristaltic movement of intestine.
- Neutralization of viruses at different steps in infectious disease processes, like Influenza virus,[5] SARS-CoV-2 virus, etc. It has higher neutralization activity than IgG.[7] IgA can neutralize the pathogen and prevent their invasion through mucosal surfaces either by its neutralizing activity or by Fc-mediated functions like antibody-dependent cellular cytotoxicity (ADCC).[1]

Immunoglobulin G

Administration of antigen to mucosal surfaces can lead to local synthesis of IgG in mucosal tissues. Local synthesis of IgG can be increased by various chemokines and cytokines produced by the immune cells in response to infection or inflammation.[1] Studies have shown a large number of IgG-producing plasma cells in the female genital tract of humans; also, high concentrations of IgG and IgA have been measured in human cervical and vaginal secretions.[8] IgG is susceptible to degradation by bacterial proteases and environment of the intestinal lumen; thus, concentration of IgG in intestinal secretions is about 30–100 times lesser than sIgA.[8] sIgG can also be transported across epithelial cells either by paracellular leakage or via IgG-receptor-mediated transport FcRN. Intact IgG present in mucosal tissues prevents systematic spread of pathogen by neutralizing the pathogen that enters the mucosa. IgG class of antibody can lead to virus neutralization and non-neutralizing antibodies can either lead to ADCC or antibody-dependent cellular phagocytosis (ADCP) via its Fc domain.[7]

Tissue Resident Memory Lymphocytes

Tissue resident memory T cells (TRM) are present as stable populations within nonlymphoid barrier tissues like skin, lungs, and intestine and in nonbarrier tissues including brain and liver. These are maintained within the peripheral tissues after getting mucosal vaccination or respiratory infection.

Various researches have shown the presence of TRM cells at multiple mucosal sites. These cells are thought to play an important role in response to an infection. A study has revealed that CD8+ T_{RM} cells in lungs are important for protection against respiratory viral infections but are usually short-lived. Lung resident helper T-cell population has been found to be present which supports tissue resident memory B cells (B_{RM}) and CD8 cells after influenza virus infection. These are induced locally in the lungs and might play a very important role in promoting long-lived cellular and humoral immunity after vaccination in the respiratory tract.[7]

Studies have shown that CD8+ T_{RM} are found throughout the respiratory tract (airways, parenchyma, and associated lymph nodes) after viral infection. Owing to their spatial distribution throughout the respiratory tract, these are mobilized earlier than the circulating CD8+ cells in response to re-exposure. The former leads to viral clearance by secreting interferon gamma (IFNγ), tumor necrosis factor alpha (TNF-α), and IL-2 cytokines and also by granzyme B molecules. Apart from this, the CD8+ T_{RM} also leads to cytokine-mediated activation of local and adaptive immunity.[7]

CD4+ T_{RM} are found to be more abundantly found than CD8+ T_{RM}.

Tissue resident memory B cells are found to be present and maintained in the mucosal tissues after infection. These are long-lived. Lung B_{RM} are found to reduce the viral titers in the lower respiratory tract much more than the memory B cells produced by spleen. This is because unlike the circulating memory B cells, B_{RM} tends to be associated with the tissues and thus leads to localized production of a large amount of antibody leading to pathogen clearance. Apart from this, some nonantigen-specific B_{RM} also helps in pathogen clearance by presenting exogenous antigens as immune complexes.[7]

Reactivation of long-lived T_{RM} by re-exposure of the same antigen can activate both innate and adaptive immune response throughout the body (not limited to the mucosal compartment) mediated via cytokines.

Mucosal Lymphocytes

Entry of virus into the GIT is known to elicit production of a high frequency of pCTLs in Peyer's patches.[5] Even mucosal CD4+ helper T cells are found in mucosal tissues. These support the development of plasma cells that produce IgA isotype antibody.[6] Naïve and memory lymphocytes enter the mucosa through high endothelial venules (HEVs), because of lymphocyte homing is discussed in the section, "Tissue-specific Homing of Mucosal Lymphocytes". FAE secretes chemokines which attract some of the naive and memory lymphocytes to the SED regions of Peyer's patches while some of the B and T cells migrate to M-cell pockets and express memory or maturation markers **(Fig. 3)**.

Induction of Mucosal Immune Responses

Antigen Sampling at Mucosal Surfaces

Pathogen may invade through various routes like inhalation, ingestion, and sexual route. Induction of mucosal immune response occurs at the mucosal inductive sites. In areas with organized lymphoid tissue, antigen sampling is mediated by M cells or FAE cells in the intestine. Microfold (M) cells form intraepithelial pockets (where lymphocytes migrate) and deliver antigens from the gut lumen to the pocket lymphocytes (IEL) and to subepithelial lymphoid tissues (underlying DCs) via transepithelial vesicular transport. Studies done on mouse models have shown that the FAE of mouse Peyer's patch produces some chemokines like CC-chemokine ligand 20 (CCL20) and CCL9, and lymphocytes and DCs have CCR6 (chemokine receptor) or CCR1 respectively. So the FAE cells do not transport the antigens like M cells but attract the DCs and lymphocytes at the sites of entry of pathogens, which in turn probably leads to antigen sampling locally while minimizing systemic infection.[8]

In areas like the female genital tract or oral cavity where no organized lymphoid tissues are present, antigen sampling is done by collaboration between DCs and epithelial cells. In such areas, motile DCs are present just beneath the epithelium and either can migrate into the

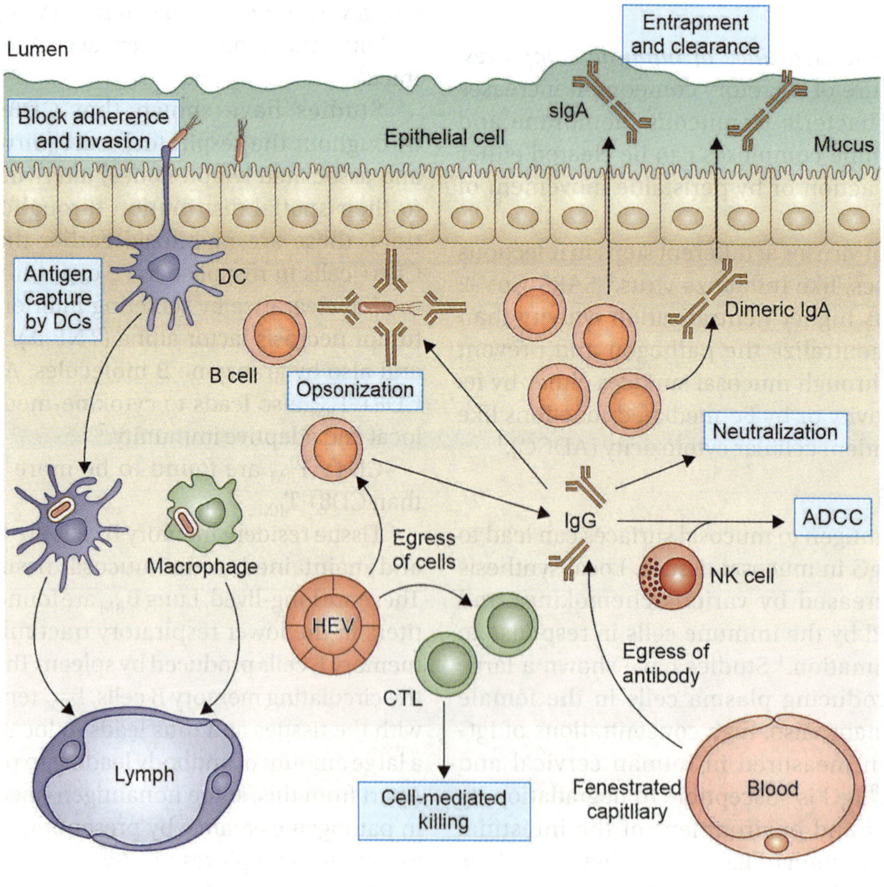

FIG. 3: Mechanism of mucosal immunity. Antigen-specific B and T lymphocytes reach the mucosa from the bloodstream via high endothelial venules (HEVs). Mucosal B cells differentiate into predominantly IgA-secreting plasma cells, which in turn is secreted into secretions as secretory IgA (sIgA).

Source: Neutra MR, Kozlowski PA. Mucosal vaccines: the promise and the challenge. Nature Rev Immunol. 2006;6(2):148-58.

narrow interepithelial spaces or can even extend their dendrites directly into the lumen (across the epithelial cells) and sample the luminal antigens **(Fig. 4)**.[8]

Antigen Presentation

Sampled antigens are either transported to the APCs or are directly captured by the APCs. APCs present the processed antigens to the CD4+ and CD8+ T cells. In case of some antigens, antigen processing and presentation can be directly done by epithelial cells to the neighboring intraepithelial T cells, including antigen nonspecific T cells (NKT cells). This can lead to a state of "*oral tolerance*" or suppression of specific immune response.[9] Active immunity is also produced depending upon the type of antigen, type of APC, and local environment.[9] Tissue resident DCs and macrophages serve as APCs, but in inflammatory condition or during an active infection, other APCs are also recruited that can present absorbed antigens and lead to effector immune responses. Thus, a local inflammatory condition produced by the mucosal vaccines can contribute to increased adaptive immunity.[4] Inflammatory conditions favor immune response, which are triggered by the stimulation of mucosal innate immunity (PRR binding to toll-like receptor ligands on mucosal APCs). Studies have shown that during inflammation, monocytes present in the gut and lungs can migrate to lymph nodes and prime T-cell responses, while recruited monocytes and immature macrophages can secrete cytokines that lead to Th1- and Th17-mediated immune responses. Similarly in the nasal mucosa, the resident conventional DCs (cDCs) are essential to maintain nonresponsiveness to harmless inhaled antigens, but during viral infection, monocytes and monocyte-derived DCs (moDCs) are recruited which helps in priming T cells. Thus, mucosal vaccines can promote protective mucosal immunity by activating monocytes and moDCs. **Figure 4** shows various ways of antigen sampling.

Mucosal Immune Response

Following antigen processing and presentation, T and B cells are activated to mount a mucosal immune response. Studies on the mice model have shown that antigens sampled by M cells are captured by DC in the subepithelial dome (SED) regions of Peyer's patches. These DCs are phenotypically immature, but after antigen capturing most of them move to interfollicular T-cell zones, leading to expression of major histocompatibility complex (MHC) molecules and maturation markers. Some of these might also carry the antigen to the draining lymph nodes, thus interfacing with the systemic immune response.[1] DCs in intraepithelial and subepithelial regions can either lead to immune response and memory response or lead to immune tolerance by interacting with local lymphocytes, or they could exit the mucosa through the lymphatics and present antigens to naïve T cells in the organized lymphoid tissues in the draining lymph nodes and naïve T cells differentiated into Th1, Th2, Th17, and Treg cells. B-cell activation occurs at various mucosal sites and in turn leads to B-cell differentiation to produce secretory IgA and antigen-specific IgG.[1] Th17 cells (subset of helper T cell) play an important role in mucosal immunity. These mostly secrete IL-17 and the latter has been shown to promote

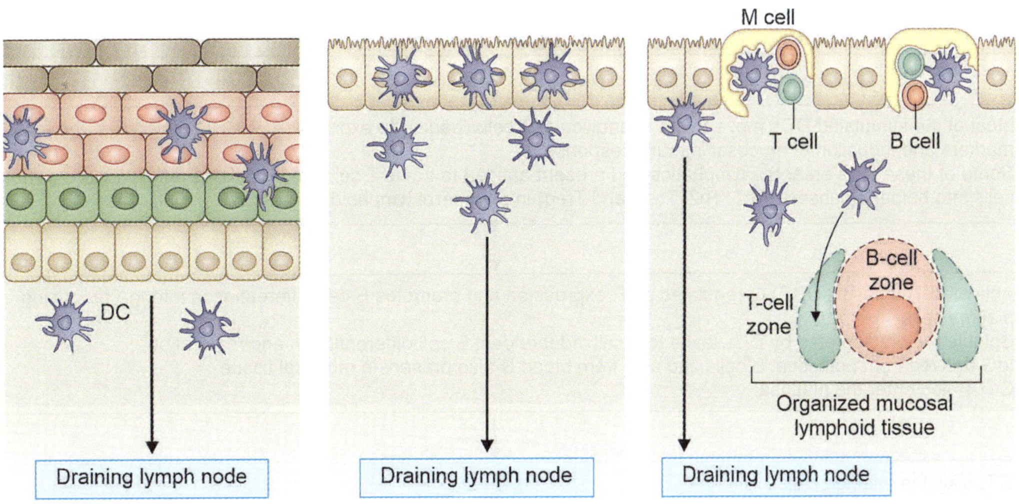

FIG. 4: Antigen sampling at mucosal epithelial surfaces. Dendritic cells (DCs) may accumulate directly beneath the epithelium, migrate into the epithelium, and even extend their dendrites and capture luminal antigens. These DCs then migrate to nearby draining lymph nodes to present antigen to T cells. In areas with organized lymphoid tissues, M cells sample antigens and deliver to subepithelial DCs and present antigens to T cells in the organized lymphoid tissues.

Source: Neutra MR, Kozlowski PA. Mucosal vaccines: the promise and the challenge. Nature Rev Immunol. 2006;6(2):148-58.

mucosal immunity following vaccination by mucosal vaccines in two ways: By upregulating the expression of pIgR in mucosal epithelial cells (thus increased sIgA) and by promoting T-cell-independent B-cell maturation and differentiation (refer to **Flowchart 1**).

sIgA has been shown to be induced following vaccination by two doses of ETVAX vaccine (oral multivalent inactivated vaccine against four stains of Enterotoxigenic *Escherichia coli*).[1] Induction of sIgA is seen to be more pronounced in vaccines utilizing viral vectors and weakened viruses, for example following intranasal live attenuated influenza vaccine and after Vaxart norovirus vaccine which is composed of stable adenovirus type 5 vectors.[4] A study by Komban et al. has found that sIgA production can be induced without depending on cDC for antigen transfer. The study found that some B cells (CC26+CCR1+GL7 B cells) in the SED of Peyer's patches can directly sample the antigens from the M cells and leads to trafficking to germinal centers where activation and population expansion take place. In the female genital tract and the lower genital tract, IgG and not IgA plays a major role in providing mucosal immunity, while in URT it is IgA which is relatively more important.[1]

In most cases, induction of mucosal immune response (and not oral tolerance) is dependent on proper antigen presentation by mucosal DCs, but in some cases if a very high amount of mucosal antigen is administered, then mucosal IgA response can be elicited even in the absence of DCs.[9]

Tissue-specific Homing of Mucosal lymphocytes

Homing of lymphocytes refers to a process where the lymphocytes circulate through the bloodstream and re-enter secondary lymphoid tissues. Activated lymphocytes express some homing factors that guide their migration between mucosal and systemic sites, such that the systemic immune cells can provide both systemic and local mucosal immunity and mucosal immune cells can contribute toward systemic immunity along with mucosal immunity. For example, IL-17 produced by Th17 cells promotes both local and systemic antibody production. Sensitized

Antigen reaches mucosal surfaces either through inhalation, ingestion or sexual route via infection or vaccination

↓

Innate immune system with epithelial cells, along with its tight cell junction, mucociliary clearance mechanism, and AMPs forms the first line of defense against any pathogen

↓

Adaptive immune response: Antigen is sampled by immune cells such as by M cells, or directly by dendrites of DCs or FAE and small intestinal goblet cells

↓

Antigen capturing and processing by DCs and macrophages, leading to activation of these APCs, cells, B cells and IgA class switch recombination

↓

- Most of the stimulated DCs move to the interfollicular T cells leading to expression of MHC molecules and maturation markers and induction of mucosal immune response
- Some of these DCs enter the lymphatics and present antigen to naïve T cells and mediates differentiation of naïve T cells into helper T subsets (Th1, Th2, Th17 and Treg) in peripheral lymphoid tissue

↓

- Activated Th subset (Th17) upregulates pIgR expression and promotes B cell differentiation into IgA producing plasma cells
- Soluble factors secreted by DCs leads to T cell independent B cell differentiation and maturation
- IgG derived from both local B cells and also from blood is also present in mucosal tissue
- CTLs also enter the mucosa

↓

- CTLs kill the infected cells
- IgG mediates neutralization or Fc receptor-mediated ADCC
- IgA converts to sIgA, which in turn leads to either direct neutralization, or Fc receptor-mediated ADCC or pathogen clearance by enhancing immune complexes and by immune exclusion

FLOWCHART 1: Mechanism of mucosal immunity.

(AMPs: antimicrobial peptides; APCs: antigen-presenting cells; CTLs: cytotoxic lymphocytes; DCs: dendritic cells; FAE: follicle-associated epithelium)

B cells, T cells, and IgA precursors leave the site of initial encounter (organized lymphoid tissue), transit through the lymph whereby they enter the systemic circulation, and then seed selected mucosal sites (preferentially in the mucosa of origin) and here they differentiate into effector cells or memory cells. Selectins and integrins present on the lymphocytes make up the homing receptors, with its specific ligands (addressins) present on HEV and venule endothelial cells. Naïve lymphocytes express α4β7 integrins and its specific ligand cell adhesion molecules (MAdCAM-1) addresin is present on HEVs of Peyer's patches and lamina propria in GIT. Memory lymphocytes have higher levels of α4β7 integrins; thus homing takes place to Peyer's patches and GIT lamina propria. This is why mucosal lymphocytes preferentially traffic to the mucosal lymphoid tissues rather than the peripheral organs. No lung-specific integrins have yet been identified.

FACTORS AFFECTING MUCOSAL IMMUNITY

This section will help the readers know about the factors that can affect mucosal immunity and hence their importance in designing mucosal vaccines.

Vitamins

Retinoic acid (RA) is the bioactive form of vitamin A and plays an essential role in inducing mucosal immune response by inducing the gut homing receptor molecules (α4β7 and CCr9) on activated T lymphocytes for migrating through the lymphatics, the bloodstream, and into GIT lamina propria. It also helps in TI immunoglobulin class switching in B cells to increase IgA production by inducing FoxP3 Treg cells. Thus, vitamin A-deficient individuals are more susceptible to disease and show poor vaccination response and increased mortality. Vitamin A and zinc can affect the response to oral adjuvants and vaccines. Evidences from studies on nonhuman models (rats, chicks) have shown that supplementation with vitamin A is associated with increased IgA production even after parenteral immunization. This finding still needs human investigations. Even vitamin D supplementation is demonstrated to show an improved humoral response to influenza vaccine in children with vitamin D deficiency.[3]

Microbiome

Microbial homeostasis is needed to maintain the gut barrier, and any alteration in it is associated with intestinal microbial dysbiosis and ultimately an abnormal gut mucosal barrier. As mentioned above, it is the microbiota which plays an important role in innate mucosal immunity by producing AMPs and thus influences immune response to both parenteral and oral vaccines. Studies done on germ-free (absence of microbiota) mice showed decreased size and number of Peyer's patches, lamina propria CD4+ T cells, IgA, and IgG and also lacked well-developed GALT. Another study done on humans (adults) showed the effect of complex microbiota on immune response against oral *Salmonella Typhi* vaccine. Adults with a diverse gut microbiome showed a multiphasic CMI, which indicates a stronger immune response in such adults.[3]

ADVANTAGES OF MUCOSAL VACCINATION OVER SYSTEMIC VACCINATION

Tissue Resident Memory Lymphocytes

Tissue resident memory lymphocytes (T_{RM} and B_{RM}) are induced in MALT after mucosal vaccination to provide durable immunity, but these memory subsets are not observed after parenteral immunization, as studied in animal models for influenza and SARS-CoV-2.[1,7] These are analogous to mucosal antibodies. Mucosal vaccination promotes retention of memory B and T cells within MALTs, providing niches for local antigen encounter and rapid recall responses, providing first-line protection against pathogen invasion and dissemination. In case pathogens leak into the body through the mucosal barrier, mucosal vaccine-induced systemic immunity provides a second layer of protection against pathogens.

Easier Delivery and Rapid Response

Mucosal vaccines are given across mucosal surfaces like nose, mouth, and lungs; thus, their delivery is easier than the parenteral routes of immunization, as they do not require needles and hence trained health professionals. This leads to better adherence, thus making mass vaccination during epidemics/pandemics easier.[3] It also provides a quicker response.

Stimulation of Both Mucosal and Systemic Immunity

Due to the cross talk between mucosal and systemic compartments, mucosal vaccines can induce not only mucosal immunity but also systemic immunity as described above in detail. MALT does not have any afferent lymphatics to carry antigens from systemic circulation to MALT. Thus, MALT can only be induced by the exposure of antigens from epithelial surfaces (mediated either by M cells or directly by DCs). So the traditional parenteral route-based vaccinations cannot induce mucosal immunity. Thus, the former provides better protection because infections mostly happen across mucosal surfaces. Parenteral vaccines can induce strong systemic humoral response but induces only weak CMI. As opposed to this, mucosal vaccination can distribute the antigens widely and thus induce both mucosal and CMI and humoral immunity. Studies done with reovirus and rotavirus oral vaccines as early as in 1987 had shown a high frequency of virus-specific CTLs present in Peyer's patches and in MALT, indicating that live oral vaccines can induce antigen-specific CTL in mucosal inductive as well as effector sites for providing mucosal immunity and in systemic lymphoid tissues also, thus providing a double layer of immunity.[5]

Immune Response not Limited to a Single Mucosal Site

Even though mucosal immune responses are compartmentalized, there still occurs cross talk between different mucosae; thus, vaccination at a single mucosal site can promote immune responses at distant mucosal sites too.[4]

Mucosal Vaccines as First Site of Contact

As the mucosal vaccines act at the first site of contact with the pathogen, these are considered to provide protection not only against the disease but also against the infection. This is unlike parenteral vaccination which protects only against the disease and not against infection.[3]

The additional advantages of mucosal vaccination, apart from those discussed above, comprise (1) Eco-friendly—generating less of biomedical waste, (2) reduced costs, (3) safety—no needle-stick injury or transmission of blood-borne infection, and (4) reduced morbidity—least physical or psychological discomfort **(Figs. 5 and 6)**.

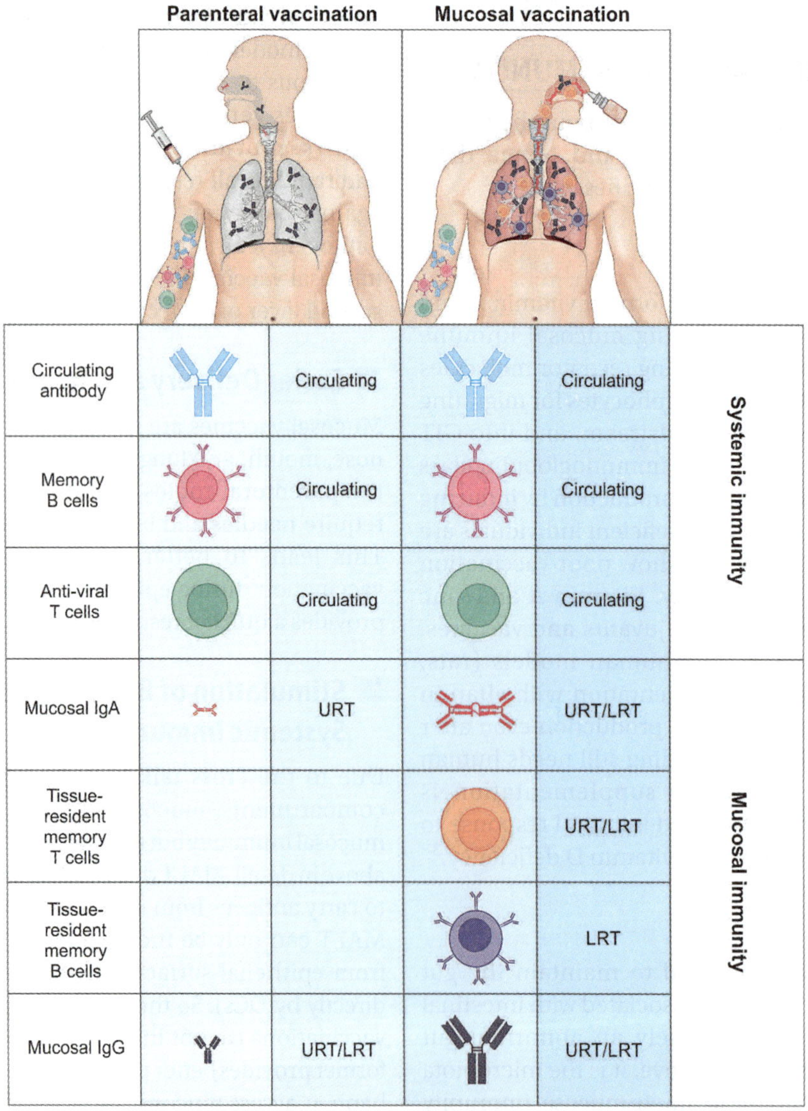

FIG. 5: A comparison of immune response to mucosal and systemic immunity.

Source: Pilapitiya D, Wheatley AK, Tan HX. Mucosal vaccines for SARS-CoV-2: triumph of hope over experience. EBioMedicine. 2023;92:104585.

CHALLENGES IN MUCOSAL VACCINE DESIGN AND WAY FORWARD

Even though the mucosal vaccines have major advantages over the traditional parenteral vaccinations, still there are only eight oral **(Table 1)** and one intranasal vaccine licensed for use in humans.[4] Various other mucosal routes like vaginal, rectal, ocular, and sublingual routes still need to be studied in greater detail. This is because of the various challenges faced during designing a mucosal vaccine.

Correlates of Protection

One of the major challenges in mucosal immunization is the identification of the measurable signs of immunity (correlates of protection) in the recipient.[1] A better understanding of the mucosal immunity is needed to identify the components which can be a true representative of durable and effective immunity at mucosal sites after natural infection or immunization. Basic research is needed to reveal the specific immune cells which are critical for mounting mucosal immunity and the molecular mechanism behind mucosal immunity.[1]

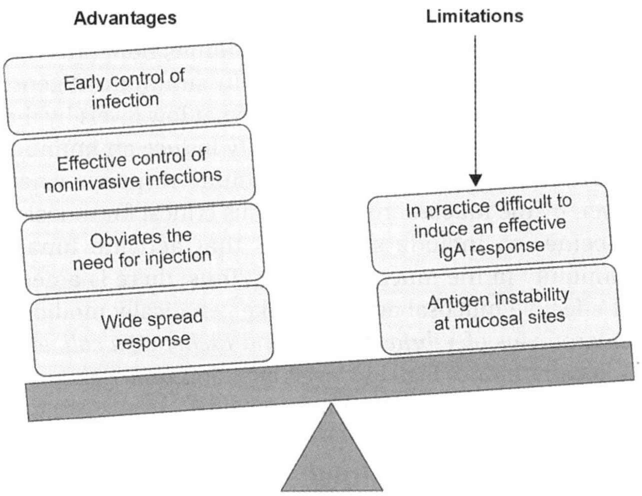

FIG. 6: Advantages and limitations of mucosal and systemic immunity.

Better Understanding of Mucosal Microenvironment

Since the mucosal microbiome affects the biophysiological features of the mucosal barrier, and hence its role in mucosal immunity, it is essential to have a clear understanding of the host mucosal microenvironment. Lack of clean water, sanitation, and hygiene might compromise the microbiome and increase colonization of enteric pathogens. These factors hamper the efficacy of oral live vaccines.[3]

Improved Animal Models Needed

The small animal models used for research may not be adequate, and their results might not correctly predict immune response in humans. This is because of various reasons: firstly simply because of the difference in the size of organs and mucosal tissues, secondly because the small animals used are usually not the native host for which mucosal vaccines are being tried, and thirdly because the mucosal structure of small animals varies from that of humans. For example, studies on intranasal influenza vaccine have been mostly done on mouse models, which are neither the natural host of influenza nor do they have the sialic receptors required for binding and entry of the influenza virus.

TABLE 1: Available licensed mucosal vaccines.

Infection	Type of vaccine	Brand name	Route of administration (Formulation)
Influenza	Live attenuated	FluMist, Fluenz Tetra	Nasal (spray)
Poliomyelitis	Live attenuated	bOPV, mOPV	Oral
Rotavirus	Live attenuated	Rotarix, RotaTeq	Oral
Typhoid	Live attenuated (Ty21a)	Vivotif	Oral (enteric coated capsule)
Cholera	Live attenuated (01 Serogroup—Inaba)	Vaxchora	Oral
	Heat and formaldehyde inactivated (01 Serogroup—Inaba +Ogawa) +0139	Euvichol, Shanchol	Oral
	Heat and formaldehyde inactivated (01 Serogroup—Inaba +Ogawa +0139 +CTB)	Dukoral	Oral
Recurrent UTI	Whole-cell inactivated	Uromune	Oral (Sublingual)—spray

Route of Immunization

Different routes of vaccination induce different responses in terms of potency and longevity because of the variation in the cellular makeup of different lymphoid structures at different sites. For example, oral immunization stimulates immune responses in the GIT along with oral mucosa, NALT, and mammary glands. The intranasal route induces antibody production in NALT, BALT of LRT, urogenital tract, and salivary glands. Thus, depending on the mucosal target site, the route should be carefully chosen **(Fig. 7)**.[10]

Dose of Vaccine

Mucosal vaccines given by the oral route can either be diluted in mucosal secretions, get captured in mucosal gels, broken down by proteases and nucleases, and excluded by epithelial barrier leading to immune tolerance, or those administered through the nasal route may be cleared by clearance mechanisms (e.g., peristalsis, mucociliary movement, sneezing). Thus, a large dose is needed to actually be able to elicit a mucosal immune response. The dose which actually reaches the mucosa cannot be determined.[8] Also, the presence of physiological and biological barrier (e.g., gastric acid, mucins, serous secretions, and tight junctions) mechanisms makes it difficult for mucosal vaccines to elicit antigen-specific immune responses. In addition, the vaccine needs to be prepared in such a way that it closely mimics the pathogen for which it is given.

Size

Size is a very important determinant in the designing of mucosal vaccines in order to be able to induce T- and B-cell responses. Soluble protein antigens of size 0.02–2 µm can enter the lamina propria via goblet cell-associated passageways. Nanosized particles of 20–40 nm enter via endocytosis through enterocytes, while large-sized inert particles of >100 nm are taken up by the M cells. Apart from the route of entry, different-sized antigens lead to different immunity. Nanoparticles predominantly induce T-cell responses, while larger particles tend to induce humoral response more effectively. Antigens < 5 µm via the intranasal route are transported across the nasal mucosa and delivered to BALT, while particles > 10 µm in size are taken up by the alveolar macrophages and DCs.[10]

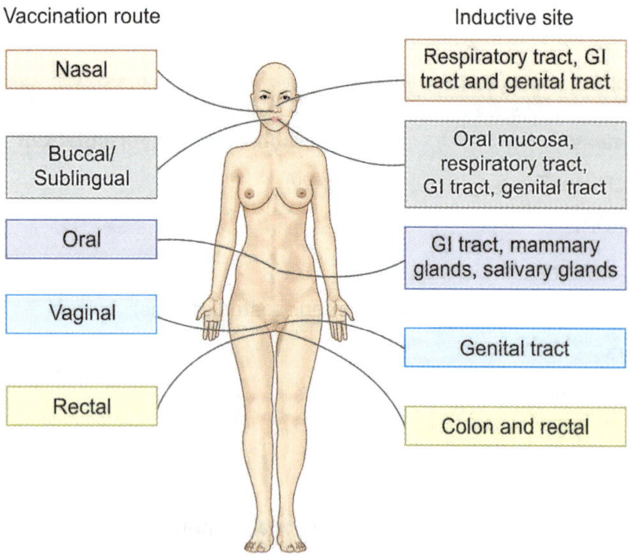

FIG. 7: Mucosal immunization routes and their inductive sites.

Need for Adjuvants/Vaccine Carriers

Depending upon the route of mucosal administration of vaccine, the vaccine needs to be protected from degradation so as to have the desired immune effect at a reasonable dose. This can be achieved with the use of safe and effective mucosal adjuvants. Soluble, nonadherent, nonliving macromolecules, protein subunit antigens, and nonmicrobial particles are taken at low levels by the intestine, and such antigens usually induce an immune tolerance or a weak adaptive immune response when given by the mucosal route. It is thus critical for mucosal vaccines to include substances that activate innate immunity in the mucosal barrier. Thus, there is a need of effective mucosal adjuvants like genetically modified enterotoxins of *Vibrio cholerae* and *Escherichia coli,* etc., adjuvants induce high IgA levels and long-lasting memory when given by mucosal routes.

Breaching the Epithelial Barrier

Live pathogens are more effective as mucosal vaccines or vaccine vectors because of their ability to survive in luminal environments and also because they can invade organized mucosal lymphoid tissue. For example, live attenuated poliovirus vaccine and live attenuated *Salmonella typhi* are amongst the most efficient oral mucosal vaccines. But nonliving mucosal vaccines will not have comparable efficiency.

Tropical Barriers

Several live oral vaccines, including oral polio vaccine, have shown poor response in developing countries than in developed countries. This is mainly because of "tropical enteropathy" or "chronic environmental enteropathy" (CEE), characterized by disturbances in digestive and absorptive functions, leading to malabsorption. Deficiencies in Vitamin A and zinc also affect the vaccination response. Seroconversion following oral poliovirus is more in a developed country like USA than in a developing nation like India.[3] In developing countries, there are high chances of gut infection with soil-transmitted helminths and concomitant bacterial and viral infection. These infections lead to persistent activation of the gut's innate immune response, thus affecting the immune response of oral vaccines. Strategies for overcoming these causes of immune hyporesponsiveness to oral vaccines include co-administration of vaccines with agents like Vitamin A, zinc, and probiotics to improve gut mucosal barrier and treatment of any kind of intestinal helminthic infection before oral vaccination.

Interference with Other Vaccines

Neonates of mothers who are constantly exposed to enteric pathogens have high titers of antibodies against such organisms in their intestines, transferred via breastfeeding. These passively transferred antibodies against enteric pathogens can hamper the efficacy of oral vaccines. This can be overcome to some extent by withdrawing breastmilk shortly before oral vaccination. Studies have shown lower efficacy of oral rotavirus vaccines in the presence of recent polio vaccination. Thus, it becomes essential to study the vaccine calendar so that the effect of one is not hampered by another vaccine.

Others

A major concern regarding live nasal vaccines is that they may transport in a retrograde fashion and reach the brain through olfactory nerves, as seen with live attenuated adenovirus.[8] This is more important for live or viral vectored intranasal vaccines.[1]

RECENT TECHNOLOGY AND MATERIALS FOR MUCOSAL DELIVERY OF SUBUNIT, DNA, AND MRNA VACCINES

- *Mucoadhesive/Mucopenetration*: This is a versatile and adaptable strategy (modifiable surface chemistry and carrier size of synthetic polymers) with stable and controlled release for enhanced antigen update in APC resulting in improved antigen-specific immune responses. However, inconsistent reproducibility in case of synthetic polymers, nonspecific interactions, and antigen loading efficiency are a concern.
- *Mucosal adjuvant*: It has the advantage of increased antigen presentation, co-stimulation of immunomodulatory signals, prolonged immune response, and less of vaccine dose and frequency. However, toxicity may be a concern.
- *Cell targeted vehicles*: They have the advantage of specific immunomodulation. However, they have low efficacy by the oral route.
- *Recombinant viral vehicle*: It is a safe and versatile strategy with high loading capacity, intracellular delivery, and intrinsic immunogenicity. However, it is expensive and difficult to make. It often requires additional adjuvants.
- *Recombinant viral vehicle*: It is a safe and inexpensive strategy with the advantage of a natural adjuvant property. The challenges are antigen presentation and stabilization.

REFERENCES

1. Song Y, Mehl F, Zeichner SL. Vaccine Strategies to Elicit Mucosal Immunity. Vaccines. 2024;12(2):191.
2. Yang J, Yan H. Mucosal epithelial cells: the initial sentinels and responders controlling and regulating immune responses to viral infections. Cellular & Molecular Immunology. 2021;18(7): 1628-30.
3. Correa VA, Portilho AI, De Gaspari E. Vaccines, adjuvants and key factors for mucosal immune response. Immunology. 2022;167(2):124-38.
4. Lavelle EC, Ward RW. Mucosal vaccines—fortifying the frontiers. Nature Reviews Immunology. 2022;22(4):236-50.
5. Boyaka PN, McGhee JR, Czerkinsky C, Mestecky J. Mucosal vaccines: an overview. Mucosal Immunol. 2005:855-74.
6. McGhee JR, Fujihashi K. Inside the mucosal immune system. PLoS Biol. 2012;10(9):e1001397.
7. Pilapitiya D, Wheatley AK, Tan HX. Mucosal vaccines for SARS-CoV-2: triumph of hope over experience. EBioMedicine. 2023;92:104585.
8. Neutra MR, Kozlowski PA. Mucosal vaccines: the promise and the challenge. Nature Rev Immunol. 2006;6(2):148-58.
9. Czerkinsky C, Holmgren J. Mucosal delivery routes for optimal immunization: targeting immunity to the right tissues. Mucosal vaccines: modern concepts, strategies, and challenges. Curr Top Microbiol Immunol. 2010;354:1-8.
10. Miquel-Clopés A, Bentley EG, Stewart JP, Carding SR. Mucosal vaccines and technology. Clin Exp Immunol. 2019;196(2):205-14.

CHAPTER 5

Broad-spectrum Effects of Vaccines

Neelima Tirkey, Anuj Bhatnagar

INTRODUCTION

Vaccines are the most effective measures for protection from infectious diseases. They influence seasonal changes of the disease and greatly contribute to the well-being of communities. Vaccines are available for some specific diseases, but no vaccine can be used universally for all infectious diseases. Genetic diversity among microorganisms affects the antigenic variation, which may decrease the effectiveness of specific vaccines.

Vaccines have long been recognized as a cornerstone of public health, providing targeted protection against specific infectious diseases.[1]

Beyond their well-established role in inducing pathogen-specific immunity, vaccines have been found to stimulate a range of nonspecific or heterologous effects on the immune system. These effects can be beneficial or, in some cases, detrimental.

NONSPECIFIC EFFECTS OF VACCINE

These effects involve enhancing the overall immune response, potentially providing protection against a broader range of pathogens.

For example, some vaccines have been shown to reduce the incidence of unrelated infections, suggesting a more generalized boost to immune function.

Type of Nonspecific Effects and Its Characteristics

- *Enhanced immune response*: Some vaccines can boost the overall immune system, making it more effective in fighting off other infections. For instance, the Bacillus Calmette-Guérin (BCG) vaccine, primarily used against tuberculosis, has been shown to reduce the incidence of respiratory infections and sepsis in children. This is thought to be due to the vaccine's stimulation of innate immunity.
- *Heterologous effects*: Vaccines can induce cross-reactive immune responses, meaning they might offer protection against pathogens not specifically targeted by the vaccine. Observational studies have suggested that some vaccines might lower overall mortality rates. For example, in some regions, BCG vaccination has been associated with reduced mortality from various infections in children, potentially due to its broad immune system effects. The measles vaccine has also been associated with reduced mortality from other infectious diseases.
- *Trained immunity*: Certain vaccines can induce a state of "trained immunity," where the innate immune system (the body's first line of defense) is primed to respond more robustly to various pathogens.[2]
- *Potential negative effects*: While many nonspecific effects (NSEs) are beneficial, some vaccines might temporarily weaken the immune system's response to other infections. For example, some studies have suggested that certain live vaccines could transiently suppress immune responses to unrelated infections.
- *Age and timing*: For instance, the sequence in which vaccines are given can influence their NSEs on the immune system.
- *Gender differences*: Research has indicated that NSEs of vaccines might differ between males and females, potentially due to differences in immune system functioning between genders.
- *Mechanisms*: The mechanisms behind these NSEs are still being studied but may include changes in immune cell function, alterations in the production of cytokines (immune signaling molecules).

INDIRECT EFFECTS OF THE VACCINES ON THE IMMUNE SYSTEM

The indirect effects of vaccines, also known as herd immunity or community immunity, occur when a significant portion of a population becomes immune to an infectious disease, thereby providing a measure of protection for individuals who are not immune.

Indirect Effect of Vaccines

Vaccines can have indirect effects by reducing the transmission of diseases within the community. This phenomenon known as herd immunity, occurs when a significant portion of the population is immunized, thereby protecting even those who are not vaccinated. This indirect protection is particularly important for vulnerable populations such as infants, elderly individuals, and those with compromised immune systems.

The indirect effects are:

- *Bacillus Calmette–Guérin vaccine*: Studies on the NSEs of the BCG vaccine, originally developed for tuberculosis (TB) prevention, suggest that it may offer broader immunological benefits. Here are a few notable findings:
  - *Reduction in infant mortality*: Some studies indicate that BCG vaccination can reduce all-cause mortality in infants, primarily by protecting against respiratory infections and sepsis.[3,4,5]
  - *Protection against other infections*: This effect is thought to be due to "trained immunity," where innate immune cells develop a memory-like response to pathogens after BCG vaccination.[6,7]
  - *Potential effects on COVID-19*: There has been interest in whether the BCG vaccine could provide some protection against COVID-19. Early observational studies suggested a correlation between countries with widespread BCG vaccination and lower COVID-19 morbidity and mortality. However, randomized controlled trials are ongoing to provide more definitive answers.[8]
  - *Autoimmune diseases and allergies*: Some research indicates that BCG vaccination might have a role in modulating immune responses, potentially reducing the incidence of autoimmune diseases like type 1 diabetes and certain allergies.
  - *Oncogenic research*: BCG may be used as an immunotherapy for bladder cancer. Its administration into the bladder has been shown to trigger an immune response that helps to destroy cancer cells.

    These findings illustrate that the BCG vaccine may have broad immunomodulatory effects beyond its original purpose of preventing tuberculosis.
- *Hepatitis-B vaccine (Hep-B)*: The hepatitis B vaccine, primarily designed to prevent hepatitis B virus (HBV) infection, has also been studied for its potential NSEs. Here are some notable findings:
  - *Reduction in infant mortality*: Studies suggest that hepatitis B vaccination at birth may reduce overall infant mortality, not just from HBV but from other infectious diseases as well. This effect is thought to be due to the vaccine's impact on the immune system, possibly enhancing the body's defense against various pathogens.
  - *Impact on other infections*: Some research indicates that the hepatitis B vaccine might protect against non-HBV infections. For instance, a study in Guinea-Bissau observed lower all-cause mortality in children who received the hepatitis B vaccine compared to those who did not.
  - *Modulation of immune responses*: The hepatitis B vaccine has been shown to modulate immune responses, which could potentially lead to a decreased risk of certain infections and improved outcomes in various health conditions.
  - *Potential effects on autoimmune diseases*: There is some evidence that hepatitis B vaccination may influence the development of autoimmune diseases, although the findings are mixed and more research is needed to draw definitive conclusions.
  - *Overall health benefits*: Some studies have suggested broader health benefits of hepatitis B vaccination, such as improved overall survival rates and reduced incidence of certain diseases, although the mechanisms behind these effects are not fully understood.

    While the evidence for NSEs of the hepatitis B vaccine is still emerging and less robust compared to the BCG vaccine, these studies provide a foundation for further investigation into its broader immunological impacts.
- *Oral polio vaccine (OPV)*: The OPV, primarily developed to prevent poliomyelitis, has been studied for its NSEs on overall health and immunity. Here are some key findings:
  - *Reduction in all-cause mortality*: Several studies have suggested that OPV may reduce all-cause mortality in children, not just mortality due to poliovirus.[9] This effect is thought to be due to the vaccine's ability to boost the immune system's response to a range of pathogens. For instance, a study in Guinea-Bissau found that children who received OPV had lower mortality rates compared to those who did not.
  - *Protection against other infections*: OPV has been associated with a decreased incidence of other infectious diseases, such as respiratory infections and diarrhea. This effect is hypothesized to result from the stimulation of the innate immune system,

leading to enhanced protection against various pathogens.

- *Impact on hospitalizations*: Research has indicated that OPV may reduce hospitalizations for non-polio infections. A study in Denmark observed fewer hospitalizations due to respiratory infections and other illnesses among children who had received OPV compared to those who had not.
- *Modulation of immune responses*: OPV has been shown to induce a broad immune response, which may provide cross-protection against different types of pathogens. This phenomenon is known as "trained immunity," where the innate immune system exhibits an enhanced response to subsequent infections.
- *Potential role in reducing autoimmune diseases*: Some studies have suggested that OPV might influence the incidence of autoimmune diseases, such as type 1 diabetes.

These findings highlight the potential nonspecific benefits of the OPV, suggesting it may contribute to improved overall health and reduced mortality in vaccinated populations.

- *Inactivated polio vaccine*: The inactivated polio vaccine (IPV), developed to prevent poliomyelitis, has also been examined for its potential NSEs on overall health and immunity. Although most research on the NSEs of polio vaccines has focused on the OPV, there are some findings related to IPV as well.
  - *Reduction in all-cause mortality*: Some studies have suggested that IPV may contribute to reduced all-cause mortality in children, like OPV.
  - Lower mortality rates among children who received IPV compared to those who did not, although the effect was more pronounced with OPV.
  - *Protection against other infections*: Research indicates that IPV might provide some level of protection against non-polio infections. This protection is likely due to the stimulation of the immune system, leading to enhanced responses to various pathogens. A study conducted in Denmark suggested that children vaccinated with IPV had a lower incidence of hospitalizations for respiratory infections compared to unvaccinated children.
  - *Impact on immune system modulation*: IPV has been shown to induce immune responses that may enhance the body's defense mechanisms against other diseases. This effect is part of the broader concept of "trained immunity," where the innate immune system develops a memory-like response to subsequent infections. This phenomenon has been observed with other vaccines as well, suggesting a potential mechanism for the NSEs of IPV.
  - *Potential influence on autoimmune diseases*: There is limited evidence suggesting that IPV might influence the risk of developing autoimmune diseases, such as type 1 diabetes. While some studies have indicated a potential protective effect, the evidence remains inconclusive and requires further research to establish a clear link.

  While the NSEs of IPV are less studied compared to those of OPV, existing research indicates potential benefits beyond its primary purpose of preventing poliomyelitis. Further studies are needed to better understand the broader immunological impacts of IPV.

- *Diphtheria, pertussis, and tetanus*: The diphtheria, pertussis, and tetanus (DPT) vaccine has been widely used to prevent these three serious diseases. However, it has also been studied for its NSEs on overall health and immunity. Here are some key findings:
  - *Impact on child mortality*: Studies have reported mixed results regarding the impact of DPT vaccination on child mortality.[10] Some research suggests that DPT vaccination may be associated with increased mortality in girls.[11] For example, a study in Guinea-Bissau found higher mortality rates among girls who received the DPT vaccine compared to those who did not, while boys showed no significant difference. This gender-differential effect has raised concerns and calls for further investigation.[4]
  - *Interactions with other vaccines*: The NSEs of the DPT vaccine may also be influenced by its interactions with other vaccines. For instance, studies have shown that children who receive the DPT vaccine along with the measles vaccine may have different health outcomes compared to those who receive the vaccines separately. In some cases, combining these vaccines has been associated with higher mortality rates, suggesting a complex interaction between different immunizations.
  - *Effect on nontargeted infections*: Some research indicates that the DPT vaccine may increase susceptibility to certain nontargeted infections. For example, a study conducted in West Africa suggested that children vaccinated with DPT had a higher risk of contracting respiratory infections and diarrhea. This effect is thought to be due to the vaccine's potential impact on the immune system's overall functionality.
  - *Gender differences*: The NSEs of the DPT vaccine appear to vary by gender. Several studies have found that girls may experience more adverse

NSEs compared to boys. For example, research in Guinea-Bissau observed higher mortality rates among girls who received DPT, raising questions about gender-specific responses to the vaccine.
    - *Immune modulation*: The DPT vaccine has been shown to modulate the immune system, potentially affecting the body's response to other pathogens. This modulation could lead to an increased risk of certain infections while protecting others. The exact mechanisms behind these effects are still under investigation, but they highlight the complexity of the immune response to vaccination.
- *Pentavalent vaccine*: Comprehensive protection against DPT, hepatitis B, and *Haemophilus influenzae* type b, reducing the overall burden of these diseases in the community.
  The pentavalent vaccine, which includes protection against diphtheria, tetanus, pertussis (whooping cough), *Haemophilus influenzae* type B (Hib), and hepatitis B, has been studied for its NSEs on overall health and immunity. Here are some key findings:
    - *Impact on child mortality*: Some studies suggest that the introduction of the pentavalent vaccine can affect child mortality rates. For example, a study in Guinea-Bissau found that the introduction of the pentavalent vaccine was associated with increased mortality rates in girls but not in boys. This raises questions about the gender-specific effects of the vaccine.
    - *Interactions with other vaccines*: The pentavalent vaccine is often given alongside other vaccines, and its NSEs can be influenced by these combinations. Research has shown that the timing and sequence of vaccinations can affect overall health outcomes. For instance, studies have suggested that receiving the pentavalent vaccine alongside the measles vaccine may influence child mortality and morbidity differently than when the vaccines are administered separately.
    - *Effect on nontargeted infections*: Some research indicates that the pentavalent vaccine may influence susceptibility to infections not directly targeted by the vaccine. A study conducted in West Africa suggested that children who received the pentavalent vaccine had higher rates of certain infections, such as respiratory infections and diarrhea, compared to those who did not receive the vaccine.
    - *Immune system modulation*: The pentavalent vaccine has been shown to modulate the immune system, potentially affecting responses to other pathogens. This modulation could result in both beneficial and adverse NSEs. For instance, some studies have observed that the vaccine can enhance the immune response to subsequent vaccinations, while others have noted increased susceptibility to certain nontargeted infections.
    - *Gender differences*: Several studies have reported gender differences in the NSEs of the pentavalent vaccine. Girls have been observed to experience different health outcomes compared to boys following vaccination. These differences highlight the need for more research to understand the underlying mechanisms and to optimize vaccination strategies accordingly.
- *Rotavirus vaccine (Rota)*: Reduced incidence of severe diarrhea and dehydration among unvaccinated children due to lower circulation of the virus in the community.
  The rotavirus vaccine, designed to protect against rotavirus infection, which causes severe diarrhea in infants and young children, has also been studied for its NSEs on overall health and immunity. Here are some key findings:
    - *Reduction in all-cause mortality and hospitalizations*: Several studies have indicated that rotavirus vaccination may reduce all-cause mortality and hospitalizations for diarrhea and respiratory infections.[12] For example, a study in Mexico found that the introduction of the rotavirus vaccine was associated with a significant reduction in diarrhea-related deaths among children under 5 years old.
    - *Impact on other gastrointestinal infections*: Research has shown that rotavirus vaccination can lead to a decrease in hospitalizations for gastroenteritis caused by pathogens other than rotavirus. This suggests that the vaccine may enhance overall gut health and immunity, protecting a broader range of gastrointestinal infections.
    - *Effect on nongastrointestinal infections*: Some studies have explored the potential impact of rotavirus vaccination on nongastrointestinal infections. For instance, research in Bangladesh observed a reduction in the incidence of respiratory infections among vaccinated children, suggesting a broader protective effect on the immune system.
    - *Modulation of the immune system*: The rotavirus vaccine has been shown to modulate the immune system in ways that may protect against various pathogens. This immunomodulation could enhance the body's overall defense mechanisms, reducing the severity and incidence of other infections.

- *Reduction in antibiotic use*: By reducing the incidence and severity of diarrhea and other infections, rotavirus vaccination may also lead to a decrease in antibiotic use. This can have broader public health benefits, including reducing the risk of antibiotic resistance.

  These studies highlight the potential nonspecific benefits of the rotavirus vaccine, suggesting that its protective effects may extend beyond just preventing rotavirus infection to improving overall child health and reducing mortality from various causes. Further research is needed to fully understand these effects and to optimize vaccination strategies accordingly.

- *Pneumococcal conjugate vaccine (PCV)*: Reduced incidence of pneumococcal disease (e.g., pneumonia, meningitis) in the population, including unvaccinated individuals, through decreased transmission of *Streptococcus pneumoniae*.

  The pneumococcal vaccine, which protects against infections caused by the bacterium *Streptococcus pneumoniae*, such as pneumonia, meningitis, and sepsis, has been studied for its potential NSEs on overall health and immunity.[13,14] Here are some key findings:
  - *Reduction in all-cause mortality and hospitalizations*: Several studies have indicated that pneumococcal vaccination can lead to reductions in all-cause mortality and hospitalizations, not just those specifically caused by *Streptococcus pneumoniae*. For instance, a study in the Gambia found that the introduction of the PCV was associated with a significant reduction in child mortality rates.
  - *Impact on other infections*: Research has shown that pneumococcal vaccination can reduce the incidence of other bacterial and viral infections, such as non-pneumococcal pneumonia and invasive bacterial infections. This may be due to a reduction in the overall bacterial load and an improvement in herd immunity.
  - *Effect on antibiotic use*: By reducing the incidence and severity of respiratory infections, the pneumococcal vaccine can lead to a decrease in antibiotic use. This is particularly important in reducing the risk of antibiotic resistance, a major public health concern.
  - *Immune system modulation*: The pneumococcal vaccine has been shown to have effects on the immune system that may enhance the body's overall defense mechanisms. This includes the potential for "trained immunity," where the innate immune system exhibits an enhanced response to subsequent infections.
  - *Reduction in hospital admissions for respiratory illnesses*: A study conducted in Denmark found that the introduction of the PCV was associated with a reduction in hospital admissions for respiratory illnesses in children, suggesting broader protective effects on respiratory health.

  These studies highlight the potential nonspecific benefits of the pneumococcal vaccine, suggesting that its protective effects may extend beyond just preventing pneumococcal infections to improving overall child health and reducing mortality from various causes. Further research is needed to fully understand these effects and to optimize vaccination strategies accordingly.

- *Measles*: Several studies have shown that the measles vaccine can have NSEs on the immune system and overall health. Here are some key findings:
  - *Reduced overall mortality*: Multiple studies have indicated that measles vaccination is associated with a reduction in overall child mortality, not just deaths from measles. For example, research conducted in West Africa showed that children who received the measles vaccine had a lower risk of dying from all causes compared to those who did not receive the vaccine.
  - *Improved immune response*: The measles vaccine has been observed to enhance the immune system's ability to fight off other infections. This is thought to be due to the vaccine's ability to induce a broad activation of the immune system, improving its responsiveness to various pathogens.
  - *Protection against other infections*: Some studies suggest that measles vaccination can reduce the incidence of other infectious diseases. For instance, a study in Bangladesh found that measles-vaccinated children had fewer episodes of respiratory infections and diarrhea compared to unvaccinated children.
  - *Reduced hospitalization and disease severity*: In addition to reducing mortality, measles vaccination has been linked to a decrease in the severity of other infections, leading to fewer hospitalizations. This effect may be due to the vaccine's role in bolstering the immune system's overall effectiveness.

  These nonspecific benefits are thought to arise from the vaccine's impact on the immune system, including effects on innate immunity and the modulation of immune responses.

- *Mumps, measles, rubella vaccine (MMR)*: The measles, mumps, and rubella vaccine, primarily designed to protect against these three viral infections, has been studied for its NSEs on overall health and immunity. Here are some key findings:

- *Reduction in all-cause mortality*: Several studies have shown that the MMR vaccine is associated with a reduction in all-cause mortality in children, beyond just preventing measles, mumps, and rubella. For instance, research from Guinea-Bissau indicated that MMR vaccination was linked to lower all-cause mortality rates in children.
- *Protection against other infections*: Evidence suggests that the MMR vaccine may offer protection against a range of other infections.[15] A study in the UK found that children who received the MMR vaccine had a reduced incidence of hospital admissions for respiratory and gastrointestinal infections, indicating broader protective effects.[16]
- *Immune system modulation*: The MMR vaccine is believed to modulate the immune system, potentially enhancing the body's ability to fight off various infections. This effect is thought to be related to the vaccine's impact on the immune system's memory and its role in "training" the immune response.
- *Reduced hospitalizations*: Studies have shown that MMR vaccination is associated with a reduction in hospitalizations for nontargeted infections.[16] For example, a study in the Netherlands observed fewer hospital admissions for infections other than measles, mumps, and rubella among vaccinated children.
- *Impact on antibiotic use*: By reducing the incidence of infections, the MMR vaccine may contribute to a decrease in antibiotic use, helping to combat antibiotic resistance.

These studies suggest that the MMR vaccine may have significant NSEs that improve overall health and reduce mortality from various causes. The evidence underscores the broader benefits of the MMR vaccination beyond its primary targets. Further research is needed to fully understand these effects and to optimize vaccination strategies accordingly.

- *Japanese encephalitis vaccine (JE):* Decreased transmission of JE virus in areas where the disease is endemic, providing indirect protection to unvaccinated individuals.

The JE vaccine, which protects against the JE virus, has also been studied for its NSEs on overall health and immunity. Here are some key findings:

- *Reduction in child mortality*: Studies have shown that the JE vaccine may be associated with a reduction in all-cause mortality among children. For example, a study in India found that the introduction of the JE vaccine was linked to a decrease in child mortality, suggesting broader protective effects beyond preventing JE.
- *Protection against other infections*: Research has indicated that the JE vaccine may offer protection against other infections.[17] A study in Vietnam observed a reduction in hospitalizations for non-JE infections among children who received the JE vaccine, indicating potential broader health benefits.
- *Immune system modulation*: The JE vaccine may modulate the immune system in ways that enhance overall immunity. This effect could be related to the vaccine's impact on the immune response and its ability to "train the immune system to respond more effectively to other pathogens".
- *Impact on hospitalizations*: Some studies have found that JE vaccination is associated with a reduction in hospital admissions for infections other than JE. For instance, research in Thailand suggested that the JE vaccine contributed to a decrease in hospitalizations for other infectious diseases.

These studies indicate that the JE vaccine may have significant NSEs, potentially improving overall health and reducing mortality from various causes. Further research is necessary to fully understand these effects and to optimize vaccination strategies accordingly.

- *Haemophilus influenzae type-b vaccine*: Reduced incidence of meningitis, pneumonia, and epiglottitis, particularly protecting unvaccinated children and adults.

The *Haemophilus influenzae* type b vaccine, which protects against invasive Hib infections such as meningitis and pneumonia, has also been studied for its NSEs on overall health and immunity.[18] Here are some key findings:

- *Reduction in all-cause mortality*: Research suggests that the Hib vaccine may be associated with a reduction in all-cause mortality. For example, a study in the Gambia found that the introduction of the Hib vaccine was linked to a significant reduction in child mortality, beyond the direct protection against Hib disease.
- *Protection against other infections*: The Hib vaccine has been observed to have a broader protective effect against other infections. A study in Sweden found that the introduction of the Hib vaccine was associated with a decrease in hospital admissions for respiratory infections, indicating that the vaccine might have a broader impact on health.

  - *Impact on hospitalizations*: Studies have indicated that Hib vaccination reduces hospitalizations for other infections. For instance, research in the United States showed a decrease in hospital admissions for pneumonia and other respiratory illnesses following the introduction of the Hib vaccine.
  - *Immune system modulation*: The Hib vaccine may modulate the immune system in ways that enhance overall immunity. This effect could be related to the vaccine's impact on the immune response and its role in potentially reducing susceptibility to other infections.

  These studies highlight that the Hib vaccine may have important NSEs, including improving overall health and reducing mortality from various causes. The evidence underscores the broader benefits of Hib vaccination beyond its primary purpose. Further research is necessary to fully understand these effects and to optimize vaccination strategies accordingly.
- *Influenza*: The influenza vaccine, primarily aimed at preventing seasonal influenza, has been studied for its NSEs on overall health and immunity.[19] Here are some key findings:
  - *Reduction in all-cause mortality*: Some studies suggest that the influenza vaccine may be associated with a reduction in all-cause mortality. For example, a study in older adults showed that influenza vaccination was linked to lower overall mortality rates, not just from influenza.
  - *Protection against other respiratory infections*: Research has indicated that the influenza vaccine might offer protection against other respiratory infections.[20] A study in elderly populations found that influenza vaccination was associated with a reduced incidence of respiratory infections other than influenza.
  - *Reduced hospitalizations*: Studies have found that influenza vaccination is associated with a reduction in hospitalizations for respiratory illnesses. For instance, research in the United States has shown that seasonal influenza vaccination is linked to fewer hospital admissions for pneumonia and other respiratory conditions.
  - *Immune system modulation*: The influenza vaccine may modulate the immune system in a way that enhances the body's overall defense mechanisms. This includes potentially providing broader protection against other pathogens due to improved immune function.
  - *Impact on antibiotic use*: By reducing the incidence of influenza and potentially other infections, the influenza vaccine may lead to decreased antibiotic use, which is beneficial for combating antibiotic resistance.

  These studies suggest that the influenza vaccine may have significant NSEs, potentially improving overall health and reducing mortality from various causes. The evidence highlights the broader benefits of influenza vaccination beyond its primary purpose. Further research is needed to fully understand these effects and to optimize vaccination strategies accordingly.
- *Typhoid*: The typhoid vaccine, designed to protect against *Salmonella typhi* infection, has been studied for its NSEs on overall health and immunity. Here are some key findings:
  - *Reduction in all-cause mortality*: Some studies suggest that the typhoid vaccine may be associated with a reduction in all-cause mortality. For instance, a study in Nepal observed a reduction in child mortality in areas where the typhoid vaccine was widely used.
  - *Protection against other infections*: Research has indicated that the typhoid vaccine might offer protection against other infections.[21] For example, a study in Bangladesh found a reduction in hospital admissions for diseases other than typhoid among children who received the vaccine.
  - *Immune system modulation*: The typhoid vaccine may have effects on the immune system that enhance overall immunity. This might be related to its impact on immune function, potentially leading to better protection against a range of infections.
  - *Impact on antibiotic use*: By reducing the incidence of typhoid and potentially other infections, the typhoid vaccine might contribute to decreased antibiotic use, which is important for reducing antibiotic resistance.

  These studies suggest that the typhoid vaccine may have NSEs that improve overall health and reduce mortality from various causes. Further research is needed to confirm these effects and optimize vaccination strategies.
- *Chickenpox*: The chickenpox (varicella) vaccine, primarily designed to protect against chickenpox, has also been studied for its NSEs on overall health and immunity.[22] Here are some key findings:
  - *Reduction in all-cause mortality*: Some research has indicated that the chickenpox vaccine may be associated with a reduction in all-cause mortality. For instance, studies have observed a decrease in child mortality rates in regions where the

varicella vaccination program has been widely implemented.

- *Protection against other infections*: The varicella vaccine may offer protection against other infections. A study in the United States found that children who received the chickenpox vaccine had lower rates of hospitalizations for infections other than chickenpox, suggesting broader health benefits.
- *Reduced hospitalizations*: Research has shown that the chickenpox vaccine is linked to a reduction in hospital admissions for various infections. For example, a study conducted in Australia reported a decrease in hospitalizations for infections other than chickenpox following the introduction of the varicella vaccination program.
- *Immune system modulation*: The chickenpox vaccine may have NSEs on the immune system, potentially enhancing the body's overall defense mechanisms. This includes a potential reduction in susceptibility to other infectious diseases.
- *Impact on antibiotic use*: By preventing chickenpox and potentially other infections, the vaccine may lead to a reduction in antibiotic use, contributing to the fight against antibiotic resistance.

These studies suggest that the chickenpox vaccine may have NSEs that improve overall health and reduce mortality from various causes. The evidence underscores the broader benefits of varicella vaccination beyond its primary purpose. Further research is needed to fully understand these effects and optimize vaccination strategies.

- *Hepatitis A*: The hepatitis A vaccine, designed primarily to prevent hepatitis A virus infection, has been studied for its NSEs on overall health and immunity. Here are some key findings:
  - *Reduction in all-cause mortality*: There is some evidence suggesting that the hepatitis A vaccine may be associated with reduced all-cause mortality. Studies have shown that vaccination programs can lead to lower overall mortality rates in populations where the vaccine is widely used.
  - *Protection against other infections*: Research has indicated that the hepatitis A vaccine might provide broader protection against other infections. For example, a study conducted in Nepal found that children vaccinated against hepatitis A had reduced hospital admissions for infections other than hepatitis A.
  - *Reduced hospitalizations*: Some studies have observed that hepatitis A vaccination is linked to a reduction in hospitalizations for various infections.[23] A study in the United States found that after the introduction of hepatitis A vaccination programs, there was a decrease in hospital admissions for infections unrelated to hepatitis A.
  - *Immune system modulation*: The hepatitis A vaccine may have effects on the immune system that enhance overall immunity. This could potentially result in better protection against a range of other infections.
  - *Impact on antibiotic use*: By reducing the incidence of hepatitis A and potentially other infections, the vaccine might contribute to decreased antibiotic use, which is beneficial for reducing antibiotic resistance.

  These studies suggest that the hepatitis A vaccine may have significant NSEs, potentially improving overall health and reducing mortality from various causes. Further research is needed to confirm these effects and to optimize vaccination strategies.
- *Human papillomavirus*: The human papillomavirus (HPV) vaccine, primarily aimed at preventing HPV infections and associated cancers, has been studied for its NSEs on overall health and immunity.[24] Here are some key findings:
  - *Reduction in all-cause mortality*: Current research does not strongly indicate that the HPV vaccine has a direct effect on all-cause mortality. The focus has largely been on its primary role in preventing HPV-related diseases, such as cervical cancer, rather than on overall mortality.
  - *Protection against other infections*: Limited evidence suggests that the HPV vaccine might have indirect effects on overall health. Some studies have observed that vaccination might be associated with a reduction in other sexually transmitted infections (STIs). For example, a study in Australia found a decrease in the prevalence of other STIs among HPV-vaccinated individuals.
  - *Reduced hospitalizations*: Research has shown that the HPV vaccine may contribute to reduced hospitalizations for HPV-related conditions, which indirectly suggests a potential impact on overall health. However, evidence of broader nonspecific hospitalization effects is less well-documented.
  - *Immune system modulation*: The HPV vaccine may modulate the immune system, potentially enhancing immune responses to other infections. However, more research is needed to confirm these effects.
  - *Impact on cancer prevention*: The primary benefit of the HPV vaccine is its role in preventing HPV-related cancers, such as cervical cancer, and potentially reducing the incidence of other HPV-associated malignancies. This can indirectly affect

overall health outcomes by reducing the burden of cancer.

While the primary benefits of the HPV vaccine are well-established in preventing HPV-related cancers and diseases, evidence regarding its NSEs on overall health and other infections is still emerging. Further research is necessary to fully understand these potential broader impacts.

- *Tetanus diphtheria (Td)*: The NSEs of vaccines, including the tetanus-diphtheria vaccine (Td), refer to the broader immune system effects beyond protection against the targeted diseases. Research has shown that vaccines can sometimes provide additional benefits or risks in terms of overall health and immune function.

  For the tetanus-diphtheria vaccine specifically, studies have explored its impact on nonspecific immunity:
  - *Enhanced immune response*: Some research suggests that vaccines can enhance general immune responses, potentially providing some protection against other infections. However, evidence for Td specifically showing such effects is limited.
  - *Immune system modulation*: The Td vaccine, like other vaccines, can influence immune system balance. This may have subtle effects on susceptibility to unrelated infections, but these effects are not well-documented for Td.
  - *General health impact*: Some studies have noted that vaccination programs can lead to improved overall health outcomes in populations by reducing the burden of infectious diseases, which might indirectly influence susceptibility to other diseases.

    Overall, while the Td vaccine primarily targets tetanus and diphtheria, its NSEs are not as thoroughly studied as some other vaccines. Most research focuses on the vaccine's efficacy against the specific diseases it targets.
- *Meningococcal*: The meningococcal vaccine, which protects against meningococcal disease caused by *Neisseria meningitidis*, has been studied for its NSEs on overall health and immunity.[25] Here are some key findings:
  - *Reduction in all-cause mortality*: There is limited evidence suggesting that the meningococcal vaccine may be associated with a reduction in all-cause mortality. Most studies focus on the vaccine's effectiveness in preventing meningococcal disease rather than its impact on overall mortality.
  - *Protection against other infections*: Research has shown that the meningococcal vaccine might have broader health benefits. For instance, a study in the UK found that the introduction of the meningococcal B vaccine was associated with a decrease in the incidence of other infections, suggesting potential nonspecific protective effects.
  - *Reduced hospitalizations*: Some studies have reported a reduction in hospitalizations for infections other than meningococcal disease following the introduction of meningococcal vaccination programs. For example, research in Canada found a decline in hospital admissions for other infections among vaccinated individuals.
  - *Immune system modulation*: The meningococcal vaccine may modulate the immune system, potentially enhancing overall immunity. This effect could lead to better protection against a range of infections, though specific studies detailing this are limited.
  - *Impact on antibiotic use*: By reducing the incidence of meningococcal disease and potentially other infections, the meningococcal vaccine may contribute to decreased antibiotic use, which is beneficial for combating antibiotic resistance.

    These studies suggest that while the primary benefit of the meningococcal vaccine is in preventing meningococcal disease, there may also be broader health benefits, including reduced hospitalizations and potentially improved overall immunity. Further research is needed to fully understand and confirm these NSEs.
- *COVID*: Nonspecific effects of vaccines refer to benefits beyond their intended targets. For COVID-19 vaccines, research has explored several NSEs:
  - *Reduced mortality from other infections*: Some studies suggest that COVID-19 vaccines might reduce mortality from other infections, possibly due to improved overall immune function.
  - *Herd immunity and indirect protection*: Vaccination can contribute to herd immunity, indirectly protecting unvaccinated individuals by reducing the overall spread of the virus.
  - *Reduced severity of other illnesses*: There is some evidence that COVID-19 vaccination may lessen the severity of illnesses that are not directly related to COVID-19, potentially due to broader immune system activation.

These effects are still being studied, and while they offer promising insights, more research is needed to fully understand their mechanisms and implication.

CONCLUSION

The broad-spectrum effects of vaccines on the immune system highlight the complexity of their impact beyond direct pathogens-specific immunity. By considering both indirect and NSEs, public health officials can better evaluate the overall benefits of vaccination programs and optimize strategies for disease prevention.

Vaccines often offer benefits beyond their primary targets, significantly enhancing public health. Research indicates that various vaccines, such as those for rotavirus, pneumococcal disease, measles, MMR, JE, Hib, influenza, typhoid, chickenpox, hepatitis A, HPV, Td, meningococcal disease, and COVID-19, can have broad health impacts.

For example, rotavirus vaccination is linked to fewer deaths and hospitalizations from both gastrointestinal and respiratory illnesses. Pneumococcal vaccines have been associated with declines in hospitalizations for a range of bacterial and viral infections. Measles and MMR vaccines have been shown to reduce overall mortality and hospital admissions for conditions unrelated to their primary targets. The Hib vaccine also contributes to lower mortality and hospitalizations for infections beyond Hib-related diseases. Similarly, influenza vaccination has been correlated with improved general health and fewer hospitalizations for respiratory conditions.

Typhoid and chickenpox vaccines have been associated with reduced mortality and hospitalizations for various infections. Hepatitis A and HPV vaccines may also offer broader health benefits, including fewer hospitalizations and enhanced immune responses. While the Td and meningococcal vaccines show some evidence of nonspecific benefits, more research is needed for a comprehensive understanding. COVID-19 vaccines are increasingly recognized for their potential to improve immune function and reduce mortality from other infections.

There are enough research findings to suggest NSEs like survival benefits from live-attenuated vaccines (BCG, OPV, and measles).[3] Understanding and harnessing these NSEs could improve vaccine strategies, especially in low-resource settings where broad protection against multiple infections is highly beneficial. It also opens up new avenues for vaccine development and deployment strategies, emphasizing the need for a broader perspective on vaccine benefits beyond specific disease prevention.

REFERENCES

1. Clemens J, Holmgren J, Kaufmann SH, Mantovani A. Ten years of the Global Alliance for Vaccines and Immunization: Challenges and progress. Nat Immunol. 2010;11(12):1069-72.
2. Netea MG, Quintin J, van der Meer JW. Trained immunity: a memory for innate host defense. Cell Host Microbe. 2011;9(5):355-61.
3. Aaby P, Roth A, Ravn H, Napirna BM, Rodrigues A, Lisse IM, et al. Randomized trial of BCG vaccination at birth to low-birth-weight children: beneficial nonspecific effects in the neonatal period? J Infect Dis. 2011;204(2):245-52.
4. Roth A, Jensen H, Garly ML, Djana Q, Martins CL, Sodemann M, et al. Low birth weight infants and Calmette-Guérin bacillus vaccination at birth: community study from Guinea-Bissau. Pediatr Infect Dis J. 2004;114(2):e268-75.
5. Biering-Sørensen S, Aaby P, Lund N, Monteiro I, Jensen KJ, Eriksen HB, et al. Early BCG-Denmark and neonatal mortality among infants weighing <2500 g: a randomized controlled trial. Clin Infect Dis. 2012;65(8):1196-203.
6. Kleinnijenhuis J, Quintin J, Preijers F, Benn CS, Joosten LA, Jacobs C, et al. Long-lasting effects of BCG vaccination on both heterologous Th1/Th17 responses and innate trained immunity. J Innate Immun. 2012;4(3):256-68.
7. Netea MG, Joosten LAB, Latz E, Mills KHG, Natoli G, Stunnenberg H, et al. Trained immunity: A program of innate immune memory in health and disease. Science. 2016;352(6284):aaf1098.
8. O'Neill LAJ, Netea MG. BCG-induced trained immunity: can it offer protection against COVID-19? Nat Rev Immunol. 2020;20(6):335-7.
9. Andersen A, Fisker AB, Nielsen S, Rodrigues A, Benn CS, Aaby P. National immunization campaigns with oral polio vaccine reduce all-cause mortality: a natural experiment within seven randomized trials. Front Public Health. 2013;1:205.
10. Mogensen SW, Andersen A, Rodrigues A, Benn CS, Aaby P. The Introduction of Diphtheria-Tetanus-Pertussis and Oral Polio Vaccine Among Young Infants in an Urban African Community: A Natural Experiment. EBioMedicine. 2017:17:192-8.
11. Aaby P, Benn CS, Nielsen J, Lisse IM, Rodrigues A, Ravn H. Testing the hypothesis that diphtheria-tetanus-pertussis vaccine has negative nonspecific and sex-differential effects on child survival in high-mortality countries. BMJ Open. 2011;2(3):e000707.
12. Zaman K, Dang DA, Victor JC, Shin S, Yunus M, Dallas MJ, et al. Efficacy of pentavalent rotavirus vaccine against severe rotavirus gastroenteritis in infants in developing countries in Asia: a randomized, double-blind, placebo-controlled trial. The Lancet. 2010;376(9741):615-23.
13. Klugman KP, Madhi SA, Huebner RE, Kohberger R, Mbelle N, Pierce N. A trial of a 9-valent pneumococcal conjugate vaccine in children with and those without HIV infection. N Engl J Med. 2003;349(14):1341-8.
14. Whitney CG, Farley MM, Hadler J, Harrison LH, Bennett NM, Lynfield R, et al. Decline in invasive pneumococcal disease after the introduction of protein-polysaccharide conjugate vaccine. N Engl J Med. 2003;348(18):1737-46.
15. Esposito S, Principi N. The impact of measles, mumps and rubella vaccination on the prevention of non-targeted infections. Vaccine. 2008;26(11):1385-93.

16. Sorup S, Benn CS, Poulsen A, Krause TG, Aaby P, Ravn H. Live vaccine against measles, mumps, and rubella and the risk of hospital admissions for nontargeted infections. JAMA. 2014;311(8):826-35.
17. Halstead SB, Gibbons RV. Japanese encephalitis: a review of the clinical features, diagnosis, and vaccine development. J NeuroVirol. 2004;10(2):132-41.
18. Ploussard JD, Foster AJ. Non-specific effects of the Haemophilus influenzae type b vaccine on overall child health: evidence from observational studies. J Pediatr Infect Dis. 2013;5(4):432-9.
19. Ferguson NM, Cummings DA, Fraser C, Cajka JC, Cooley PC, Burke DS. Strategies for mitigating an influenza pandemic. Nature. 2006;442(7101):448-52.
20. Bollaerts K, Cohet C. Impact of influenza vaccination on hospitalizations for respiratory and cardiovascular diseases. Vaccine. 2014;32(37):4658-64.
21. Gonsalves J, Nair P. Reduction in hospitalizations for non-targeted infections following typhoid vaccination in endemic regions. Vaccine. 2011;29(45):8170-6.
22. Gershon AA, Steinberg SP. Non-specific effects of varicella vaccination on child health: evidence from large cohort studies. J Infect Dis. 2004;189(3):737-43.
23. Kark JA, Riedel DJ. The impact of hepatitis A vaccination on hospitalization rates for non-targeted infections. J Infect Dis. 2009;199(9):1350-6.
24. Garland SM, Brotherton JM. The impact of HPV vaccination on HPV-related disease: a review of recent evidence. Vaccine. 2016;34(42):4881-90.
25. Sings HJ, McIntyre PB. Meningococcal vaccination and its impact on overall health and hospitalizations: evidence from large cohort studies. J Infect Dis. 2013;208(6):922-30.

CHAPTER 6

Evaluating Immunity: Laboratory Techniques and Innovations

Anwita Khaitan, Pentapati Siva Santosh Kumar

INTRODUCTION

Immune response evaluation provides immense help at the critical stage of vaccine design in a multitude of ways. It provides information that helps optimize antibody specificity by helping design a suitable epitope for binding. It also helps decide the optimal route of vaccination. Further, it provides immense information on the different types of immune responses to various candidate vaccines.

In this chapter, we shall talk about the important and common laboratory methods and established correlates of protection (CoPs) used to assess the immune response to candidate vaccines. The control of pathogens and disease exacerbation is a multiparametric immune response. However, in vaccination, most of the time, we test only one parameter.

Immunological response produced by the administration of vaccines is mainly through the generation of exquisitely specific and high-affinity antibodies. Immunological response produced by the administration of vaccines, which can reliably predict protection from clinically manifested disease or infection, can serve as useful CoPs. These correlates provide a much-needed objective tool to evaluate protection or susceptibility to infection or disease in vaccinated subjects. They are also useful for ensuring the consistency of vaccines across vaccine lots and in different populations and for evaluating the efficacy of vaccines in vaccine trials.

During the preclinical phases of testing a candidate vaccine, it is important to have information that helps in the design of the antigen, to inform on surrogates or CoPs, most of the time surrogates of protection, to select the antigen for in silico design, to propose may be vaccination strategies to have the right quality of the immune responses, to have information on baseline immunity, and to propose formulations that are inducing the right quality of immune responses.

Preclinical research focuses mostly on animal models for testing vaccine candidates. One tests the antigen design gathers information on immunogenicity, and sometimes uses animal protection models.

Phases I, II, and III generate more refined knowledge about vaccine candidates. In phase I trials, immunological data helps to validate the vaccination strategy, evaluate immune responses, propose a prime-boost strategy, and test the safety, the dose immunogenicity.

In phases II and III, immunological data provide more information on immunogenicity and CoPs, and the immune correlates for protection are validated at the end of the phase III trial.

Barring a few, such as tuberculosis, antibody responses have been identified for most diseases as potential correlates or surrogates of protection. Immune profiling of the target population helps to define or refine the antigen for the vaccine candidates.

While reliable and validated CoPs exist for some of the vaccines, such as the ones used against diphtheria and tetanus in the form of toxin-neutralizing antibodies, there are other instances in which reliable CoPs are lacking. This is exemplified by the case of the Bacillus Calmette–Guérin (BCG) vaccine. Although the primacy of the vaccine-specific helper T-cell response induced by BCG is undoubted, it does not serve as a correlate of protection. Novel ex vivo assays have been developed recently to enumerate T-cell responses to vaccine antigens.

Measures of vaccine effectiveness called "correlates" or "surrogates" of vaccine protection are central to the testing and licensing of vaccines, which precludes their use in clinical practice. An in-depth understanding of the pathogen structure, function, disease pathogenesis, and host-immune response is essential to devise and interpret these "correlates" or "surrogates."

Most of the current vaccines in use work predominantly through the induction of specific antibodies of high avidity.[1,2] These antibodies are produced by plasma cells that undergo affinity maturation via somatic hypermutation in germinal centers of the spleen and lymph nodes. Normal T-cells are essential for vaccine-induced protection even in cases where immunity is mediated via B-cells and antibodies—as elegantly illustrated by patients with inborn errors of immunity (IEI), who may even present with disease from live-attenuated vaccines. T-cells secrete cytokines that modulate B-cell proliferation and maturation into antibody-secreting plasma cells. Vaccine antigens and even adjuvants, in some cases, stimulate and skew the differentiation of T-helper cells. Activated T-cells, especially CD4+ helper T-cells, are indispensable for the generation of high-affinity antibodies by producing appropriate cytokines for B-cell differentiation and activation. It is also worthwhile to remember that most vaccines stimulate both T and B lymphocyte-mediated responses, which are generally not mutually exclusive.

On the contrary, antibodies also modulate the T helper type I activation via Fc receptors by facilitating a rapid uptake, processing, and presentation of pathogen-derived antigens.[3] Thus, a durable and protective T-cell response results from an effective primary antibody-mediated response.[4]

Immune responses to vaccines, which can predict protection from disease or infection, can be useful correlates of vaccine-induced protection. These correlates fulfill the need for an objective tool to evaluate protection or susceptibility to a particular disease in vaccinated individuals. Such correlates also provide a reliable means to ensure the consistency of vaccines across different vaccine lots and varying populations. Reliable and well-validated CoPs have been defined as vaccines for certain diseases such as tetanus and diphtheria. These correlates have been widely used to predict the level of protection in vaccinated individuals. However, there is a lack of any well-authenticated immunologic correlate that can predict protection in the case of certain vaccines, e.g., the BCG vaccine for tuberculosis.

MEDIATORS OF VACCINE-INDUCED IMMUNITY

The nature of the vaccine administered is the most critical determinant of the type of effector immune response generated and, thus, mediates protection. However, the major effectors of a vaccine-induced immune response include:

B lymphocytes and antibodies: High-affinity antibodies generated by vaccines prevent infection or reduce the severity of infection by:

- Decreasing the binding, adhesion, and entry of pathogens in cells, thus preventing viral replication or bacterial colonization.
- Neutralization of toxins at their site of production or periphery or blocking their diffusion from sites of production.
- Increasing phagocytic uptake and clearance of extracellular pathogens by opsonization.
- Complement activation

CD4+ helper T-cells aid in the clearance of both intracellular and extracellular pathogens by promoting the differentiation and activation of B lymphocytes, CD8+ T lymphocytes, and macrophages by providing the appropriate cytokine milieu.

CD8+ cytotoxic T lymphocytes (CTLs) help in the clearance of intracellular organisms by killing infected cells either directly by the release of perforin and granzyme or indirectly by releasing microbicidal cytokines.

CORRELATES OF PROTECTION

Terminology and Basic Concepts

A correlate of protection is defined as a laboratory parameter that is associated with protection from the occurrence of clinical disease after sufficient and controlled trials.[5] However, there has been much confusion about the terminology, which has been partly resolved recently.[6]

Plotkin's Nomenclature

- *Correlate of protection (CoP)*: The CoP is a measure used to determine the protective efficacy of a particular vaccine, for example, anti-tetanus toxin titers induced after tetanus toxoid administration.
- *Mechanistic correlate of protection (mCoP)*: The term mCoP is used when the immune response measured is the unequivocal mechanism of protection against a particular pathogen; e.g., antidiphtheria toxin antibody titer induced after vaccination with diphtheria toxoid is a mCoP as it is a causal mechanism for protection against the disease.
- *Nonmechanistic correlate of protection (nCoP)*: The term nCoP is used when the immune marker measured is not the actual mechanism of protection against the pathogen. For instance, serum IgA levels induced after rotavirus vaccine administration are not the causal mechanism for protection against rotavirus disease. However, they are useful proxy measurements for the assessment of vaccine protection. Hence, in a strict sense, an nCoP can be referred to as a "surrogate" of protection, whereas, in comparison, mCoP is a real "correlate" of protection.[7]

Another example to explain this concept is vaccination against encapsulated organisms, notably pneumococcus, meningococcus, and *Haemophilus influenzae*. The "opsonophagocytic" antibodies generated as a result of vaccination are protective against disease. These antibodies bind to the polysaccharide capsule, enhance recognition, and augment phagocytosis, thereby resulting in the killing of these organisms. These "bactericidal" antibodies, when measured after vaccination, give mCoP for a particular vaccine. However, more convenient is the measurement of total antibody response, which may also contain ineffective antibodies against the specific vaccine antigen, which would give an nCoP or "surrogate" marker for assessment of vaccine effectiveness.

A "co-correlate" is one among the various factors that correlate with vaccine protection. Taken together, the "co-correlates" may explain vaccine protection in a synergistic or additive manner or may be just alternative measures.

It is noteworthy to mention that the actual goal of vaccination needs to be kept in mind when analyzing these parameters. For example, antidiphtheria or anti-tetanus toxin titers are mCoPs for disease prevention following vaccination but not at all for prevention against colonization.

When the serum antibody or antitoxin titers are mCoPs, an absolute value called "absolute correlate of protection" is often stated, which would be protective. For example, after *Haemophilus influenzae type b* (Hib) conjugate vaccinations, titers >0.15 µg/L are often stated as protective against disease. Titers >5 µg/L are considered protective against colonization.[8] However, these cutoffs or thresholds or absolute CoPs, although highly desirable, may not be in the strictest sense absolute. Breakthrough infection or colonization may still occur in individuals with antibody titers higher than these values. In practice, the antibody titers should be interpreted as a continuous rather than a dichotomous variable, in which higher antibody titers would be more likely to afford protection against disease and colonization. However, an absolute value does help define therapeutic endpoints and eases out statistical analysis among other benefits.

Qin's Nomenclature

It differs slightly from Plotkin's nomenclature. Some important terms to be familiar with are as follows:

- *Correlate of risk (CoR)*: CoR, in contrast to Plotkin's CoP, is a broader term used in a variety of settings. In the context of vaccination, it refers to the immune response that correlates with a particular endpoint of interest. For example, considering a particular strain of influenza virus, the incidence of influenza in vaccinated individuals having different titers of antibodies against the pathogen compared to that of unvaccinated individuals who also have different titers of antibodies as a result of previous exposure to related strains. If a significant difference in the incidence of illness is found by statistical analysis, the measured immune response is a definite "CoR."
- *Surrogate of protection (SoP)*: As per Qin's nomenclature, an SoP is a CoR that reliably explains vaccine effectiveness and is defined at two levels:[9]
    i. Level 1 SoP is valid in a particular scenario, e.g., a particular population.
    ii. Level 2 SoP is valid across different scenarios.
- *Vaccine efficacy (VE)*: It is usually defined as the percentage reduction in the risk of illness, colonization, hospitalization, or any other endpoint as a result of vaccination,[9,10] calculated as follows:

$$[(\text{Incidence in unvaccinated} - \text{Incidence in vaccinated}) \div (\text{Incidence in unvaccinated})] \times 100$$

To explain the concept of VE, let us assume 100 vaccinated (cohort A) and 100 unvaccinated (cohort B) participants each. A vaccine with an efficacy of 90% administered to cohort A would mean an incidence of endpoint (say illness) in 2 out of 100 in cohort A as compared to 20 out of 100 in cohort B.

Immunological CoPs are measured to estimate VE when population studies are not carried out due to technical or ethical reasons.

General Information Regarding Correlate of Protection

- Immunologic CoPs differ even for the same vaccine for different protection endpoints, viz., protection against infection, disease, severe disease, hospitalization, or death.[11]
- Correlates are also partly determined by host characteristics such as age, gender, and the major histocompatibility complex (MHC) of the vaccine.
- Challenge dose invariably influences the CoP both quantitatively and qualitatively. An overwhelming challenge dose might hamper the immunity induced by vaccination.[12]
- CoPs against infection and recovery from infection are often not the same.[13]

IMMUNOLOGICAL FACTORS ASSOCIATED WITH VACCINE-INDUCED IMMUNITY DRIVEN BY ANTIBODIES

Most currently licensed vaccines generate a robust and lasting humoral immune response mediated by antibodies. Different characteristics of antibodies have been studied by various immunological assays in a number of vaccine trials. They include titer, isotype, function, specificity, affinity, and location.

MECHANISMS OF VACCINE IMMUNITY MEDIATED BY ANTIBODIES

Adequate Titer of Antibody

The persistence of an antibody generated by immunization in sufficient concentrations for a prolonged period has been an indicator of an effective vaccine response.[14]

Many commercially licensed vaccines elicit defined concentrations of antibodies. These can be measured by various immunological assays, including enzyme-linked immunosorbent assay (ELISA), hemagglutination assay, and neutralization assays.[15]

Table 1 summarizes the neutralization titers and the suggested minimum threshold for protection for some of the commonly used vaccines.

Immunoglobulin Isotype and Subclass

Humoral protection afforded by vaccines is mainly affected by serum immunoglobulin G (IgG), mucosal IgG, and IgA present both in the serum and the mucosal secretions. Mucosal immunoglobulins are particularly crucial for protection against infectious agents replicating on mucosal surfaces. It holds for oral polio vaccine, rotavirus vaccine, and influenza vaccine. IgA, especially mucosal IgA, present in the secretions of the gastrointestinal and respiratory tract, mediates protection predominantly by neutralization.[16,17]

Memory B-cell Response

The generation of a robust humoral memory following vaccination provides long-lasting protection against many vaccine-preventable diseases. Humoral memory against smallpox has been detected for as long as 50 years following vaccination.[18] Memory B-cell also protects against progression to chronic hepatitis following vaccination against hepatitis B.[19] Long-lived plasma cells in the bone marrow and memory B-cells can be enumerated by enzyme-linked immunosorbent spot (ELISpot) and by multicolor flow cytometry.[20]

Antibody-dependent Cell-mediated Cytotoxicity

Antibody-dependent cell-mediated cytotoxicity (ADCC) is an important mechanism through which antibodies act to limit and contain an invading pathogen. It is mediated by Fc receptors present on the surface of natural killer cells and phagocytic cells, which bind to the opsonized microbes and execute the killing of the same.

TABLE 1: Protective antibody levels and titers for different routinely administered vaccines.

Vaccine	Method of detection	Minimum threshold for protection	References
Diphtheria	Toxin neutralization	0.01–0.1 IU/mL	21,22
Tetanus	Toxin neutralization	0.1 IU/mL	23,24
Hib polysaccharide	ELISA	1 µg/mL	25
Hib conjugate	ELISA	0.15 µg/mL	26
Hepatitis A	ELISA	10 mIU/mL	27
Hepatitis B	ELISA	10 mIU/mL	28
Measles	Plaque reduction neutralization assay	120 mIU/mL	29,30
Pertussis	ELISA	5 units	31,32
Rubella	Immunoprecipitation	10–15 mIU/mL	33,34
Rabies	Neutralization	0.5 IU/mL	35
Polio	Neutralization	1/4–1/8 dilution	36,37
Smallpox	Neutralization	1/20–1/32 dilution	38,39
Varicella	FAMA, gpELISA	1/64 dilution, 5 IU/mL	40,41
Pneumococcus	ELISA	0.35 µg/mL	42,43
Tuberculosis [Bacillus Calmette–Guérin (BCG) vaccine)]	Interferon-gamma production by vaccine-specific CD4+ T-cells	Not defined	44

(Hib: *Haemophilus influenzae* type b; FAMA: fluorescent antibody to membrane antigen; gpELISA: glycoprotein enzyme-linked immunosorbent assay)

DETERMINANTS OF HUMORAL RESPONSES TO VACCINE ANTIGENS

Type of vaccine: Higher and more sustained antibody responses are elicited by live-attenuated compared to inactivated vaccines. This is due to higher antigenic load due to replication and longer persistence of vaccine antigens in the case of live-attenuated vaccines.

Nature of vaccine antigen: Protein or conjugate vaccines such as conjugated Hib vaccine result in higher, more specific, and prolonged antibody responses than polysaccharide vaccines (Hib polysaccharide vaccine). The heightened and sustained humoral response is due to the stimulation of T-cells and the induction of germinal center reaction in the lymph nodes and spleen.

Dose of the vaccine antigen: Higher doses of vaccine antigen increase the chances of antigen binding to T- and B-cells and their activation. A higher antigen dose also ensures antigen availability for association with follicular dendritic cells in the germinal centers.

Dosage schedule: Generally, a minimum gap of 3 weeks between the primary doses of a vaccine prevents undesired interference and competition between successive waves of the primary responses.

Age at immunization: Immunization at extremes of age does not generate an effective and lasting antibody response to vaccines. Immaturity in early life and immunosenescence associated with later life preclude the induction and persistence of memory B-cells and long-lived plasma cells. The effect of age is illustrated by the pneumococcal polysaccharide vaccine. Children under 2 years and elderly individuals do not develop protective titers of antibodies after vaccination. This is due to impaired T-cell independent humoral response to polysaccharide antigens in these subjects.

CORRELATES OF CELL-MEDIATED VACCINE RESPONSES

The development of antibodies is a weak correlate of protection in the case of intracellular pathogens, and appropriate cell-mediated immune responses are probably more important. Conventionally delayed-type hypersensitivity (DTH) responses have been used to assess cell-mediated immune responses in the case of intracellular infections and vaccination. However, it has been shown that DTH responses to vaccines are imprecise CoPs.[45] The immunogenicity of vaccines for intracellular pathogens is better estimated by measuring antigenic specific helper and cytotoxic T-cells. The functional status of these antigen-specific T-cells can also be determined by assaying the cytokines secreted by these cells upon activation. In recent years, ex vivo assays have been developed which can enumerate the frequency and the phenotype of antigen-specific T-cells. These assays can also estimate the proliferative population and the lytic activity of these antigen-specific T-cells.

MAJOR EFFECTORS OF CELL-MEDIATED RESPONSES TO VACCINE ANTIGENS (TABLE 2)

CD4+ Helper T-cells

CD4+ helper T-cells are the key orchestrators of the cellular immune response. After antigen recognition in the context of MHC class II molecules, helper T-cells differentiate into different functional subsets depending upon the appropriate cytokine milieu. These cells provide growth factors and signals for the generation and maintenance of CD8+ cytotoxic T-cells.[46] In addition, helper T-cells can also act as immune effectors by secretion of various cytokines such as interferon-gamma (IFN-γ) and tumor necrosis factor-alpha (TNF-α).

Interferon-gamma is the signature cytokine of the Th1-type immune response. The secretion of IFN-γ has been shown to play a crucial role in vaccine-induced protection to several infections.[47] This has been best exemplified by the generation of specific CD4+ T-cells, which secrete IFN-γ after stimulation with specific antigen.[48] TNF-α is another cytokine secreted by effector T-cells that mediate killing of intracellular bacteria, viruses, and parasites.[49] Interleukin-2 (IL-2) has also been ascribed a role in host defense against a variety of intracellular pathogens.[50] It has also been aptly demonstrated that T-cells capable of producing multiple cytokines in response are better correlates of vaccine-induced protection against chronic bacterial and viral infections compared to T-cells producing only a single cytokine.[51,52]

CD8+ Cytotoxic T-cells

Cytotoxic T-cells contribute to the protection afforded by vaccines not by preventing infection but by limiting and clearing off intracellular pathogens. CD8+ cytotoxic T-cells possess the ability to directly lyse infected cells by the release of perforin or granzyme or indirectly by releasing antimicrobial cytokines. Advances in immunological techniques in recent years have enabled rapid enumeration and isolation of antigen-specific cytotoxic T-cells. Antigen-specific CTLs are currently detected by tetramer staining,[53] ELISA,[54] ELISpot,[55] and by using transgenic mice.[56] Additionally, cell proliferation assays using carboxyfluorescein succinimidyl ester (CFSE)

TABLE 2: Methods for estimation of cell-mediated immune responses to vaccines.

Assay method	Sample	Result
Cytokine release assays	PBMCs/whole blood	Total cytokine production by cells in whole blood or cultured PBMCs
ELISpot	PBMCs	Detection of the number of cells secreting a particular cytokine or two cytokines
Multiplex bead arrays	Serum, plasma, culture supernatants	Detection of multiple cytokines in small volumes of samples
Intracellular cytokine detection	Whole blood or PBMCs	Can detect multiple cytokines in different cell populations using different surface markers and cytokine antibodies by flow cytometry
CFSE-labeling assay	PBMCs	A two-fold reduction in fluorescence intensity with each successive division in the proliferative cell population of interest by flow cytometry
Cytotoxic assay	PBMCs	Cr51 or Eu or S35 release, GAPDH release assay, flow cytometry-based perforin assay or granzyme assay
MHC tetramer assays	Whole blood or PBMCs	Enumeration of epitope-specific CD4+ and CD8+ T-cells by flow cytometry, limited utility in determining the functionality of T-cells

(CFSE: carboxyfluorescein succinimidyl ester; ELISpot: enzyme-linked immunosorbent spot; GAPDH: glyceraldehyde-3-phosphate dehydrogenase; MHC: major histocompatibility complex; PBMCs: peripheral blood mononuclear cells)

have facilitated the tracking and monitoring of antigen-specific CTLs. Together, these assays are useful tools for enumerating frequencies of CTLs and determining the effector function of specific CTLs, i.e., secretion of cytokines, chemokines, and lytic killing of target cells.

Memory T-cells

To afford effective and long-lasting protection following vaccination, the vaccine must produce a clone of long-lived memory T-cells, which can recognize and expand rapidly upon encountering the putative pathogen.[57] Memory T-cells of both CD4+ and CD8+ subsets are classified into two major subsets—effector memory cells and central memory cells. Effector memory T-cells exhibit high cytolytic activity but are limited in their proliferative capacity. They are short-lived and present mainly in nonlymphoid tissues. Central memory T-cells, in contrast, have a high proliferative potential with little cytolytic activity. They are present in lymphoid organs and have a longer life span than effector memory T-cells.[58] Memory T-cells have been shown to persist for >50 years in humans after immunization.[59] Central memory T-cells of both CD4+ and CD8+ subtypes are associated with protection in various studies.[60,61]

INNATE EFFECTORS OF VACCINE-INDUCED IMMUNITY

Invariant Natural Killer T-cells

Invariant natural killer T-cells (iNKTs) are an essential subset of T-cells at the interface of the innate and adaptive immune system. These cells have characteristics of both innate and adaptive immune cells. Thus, they do not require prior exposure to the antigen for activation and respond rapidly to invading pathogens. On the other hand, they express T-cell receptors, albeit with limited antigenic diversity. They also display antigenic memory a feature generally ascribed to adaptive immune cells. These cells can recognize lipids and glycolipids in the context of CD1 molecules. Besides, iNKTs also direct the maturation of dendritic cells and B lymphocytes. Invariant NKTs have been shown to facilitate the development of effector and memory T-cells in vaccinated individuals.[62,63]

γδ T-cells

The γδ T-cells are another subset of T-cells, predominantly present on the mucosal surfaces of the body. Stimulation of γδ T-cells by vaccination has been shown to afford early protection against infection by mucosal administration of vaccines or following a mucosal challenge with pathogenic viruses.[64,65]

CORRELATE FOR PROTECTION AFFORDED BY BACILLUS CALMETTE–GUÉRIN VACCINE

In the case of the BCG vaccine, which is the most efficacious among all tuberculosis vaccines developed to date, no reliable mCoP is available. As tuberculosis is endemic, many children may go on to receive the BCG vaccine after already being colonized or asymptomatically infected. Therefore, the immune response may not truly reflect the effect of the vaccine. An intact IL-12–IFN-γ immune axis is essential for protection against *Mycobacterium* as reflected by the disorders classified under Mendelian susceptibility to mycobacterial disease (MSMD). IFN-γ is a key protective cytokine, and its measurement has the potential to serve rather than vaccine protection. Antigen-specific central memory T-cells (TCM), effector memory T-cells, Th17 cells, stem cell memory T-cells, CD4+ T-cells expressing various combinations of IFN-γ, and TNF-α IL-2 (e.g., antigen-specific CD4+ IFN-γ+ TNF-α+ IL-2+ cells, CD4+ TNF-α+ cells, CD4+ IL-2+ cells, etc.) are potential CoPs.[66-68]

NEWER VACCINES AND NEED TO DEVELOP NOVEL CORRELATES OF PROTECTION

Even when a well-established mCoP is available, newer mCoPs are required, as new vaccines targeting a different antigen of pathogen or different antigenic epitopes are developed. For example, hemagglutinin stalk vaccines for the prevention of influenza generate the production of antihemagglutinin stalk antibodies that are protective in humans and can serve as CoP.[69] These are non-neutralizing antibodies that cannot be assessed accurately by the conventional hemagglutinin inhibition assay and need ELISA for measurement. Vaccines such as these, targeting a conserved region, are unlikely to be affected by an antigenic drift that results in loss of efficacy of traditional influenza vaccines.

The example of vaccines against enterotoxigenic *Escherichia coli* can illustrate the complexity of CoPs for vaccines in development and testing. Multivalent vaccines against heat-labile toxin B (LTB) subunit and various colonization factor antigens have been tested and may provide up to 80% protection for susceptible individuals. Possible CoPs include IFN-γ, IL-17A-secreting T-cells responsive to LTB, activated follicular helper (Tfh) like CD4+ cells expressing CXCR5 and gut homing marker β7 integrin, and other lymphocyte subpopulations.[70]

CORRELATES OF PROTECTION: THINKING BEYOND VACCINE PROTECTION

Established CoPs can serve as measures of immune function in patients with IEI. Even with normal or elevated levels of various immunoglobulin isotypes, patients with primary immunodeficiency disease may have low functional antibodies, i.e., antibodies directed against pathogens, despite optimal vaccination. Notable examples include hyper-IgM syndromes, Wiskott–Aldrich syndrome, and specific antibody deficiency. We have measured IgG antidiphtheria toxin antibody, IgG anti-tetanus toxin, and anti-pneumococcal antibodies in children and adults with primary antibody deficiencies such as common variable immunodeficiency (CVID), IgG subclass deficiencies, and specific antibody deficiency. IgG anti-diphtheria toxin antibody levels <0.1 IU/mL were estimated in most of these children, with levels as low as <0.01 IU/mL. Such measurements can also be done before and after boosting with vaccines to confirm the impaired antibody response. Measurement of functional antibodies is, in fact, a valuable tool in the evaluation of children suspected to have an IEI.[71]

CONCLUSION

Immunological CoPs are valuable measures for assessing VE. Established and validated correlates of vaccine protection also serve as useful indicators of immune function in patients suspected of having IEI.

REFERENCES

1. Plotkin SA. Vaccination against the major infectious diseases. C R Acad Sci III. 1999;322(11):943-51.
2. Plotkin SA. Immunologic correlates of protection induced by vaccination. Pediatr Infect Dis J. 2001;20(1):63-75.
3. Joller N, Weber SS, Oxenius A. Antibody – Fc receptor interactions in protection against intracellular pathogens. Eur J Immunol. 2011;41(4):889-97.
4. Igietseme JU, Eko FO, He Q, Black CM. Antibody regulation of T-cell immunity: implications for vaccine strategies against intracellular pathogens. Expert Rev Vaccines. 2004;3(1):23-34.
5. Center for Biologics Evaluation and Research. (1997). Guidance for Industry for the Evaluation of Combination Vaccines for Preventable Diseases: Production, Testing and Clinical Studies. [online] Available from https://www.fda.gov/regulatory-information/search-fda-guidance-documents/guidance-industry-evaluation-combination-vaccines-preventable-diseases-production-testing-and. [Last accessed March, 2025]
6. Plotkin SA, Gilbert PB. Nomenclature for Immune Correlates of Protection After Vaccination. Clin Infect Dis. 2012;54(11):1615-7.
7. Plotkin SA. Vaccines: Correlates of Vaccine-Induced Immunity. Clin Infect Dis. 2008;47(3):401-9.
8. Fernandez J, Levine OS, Sanchez J, Balter S, LaClaire L, Feris J, et al. Prevention of *Haemophilus influenzae* Type b Colonization by Vaccination: Correlation with Serum Anti-Capsular IgG Concentration. J Infect Dis. 2000;182(5):1553-6.
9. Qin L, Gilbert PB, Corey L, McElrath MJ, Self SG. A Framework for Assessing Immunological Correlates of Protection in Vaccine Trials. J Infect Dis. 2007;196(9):1304-12.
10. The Department of Immunization, Vaccines and Biologicals. (2013). Correlates of vaccine-induced protection: methods and implications. [online] Available from https://www.who.int/publications/i/item/WHO-IVB-13.01. [Last accessed March, 2025]
11. Slifka MK. Immunological memory to viral infection: Commentary. Curr Opin Immunol. 2004;16(4):443-50.

12. Plotkin SA, Starr SE, Friedman HM, Gönczöl E, Weibel RE. Protective Effects of Towne Cytomegalovirus Vaccine Against Low-Passage Cytomegalovirus Administered as a Challenge. J Infect Dis. 1989;159(5):860-5.
13. Permar SR, Klumpp SA, Mansfield KG, Carville AAL, Gorgone DA, Lifton MA, et al. Limited Contribution of Humoral Immunity to the Clearance of Measles Viremia in Rhesus Monkeys. J Infect Dis. 2004;190(5):998-1005.
14. Siegrist CA. 2 - Vaccine Immunology. In: Plotkin SA, Orenstein WA, Offit PA, Edwards KM (Eds). Plotkin's Vaccines, 7th edition. Amsterdam: Elsevier; 2018. pp. 16-34.e7.
15. Plotkin SA. Correlates of Protection Induced by Vaccination. Clin Vaccine Immunol. 2010;17(7):1055-65.
16. Azevedo MSP, Yuan L, Iosef C, Chang KO, Kim Y, Nguyen TV, et al. Magnitude of serum and intestinal antibody responses induced by sequential replicating and nonreplicating rotavirus vaccines in gnotobiotic pigs and correlation with protection. Clin Diagn Lab Immunol. 2004;11(1):12-20.
17. Torrieri-Dramard L, Lambrecht B, Ferreira HL, Van Den Berg T, Klatzmann D, Bellier B. Intranasal DNA Vaccination Induces Potent Mucosal and Systemic Immune Responses and Cross-protective Immunity Against Influenza Viruses. Mol Ther. 2011;19(3):602-11.
18. Crotty S, Felgner P, Davies H, Glidewell J, Villarreal L, Ahmed R. Cutting Edge: Long-Term B Cell Memory in Humans after Smallpox Vaccination. J Immunol. 2003;171(10):4969-73.
19. Lin YC, Chang MH, Ni YH, Hsu HY, Chen DS. Long-Term Immunogenicity and Efficacy of Universal Hepatitis B Virus Vaccination in Taiwan. J Infect Dis. 2003;187(1):134-8.
20. Longwe H, Gordon S, Malamba R, French N. Characterising B cell numbers and memory B cells in HIV infected and uninfected Malawian adults. BMC Infect Dis. 2010;10(1):280.
21. Björkholm B, Böttiger M, Christenson B, Hagberg L. Antitoxin Antibody Levels and the Outcome of Illness during an Outbreak of Diphtheria among Alcoholics. Scand J Infect Dis. 1986;18(3):235-9.
22. Gowin E, Wysocki J, Kałużna E, Świątek-Kościelna B, Wysocka-Leszczyńska J, Michalak M, et al. Does vaccination ensure protection? Assessing diphtheria and tetanus antibody levels in a population of healthy children: A cross-sectional study. Medicine (Baltimore). 2016;95(49):e5571.
23. Edsall G. Specific prophylaxis of tetanus. J Am Med Assoc. 1959;171:417-27.
24. Bizzini B. 2 - Tetanus. In: Germanier R (Ed). Bacterial Vaccines. Boston: Academic Press; 1984. pp. 37-68.
25. Käyhty H, Peltola H, Karanko V, Mäkelä PH. The protective level of serum antibodies to the capsular polysaccharide of Haemophilus influenzae type b. J Infect Dis. 1983;147(6):1100.
26. Käyhty H. Difficulties in Establishing a Serological Correlate of Protection After Immunization with Haemophilus Influenzae Conjugate Vaccines. Biologicals. 1994;22(4):397-402.
27. Nalin DR, Kuter BJ, Brown L, Patterson C, Calandra GB, Werzberger A, et al. Worldwide experience with the CR326F-derived inactivated hepatitis A virus vaccine in pediatric and adult populations: an overview. J Hepatol. 1993;18 Suppl 2:S51-5.
28. Jack AD, Hall AJ, Maine N, Mendy M, Whittle HC. What Level of Hepatitis B Antibody Is Protective? J Infect Dis. 1999;179(2):489-92.
29. Chen RT, Markowitz LE, Albrecht P, Stewart JA, Mofenson LM, Preblud SR, et al. Measles Antibody: Reevaluation of Protective Titers. J Infect Dis. 1990;162(5):1036-42.
30. Samb B, Aaby P, Whittle HC, Seck AM, Rahman S, Bennett J, et al. Serologic status and measles attack rates among vaccinated and unvaccinated children in rural Senegal. Pediatr Infect Dis J. 1995;14(3):203-9.
31. Storsaeter J, Hallander HO, Gustafsson L, Olin P. Levels of anti-pertussis antibodies related to protection after household exposure to *Bordetella* pertussis. Vaccine. 1998;16(20):1907-16.
32. Taranger J, Trollfors B, Lagergård T, Sundh V, Bryla DA, Schneerson R, et al. Correlation between Pertussis Toxin IgG Antibodies in Postvaccination Sera and Subsequent Protection against Pertussis. J Infect Dis. 2000;181(3):1010-3.
33. Skendzel LP. Rubella Immunity: Defining the Level of Protective Antibody. Am J Clin Pathol. 1996;106(2):170-4.
34. Matter L, Kogelschatz K, Germann D. Serum Levels of Rubella Virus Antibodies Indicating Immunity: Response to Vaccination of Subjects with Low or Undetectable Antibody Concentrations. J Infect Dis. 1997;175(4):749-55.
35. World Health Organization. Rabies vaccines: WHO position paper = Vaccins antirabiques Note d'information de l'OMS. Wkly Epidemiol Rec Relevé Épidémiologique Hebd. 2007;82(49–50):425-35.
36. Faden H, Modlin JF, Thoms ML, McBean AM, Ferdon MB, Ogra PL. Comparative Evaluation of Immunization with Live Attenuated and Enhanced-Potency Inactivated Trivalent Poliovirus Vaccines in Childhood: Systemic and Local Immune Responses. J Infect Dis. 1990;162(6):1291-7.
37. Marine WM, Chin TD, Gravelle CR. Limitation of fecal and pharyngeal poliovirus excretion in Salk-vaccinated children. A family study during a type 1 poliomyelitis epidemic. Am J Hyg. 1962;76:173-95.
38. Sarkar JK, Mitra AC, Mukherjee MK. The minimum protective level of antibodies in smallpox. Bull World Health Organ. 1975;52(3):307-11.
39. Mack TM, Noble J, Thomas DB. A prospective study of serum antibody and protection against smallpox. Am J Trop Med Hyg. 1972;21(2):214-8.
40. Li S, Chan ASFI, Matthews H, Heyse JF, Chan CY, Kuter BJ, et al. Inverse relationship between six week postvaccination varicella antibody response to vaccine and likelihood of long term breakthrough infection. Pediatr Infect Dis J. 2002;21(4):337.
41. White CJ, Kuter BJ, Ngai A, Hildebrand CS, Isganitis KL, Patterson CM, et al. Modified cases of chickenpox after varicella vaccination: correlation of protection with antibody response. Pediatr Infect Dis J. 1992;11(1):19-23.
42. Lee L. Correlates of immunity for pneumococcal conjugate vaccines. Vaccine. 2003;21(17–18):2190-6.
43. Siber GR, Chang I, Baker S, Fernsten P, O'Brien KL, Santosham M, et al. Estimating the protective concentration of anti-pneumococcal capsular polysaccharide antibodies. Vaccine. 2007;25(19):3816-26.
44. Fletcher H. Correlates of Immune Protection from Tuberculosis. Curr Mol Med. 2007;7(3):319-25.
45. Comstock GW. Field trials of tuberculosis vaccines: How could we have done them better? Control Clin Trials. 1994;15(4):247-76.
46. Sun JC, Williams MA, Bevan MJ. CD4+ T cells are required for the maintenance, not programming, of memory CD8+ T cells after acute infection. Nat Immunol. 2004;5(9):927-33.
47. Flynn JL, Chan J, Triebold KJ, Dalton DK, Stewart TA, Bloom BR. An essential role for interferon gamma in resistance to *Mycobacterium tuberculosis* infection. J Exp Med. 1993;178(6):2249-54.
48. Kawamura I, Tsukada H, Yoshikawa H, Fujita M, Nomoto K, Mitsuyama M. IFN-gamma-producing ability as a possible marker for the protective T cells against *Mycobacterium bovis* BCG in mice. J Immunol. 1992;148(9):2887-93.
49. Bloom BR, Flynn J, McDonough K, Kress Y, Chan J. Experimental Approaches to Mechanisms of Protection and Pathogenesis in M. tuberculosis Infection. Immunobiology. 1994;191(4–5):526-36.

50. Williams MA, Holmes BJ, Sun JC, Bevan MJ. Developing and maintaining protective CD8+ memory T cells. Immunol Rev. 2006;211(1):146-53.
51. Darrah PA, Patel DT, De Luca PM, Lindsay RWB, Davey DF, Flynn BJ, et al. Multifunctional TH1 cells define a correlate of vaccine-mediated protection against Leishmania major. Nat Med. 2007;13(7):843-50.
52. Rosa DS, Ribeiro SP, Almeida RR, Mairena EC, Postól E, Kalil J, et al. A DNA Vaccine Encoding Multiple HIV CD4 Epitopes Elicits Vigorous Polyfunctional, Long-Lived CD4+ and CD8+ T Cell Responses. PLoS One. 2011;6(2):e16921.
53. Leisner C, Loeth N, Lamberth K, Justesen S, Sylvester-Hvid C, Schmidt EG, et al. One-Pot, Mix-and-Read Peptide-MHC Tetramers. PLoS One. 2008;3(2):e1678.
54. Sylvester-Hvid C, Kristensen N, Blicher T, Ferré H, Lauemøller SL, Wolf XA, et al. Establishment of a quantitative ELISA capable of determining peptide – MHC class I interaction. Tissue Antigens. 2002;59(4):251-8.
55. Malyguine A, Strobl S, Zaritskaya L, Baseler M, Shafer-Weaver K. New Approaches for Monitoring CTL Activity in Clinical Trials. In: Shurin MR, Smolkin YS (Eds). Immune-Mediated Diseases. New York, NY: Springer; 2007. pp. 273-84.
56. Choi EM, Palmowski M, Chen J, Cerundolo V. The use of chimeric A2Kb tetramers to monitor HLA A2 immune responses in HLA A2 transgenic mice. J Immunol Methods. 2002;268(1):35-41.
57. Kaech SM, Wherry EJ, Ahmed R. Effector and memory T-cell differentiation: implications for vaccine development. Nat Rev Immunol. 2002;2(4):251-62.
58. Sallusto F, Lenig D, Förster R, Lipp M, Lanzavecchia A. Two subsets of memory T lymphocytes with distinct homing potentials and effector functions. Nature. 1999;401(6754):708-12.
59. Hammarlund E, Lewis MW, Hansen SG. Duration of antiviral immunity after smallpox vaccination. Nat Med. 2003;9:1131-7.
60. Vaccari M, Trindade CJ, Venzon D, Zanetti M, Franchini G. Vaccine-Induced CD8+ Central Memory T Cells in Protection from Simian AIDS. J Immunol. 2005;175(6):3502-7.
61. Castiglioni P, Hall de S, Jacovetty EL, Ingulli E, Zanetti M. Protection against Influenza A Virus by Memory CD8 T Cells Requires Reactivation by Bone Marrow-Derived Dendritic Cells. J Immunol. 2008;180(7):4956-64.
62. Dondji B, Deak E, Goldsmith-Pestana K, Perez-Jimenez E, Esteban M, Miyake S, et al. Intradermal NKT cell activation during DNA priming in heterologous prime-boost vaccination enhances T cell responses and protection against Leishmania. Eur J Immunol. 2008;38(3):706-19.
63. Guillonneau C, Mintern JD, Hubert FX, Hurt AC, Besra GS, Porcelli S, et al. Combined NKT cell activation and influenza virus vaccination boosts memory CTL generation and protective immunity. Proc Natl Acad Sci. 2009;106(9):3330-5.
64. Tenner-Racz K, Hennig CS, Überla K, Stoiber H, Ignatius R, Heeney J, et al. Early protection against pathogenic virus infection at a mucosal challenge site after vaccination with attenuated simian immunodeficiency virus. Proc Natl Acad Sci. 2004;101(9):3017-22.
65. Price S, Davies M, Villarreal-Ramos B, Hope J. Differential distribution of WC1+ γδ TCR+ T lymphocyte subsets within lymphoid tissues of the head and respiratory tract and effects of intranasal *M. bovis* BCG vaccination. Vet Immunol Immunopathol. 2010;136(1):133-7.
66. Rodo MJ, Rozot V, Nemes E, Dintwe O, Hatherill M, Little F, et al. A comparison of antigen-specific T cell responses induced by six novel tuberculosis vaccine candidates. PLOS Pathog. 2019;15(3):e1007643.
67. Thakur A, Pedersen LE, Jungersen G. Immune markers and correlates of protection for vaccine induced immune responses. Vaccine. 2012;30(33):4907-20.
68. Counoupas C, Triccas JA. The generation of T-cell memory to protect against tuberculosis. Immunol Cell Biol. 2019;97(7):656-63.
69. Ng S, Nachbagauer R, Balmaseda A, Stadlbauer D, Ojeda S, Patel M, et al. Novel correlates of protection against pandemic H1N1 influenza A virus infection. Nat Med. 2019;25(6):962-7.
70. Holmgren J, Parashar UD, Plotkin S, Louis J, Ng SP, Desauziers E, et al. Correlates of protection for enteric vaccines. Vaccine. 2017;35(26):3355-63.
71. Orange JS, Ballow M, Stiehm ER, Ballas ZK, Chinen J, De La Morena M, et al. Use and interpretation of diagnostic vaccination in primary immunodeficiency: A working group report of the Basic and Clinical Immunology Interest Section of the American Academy of Allergy, Asthma & Immunology. J Allergy Clin Immunol. 2012;130(3):S1-24.

CHAPTER 7

Enhancing Vaccine Efficacy: The Role of Adjuvant

Abhishek Kumar

INTRODUCTION

Overview of Vaccine Efficacy

Vaccination has been shown to be one of the most successful public health initiatives in history, considerably lowering the global burden of infectious illnesses. But attaining the best possible vaccination efficacy is still a constant struggle, particularly when it comes to viruses that have sophisticated immune evasion mechanisms or that cause illnesses with high rates of morbidity and mortality. Adjuvants, which are compounds that are included in vaccines to strengthen the immunological response, are essential in overcoming these obstacles because they focus and intensify the immune system's response to the target antigen. This chapter covers many adjuvant forms that are now in use or under development, gives a thorough description of the mechanisms underpinning adjuvant-mediated improvement of vaccination efficacy, and investigates their applicability in vaccine development against a variety of infectious diseases.

Important topics discussed:

- *Mechanism of action*: Adjuvants exert their effects through a variety of processes, such as enhancing the absorption and presentation of antigens, stimulating innate immune responses, and modifying the adaptive immunological response. Comprehending these pathways is crucial in creating adjuvants customized for certain vaccinations and diseases.
- *Types of adjuvants*: This chapter discusses the many adjuvant classes, including oil-in-water emulsions, aluminum salts, toll-like receptor (TLR) agonists, and adjuvants based on nanoparticles, emphasizing their special qualities and uses in the development of vaccines.
- *Clinical significance*: The production of vaccines has been revolutionized by adjuvants, which have made it possible to create highly immunogenic formulations against difficult targets such as hepatitis B, influenza, and human papillomavirus. They also have potential for use in next-generation vaccine platforms, such as messenger RNA (mRNA) and viral vector-based vaccines, and newly developing infectious illnesses.
- *Safety and regulatory considerations*: Adjuvants offer advantages, but before they can be used on humans, they must pass stringent safety testing. The regulatory frameworks for adjuvant approval and the significance of striking a balance between safety and efficacy in vaccine development are covered in this chapter.
- *Future directions*: New adjuvants with better safety and efficacy profiles are in the works as our knowledge of the immune system develops. The chapter examines new developments in adjuvant research and how they might affect the development of vaccines in the future, including the application of synthetic biology and structure-based design techniques.

Importance of Adjuvants in Vaccine Development

Adjuvants, which improve and alter the immune response to the given antigen, are essential ingredients in vaccination formulations. The creation of more robust and effective immunity is made possible by their incorporation into vaccines, which greatly enhances the effectiveness of contemporary immunization campaigns. This section highlights the types, modes of action, and clinical significance of adjuvants, highlighting their crucial roles in vaccine development.

Modulating Immune Profiles

Different vaccine targets require tailored immune responses, such as a balanced Th1/Th2 response or a specific cytotoxic T lymphocyte (CTL) activation. Adjuvants can be designed to steer the immune system toward the desired profile. For instance, oil-in-water emulsions such as MF59 enhance Th2 responses, while adjuvants such as monophosphoryl lipid A (MPLA), derived from bacterial components, favor Th1-dominated immunity critical for combating intracellular pathogens such as *Mycobacterium tuberculosis*.[1]

Dose Sparing and Antigen Economy

By boosting immune responses, adjuvants allow the use of smaller antigen doses, making vaccine production more cost-effective. This attribute is especially vital during pandemics or when addressing diseases affecting low-resource settings. For example, the use of adjuvants such as AS03 in influenza vaccines during the 2009 H1N1 pandemic enabled dose-sparing strategies, allowing for the immunization of a larger population.

Broadening Population Coverage

Certain populations, such as the elderly or immunocompromised individuals, exhibit weaker immune responses to vaccines. Adjuvants play an essential role in enhancing vaccine efficacy in these groups by overcoming immunosenescence and suboptimal immune activation. For instance, the addition of MF59 to influenza vaccines has been shown to improve immune responses in older adults.

Types of Adjuvants in Current Use

- *Traditional adjuvants*: Aluminum-based adjuvants remain widely used in vaccines such as the diphtheria-tetanus-pertussis (DTP) combination and hepatitis B vaccines.
- *Novel adjuvants*: Advances in immunology have led to the development of adjuvants such as AS01, a liposome-based formulation used in the malaria vaccine RTS,S, and CpG oligodeoxynucleotides, which mimic bacterial DNA to stimulate innate immune receptors.

Conclusion

Adjuvants are indispensable in the development of effective, safe, and accessible vaccines. By amplifying and directing the immune response, enabling antigen economy, and addressing the needs of vulnerable populations, they ensure broader protection against infectious diseases. Continuous research into novel adjuvants is pivotal to addressing emerging global health challenges and the development of next-generation vaccines.

UNDERSTANDING ADJUVANTS

Definition and Function

Adjuvants are pharmacological or immunological agents added to vaccines to enhance the immune response to the antigen. The primary function of adjuvants is to improve the magnitude, quality, and duration of the immune response, enabling the use of smaller doses of antigen and providing better protection against diseases. They can also help direct the immune response toward specific pathways, such as cellular or humoral immunity, depending on the disease target. Adjuvants achieve this by acting on the innate immune system, stimulating antigen-presenting cells (APCs), and creating a local depot effect to release antigens over time.

Types of Adjuvants

Adjuvants can be broadly classified into:

- *Particulate adjuvants*: Includes aluminum salts (alum), emulsions, liposomes, and nanoparticles
- *Immunostimulatory adjuvants*: Includes molecules such as TLR agonists (e.g., CpG DNA and MPLA).
- *Combination adjuvants*: A mix of particulate and immunostimulatory agents to optimize efficacy
- *Natural adjuvants*: Derived from biological sources such as saponins or microbial components

Each type of adjuvant has unique properties tailored to different vaccine formulations and target populations.

Immunostimulatory Adjuvants

Immunostimulatory adjuvants enhance the immune response by activating innate immune receptors such as TLRs, Nod-like receptors (NLRs), or C-type lectin receptors (CLRs). Examples include:

- *CpG oligodeoxynucleotides*: TLR9 agonists that stimulate strong Th1 responses
- *MPLA*: A TLR4 agonist with reduced toxicity but effective in inducing innate immunity
- *Flagellin*: Activates TLR5 and enhances both humoral and cellular immunity

These adjuvants mimic pathogen-associated molecular patterns (PAMPs), prompting a robust immune response.

Delivery Systems

Delivery systems are adjuvants designed to improve antigen presentation by targeting immune cells or creating antigen depots. Types include:

- *Emulsions*: For example, MF59, AS03, enhancing antigen uptake by dendritic cells
- *Liposomes*: Biodegradable lipid vesicles encapsulating antigens
- *Nanoparticles*: Tailored to mimic viral particles, promoting targeted delivery to APCs
- *Virosomes*: Lipid-based systems incorporating viral membrane proteins for enhanced immunogenicity.

Delivery systems protect antigens from degradation and ensure a sustained release at the site of administration.

Formulation Adjuvants

Formulation adjuvants are included in vaccines to stabilize antigens, optimize immune responses, and improve storage properties. Common examples are:

- *Aluminum salts*: Widely used for their depot effect and safety profile
- *Oil-in-water emulsions*: Improve antigen dispersion and immune activation
- *Saponins*: Natural glycosides (e.g., QS-21) often used in combination with other adjuvants
- *Stabilizers*: Compounds such as trehalose or polysorbates to prevent antigen degradation

Formulation adjuvants must balance efficacy, safety, and manufacturability for successful vaccine deployment.

MECHANISMS OF ACTION

Enhancement of Immune Response

The enhancement of the immune response is a cornerstone of immunological research and clinical intervention. It involves strategies to amplify the body's ability to recognize and neutralize pathogens, cancer cells, or other harmful entities effectively.

Mechanisms of Immune Enhancement

- *Cytokine modulation*: Cytokines such as interleukins, interferons, and tumor necrosis factors play pivotal roles in enhancing the immune response. For instance, interleukin-2 (IL-2) promotes T-cell proliferation, boosting adaptive immunity.[2]
- *Adjuvants*: Vaccine adjuvants, such as aluminum salts and oil-in-water emulsions, are designed to enhance the immunogenicity of antigens. Adjuvants stimulate and prolong antigen availability.[1]
- *Cellular therapies*: Adoptive T-cell therapies, including CAR-T cells, have revolutionized cancer immunotherapy by enhancing cytotoxic T-cell responses against tumors.[3]
- *Genetic and epigenetic modulation*: CRISPR-based editing and histone modifications can amplify gene expression linked to immune cell activation.

Modulation of Antigen Presentation

Antigen presentation is a critical step in initiating an immune response, involving the processing and display of antigens on the surface of APCs via major histocompatibility complex (MHC) molecules.

Strategies to Modulate Antigen Presentation

- *Enhancing MHC expression*: The upregulation of MHC molecules, either by cytokines such as interferon-gamma or through genetic engineering, improves antigen presentation and T-cell activation.[4]
- *Antigen engineering*: Designing antigens with higher binding affinities for MHC molecules ensures a more robust presentation. This strategy is commonly applied in vaccine development.[5]
- *Targeted delivery to APCs*: Nanoparticle-based delivery systems and monoclonal antibodies are used to ensure the efficient delivery of antigens to dendritic cells, the most potent APCs.[6]
- *Immune checkpoint modulation*: Blocking inhibitory molecules such as PD-1/PD-L1 and CTLA-4 enhances APC functionality and antigen presentation.

Induction of Immunological Memory

The development of immunological memory is fundamental for long-lasting protection against infections and forms the basis for vaccination.

Mechanisms of Memory Induction

- *T-cell memory development*: Memory T cells arise following antigen exposure and persist in the body for years. Subtypes include central memory (Tcm) and effector memory (Tem) cells, each with distinct roles in rapid immune response.
- *B-cell memory and long-lived plasma cells*: Memory B cells and plasma cells ensure the production of high-affinity antibodies upon re-exposure to antigens. Germinal center reactions are critical for their development.
- *Vaccination strategies*: Modern vaccines, such as mRNA vaccines, are designed to mimic natural infections and efficiently induce immunological memory.
- *Adjuvant use in memory formation*: Adjuvants not only enhance initial immune responses but also play a role in the formation of robust immunological memory by promoting the persistence of antigen-specific cells.

Challenges and Future Directions

Developing vaccines and immunotherapies that effectively induce long-term immunological memory remains a challenge, especially for chronic infections and cancers. Advancements in systems immunology and bioinformatics are likely to provide novel insights.[7]

KEY CONSIDERATIONS IN ADJUVANT SELECTION

Adjuvants play a crucial role in vaccine development by enhancing the immune response to antigens. Selecting an appropriate adjuvant involves several key considerations, including its safety profile, compatibility with the antigen, intended route of administration, and targeted immune response. These factors collectively ensure the efficacy and safety of the vaccine.

Safety Profile

The safety profile of an adjuvant is a paramount consideration during selection. Adjuvants must exhibit minimal local and systemic adverse effects, such as inflammation, hypersensitivity, or autoimmunity. Preclinical and clinical evaluations assess toxicity, reactogenicity, and long-term safety. Regulatory guidelines mandate thorough toxicity studies to identify potential risks.

For example, aluminum salts (e.g., aluminum hydroxide and aluminum phosphate) are widely used due to their long-standing safety record. However, emerging adjuvants, such as saponins or lipid nanoparticles, require rigorous evaluation to ensure they meet acceptable safety standards. Identifying patient-specific factors, such as preexisting allergies or autoimmune conditions, is essential to mitigate risks.

Compatibility with Antigen

The compatibility of the adjuvant with the antigen is a critical factor for the formulation's stability and efficacy. The adjuvant must not chemically alter or degrade the antigen, as this could reduce immunogenicity or increase the risk of side effects. Furthermore, adjuvant-antigen interactions can affect vaccine delivery, antigen release kinetics, and immune activation.

For example, oil-in-water emulsions such as MF59 are particularly compatible with protein-based antigens, while liposome-based adjuvants are often used for peptide or nucleic acid vaccines. The choice of adjuvant depends on the antigen's physical and chemical properties, including solubility, stability, and charge.

Route of Administration

The route of administration influences adjuvant selection as it determines the formulation's stability, absorption, and immune response type. For instance, intramuscular and subcutaneous routes are commonly used for adjuvanted vaccines due to their ability to elicit systemic immune responses. Conversely, mucosal routes (e.g., intranasal or oral) require adjuvants that can survive harsh environments, such as low pH and enzymatic degradation.

For example, chitosan and mucosal adjuvants such as cholera toxin B subunit have shown promise for oral and intranasal vaccines. Tailoring the adjuvant to the administration route ensures optimal antigen uptake by APCs and effective immune priming.

Immunological Targets

Adjuvant selection is closely tied to the desired immune response, whether it is humoral (antibody-mediated), cellular (T-cell-mediated), or a combination of both. Different adjuvants stimulate specific arms of the immune system by targeting pattern recognition receptors (PRRs) such as TLRs or NLRs.

For example, AS01, an adjuvant system containing MPL (a TLR4 agonist) and QS-21 (a saponin), promotes a balanced Th1 and Th2 response, ideal for subunit vaccines targeting complex pathogens. Conversely, aluminum-based adjuvants predominantly stimulate Th2 responses, making them suitable for antibody-centric vaccines.

CLINICAL APPLICATIONS

Adjuvanted Vaccines in Use

Adjuvants enhance the immune response of vaccines by augmenting antigen presentation, stimulating innate immunity, and prolonging antigen release. Several adjuvanted vaccines are currently in widespread use, including:

- *Hepatitis B vaccines*:
  - *Adjuvant*: Aluminum salts (alum)
  - *Application*: Induces a strong humoral response to prevent hepatitis B virus (HBV) infection
- *Human papillomavirus (HPV) vaccines*:
  - *Adjuvant*: AS04, a combination of aluminum hydroxide and monophosphoryl lipid A
  - *Application*: Provides long-lasting immunity against oncogenic HPV strains
- *Seasonal influenza vaccines*:
  - *Adjuvant*: MF59 (oil-in-water emulsion)
  - *Application*: Enhances efficacy in older adults and immunocompromised populations
- *Shingles vaccine (Shingrix)*:
  - *Adjuvant*: AS01B, composed of QS-21 and monophosphoryl lipid A
  - *Application*: Prevents herpes zoster in adults aged 50 years and older with high efficacy
- *Malaria vaccine (RTS,S)*:
  - *Adjuvant*: AS01
  - *Application*: Provides partial protection against *Plasmodium falciparum* in children in endemic regions. Studies demonstrating efficacy adjuvanted vaccines have shown superior efficacy in various scenarios.

- *Shingrix for herpes zoster*: Clinical trials showed >90% efficacy in preventing herpes zoster across all age groups, outperforming earlier vaccines without adjuvants.
- *RTS,S Malne*: In African children, the vaccine reduced malaria cases by 39% over 4 years. The AS01 adjuvant played a critical role in generating a strong immune response in young children.
- *MF59-adjuvanted vaccine*: In older adults, studies demonstrated improved seroconversion rates and a significant reduction in influenza-related complications.

These case studies underscore adjuvants in achieving robust and durable vaccine efficacy, especially in vulnerable populations.

Future Directions and Emerging Trends

The field of adjuvanted vaccines is evolving rapidly, with innovations aimed at improving safety, efficacy, and broad applicability:

- *Next-generation adjuvants*: Use of TLR agonists and saponins to target specific immune pathways more precisely
- *mRNA vaccines with adjuvants*: mRNA vaccines, such as those for COVID-19, currently rely on lipid nanoparticles; integrating adjuvants could further enhance immune responses.
- *Combination vaccines*: The development of vaccines incorporating multiple adjuvants to elicit diverse and robust immune responses
- *Nanoparticle-based delivery systems*: Research on adjuvants coupled with nanoparticles aims to improve antigen stability and targeted delivery.
- *Personalized vaccinology*: Tailoring vaccine adjuvants to individual genetic and immunological profiles for optimal efficacy

REGULATORY AND ETHICAL CONSIDERATIONS

Approval Process for Adjuvanted Vaccines

The approval process for adjuvanted vaccines involves a thorough assessment by regulatory agencies to ensure their safety, efficacy, and quality. The inclusion of adjuvants, substances designed to enhance the immune response to the antigen, requires specific attention due to their potential for unique safety and efficacy concerns.

- *Preclinical evaluation*: Adjuvanted vaccines undergo rigorous preclinical studies, including in vitro and animal models, to assess toxicity, immunogenicity, and pharmacokinetics.
- *Clinical trials*:
  - *Phase I*: Focuses on the safety and immunogenicity of the vaccine-adjuvant combination
  - *Phase II*: Evaluates optimal dosage and continues to monitor safety
  - *Phase III*: Assesses large-scale efficacy and identifies rare adverse effects
- *Regulatory review*: Agencies such as the US Food and Drug Administration (FDA), the European Medicines Agency (EMA), and the Central Drugs Standard Control Organization (CDSCO) in India review the data. Special emphasis is placed on postmarketing surveillance plans for long-term safety monitoring.
- *Ethical oversight*: Institutional review boards (IRBs) ensure that clinical trials comply with ethical standards, including informed consent and risk-benefit analysis.

Safety Monitoring and Surveillance

Safety monitoring is critical for identifying and managing adverse events associated with adjuvanted vaccines, both during clinical trials and postlicensure.

- *Adverse event reporting systems*: Programs such as the vaccine adverse event reporting system (VAERS) in the United States and VigiBase by WHO collect data on suspected adverse events.
- *Postmarketing surveillance*: Postapproval vaccines are subject to pharmacovigilance, which includes:
  - Active surveillance through cohort event monitoring systems
  - Passive surveillance relying on healthcare providers and public reports
- *Long-term monitoring*: Some adjuvants may cause delayed or rare adverse effects, necessitating extended follow-up studies.
- *Risk communication*: Transparency in reporting adverse events and the establishment of vaccine injury compensation programs mitigate ethical concerns.

Public Perception and Acceptance

Public perception of adjuvanted vaccines plays a pivotal role in the success of immunization programs. Misinformation and mistrust can pose significant challenges.

- *Addressing vaccine hesitancy*:
  - Clear communication of the benefits and risks of adjuvanted vaccines
  - Tailoring messages to address cultural and social concerns
- *Community engagement*:
  - Involving community leaders and healthcare workers to build trust
  - Using participatory approaches to involve stakeholders in decision-making
- *Combatting misinformation*: Leveraging social media platforms and digital campaigns to counteract vaccine-related misinformation

- *Ethical communication*: Providing balanced, evidence-based information while respecting individual autonomy fosters informed decision-making.

CHALLENGES AND FUTURE DIRECTIONS

Overcoming Formulation Challenges

Adjuvant formulation is a critical aspect that determines its stability, safety, and efficacy. A major challenge is ensuring that adjuvants maintain their stability during storage while being compatible with various antigens. Complex adjuvant systems such as emulsions and nanoparticles often require precise manufacturing and storage conditions, which can increase production costs and limit accessibility in resource-poor settings.[8] Additionally, ensuring uniformity and reproducibility of adjuvant-based vaccines remains a concern for large-scale manufacturing.

Future directions to address these challenges include the development of innovative delivery systems, such as lipid nanoparticles, which provide a more stable matrix for adjuvants and antigens. Moreover, advances in lyophilization techniques can help improve the shelf life of adjuvant formulations, enabling broader global distribution.

Designing Adjuvants for Specific Populations

Adjuvants often exhibit variable efficacy across different populations due to genetic, age-related, or environmental factors. For example, older adults with immunosenescence may respond suboptimally to traditional adjuvants, whereas neonates and infants may require adjuvants tailored to their developing immune systems.[9] Furthermore, individuals with autoimmune disorders or other comorbidities present unique challenges in balancing efficacy with safety.

To address these challenges, researchers are exploring personalized adjuvant strategies that incorporate biomarkers to predict immune responses. Targeted delivery systems, such as dendritic cell-targeting adjuvants, are also being investigated to enhance immune activation while minimizing systemic side effects in specific populations.

Advancements in Adjuvant Research

The rapid progress in immunology and biotechnology is driving the development of next-generation adjuvants. Advances in systems biology and computational modeling have enabled the prediction of immune responses to adjuvant-antigen combinations, expediting the design process. Synthetic biology is emerging as a promising avenue, allowing the customization of adjuvants with precise molecular architectures to elicit desired immune responses.

Additionally, novel adjuvants, such as TLR agonists and saponin-based systems, are being explored to stimulate robust and long-lasting immunity. The integration of nanotechnology has further expanded possibilities, enabling the creation of multifunctional adjuvants that can simultaneously deliver antigens and immune-modulatory molecules. Despite these advancements, translating these innovations into safe and widely accepted clinical applications remains a formidable challenge.

CONCLUSION

Adjuvants are critical components in modern vaccine formulations, playing a pivotal role in enhancing immune responses to antigens. Their importance in vaccine development lies in their ability to improve immunogenicity, especially for subunit, recombinant, and inactivated vaccines that may otherwise elicit weak or insufficient immune responses. By stimulating both the innate and adaptive arms of the immune system, adjuvants help ensure robust and long-lasting immunity.

Adjuvants contribute significantly to dose-sparing strategies, reducing the antigen amount required for effective vaccination. This not only lowers production costs but also facilitates rapid scalability during outbreaks or pandemics. Additionally, they enable vaccines to induce immunity across diverse population groups, including the very young, elderly, and immunocompromised, who often exhibit weaker immune responses.

The choice of an adjuvant is also central to tailoring immune responses to specific pathogens. For instance, some adjuvants enhance the production of neutralizing antibodies, while others skew the immune response toward a Th1 or Th2 profile, depending on the disease being targeted. Moreover, adjuvants can support the induction of mucosal immunity and memory cell development, which are key features for long-term protection.

Adjuvant research has evolved significantly, with advances in immunology and molecular biology driving the design of novel adjuvants with improved safety and efficacy profiles. This progress has opened avenues for the development of next-generation vaccines against complex diseases such as human immunodeficiency virus (HIV), tuberculosis, and cancer, which require more sophisticated immune responses.

In summary, adjuvants are indispensable for the success of many vaccines. Their ability to potentiate immune responses, optimize antigen use, and customize immunity profiles has transformed the landscape of vaccinology. Ongoing innovations in adjuvant technology continue to enhance the potential of vaccines, addressing global health challenges with greater precision and impact.

REFERENCES

1. Petrovsky N, Aguilar JC. Vaccine adjuvants: Current state and future trends. Immunol Cell Biol. 2004;82(5):488-96.
2. Rosenberg SA. Progress in human tumour immunology and immunotherapy. Nature. 2001;411(6835):380-4.
3. June CH, O'Connor RS, Kawalekar OU, Ghassemi S, Milone MC. CAR T cell immunotherapy for human cancer. Science. 2018; 359(6382):1361-5.
4. Schumacher TN, Schreiber RD. Neoantigens in cancer immunotherapy. Science. 2015;348(6230):69-74.
5. Wang S, Mboudjeka I, Goguen JD, Lu S. Antigen engineering can play a critical role in the protective immunity elicited by Yersinia pestis DNA vaccines. Vaccine. 2010;28(8):2011-9.
6. Khalil DN, Smith EL, Brentjens RJ, Wolchok JD. The future of cancer treatment: Immunomodulation, targeted therapy, and advanced technologies. Nat Rev Clin Oncol. 2016;13(5):273-90.
7. Pulendran B, Ahmed R. Translating innate immunity into immunological memory: Implications for vaccine development. Cell. 2006;124(4):849-63.
8. Tavano R, Zuliani C, Campi G, Fattoretti G. Formulation challenges in vaccine adjuvants development. J Drug Delivery Sci Technol. 2020;60:101980.
9. Dowling DJ, Levy O. Ontogeny of early life immunity. Trends Immunol. 2014;35(7):299-310.

CHAPTER

8

Approaches to Measuring Vaccine Efficacy and Effectiveness

Madhu Gupta, Athulya V Ajith, Aritrik Das

SUMMARY

Vaccination is one of the most cost-effective public health interventions, significantly reducing morbidity and mortality from preventable diseases. Before a vaccine is licensed, it undergoes several phases of clinical trials, beginning with preclinical and early-phase trials that assess safety and immunogenicity. Phase III trials mainly measure vaccine efficacy—how well a vaccine prevents disease under ideal conditions. Upon licensure, phase IV studies evaluate vaccine effectiveness in real-world conditions. Accurately estimating vaccine efficacy is critical as it informs herd immunity thresholds and public health strategies. Overestimating or underestimating efficacy can lead to resource misallocation or prolonged vaccination campaigns, respectively. Demonstrating vaccine effectiveness, particularly in reducing disease burden, is essential for gaining policy support, securing funding, and ensuring widespread uptake. Methodologically rigorous trials, such as randomized controlled trials, are necessary to estimate efficacy, while cohort and case-control studies help determine effectiveness post-licensure. In this chapter, we have discussed the methodological approaches in evaluating vaccine efficacy and effectiveness, underscoring their importance in vaccine development and public health policy.

INTRODUCTION

Vaccination has been widely accepted as one of the most cost-effective public health interventions that can be implemented by a country, with the aim to reduce morbidity and mortality resulting from vaccine-preventable diseases.[1] Each candidate vaccine undergoes various phases of clinical testing before being licensed for general use. One of the most vital considerations in this regard is vaccine safety. Preclinical animal studies and phase I and II clinical trials are primarily designed to evaluate safety and immunogenicity.[2] Phase III studies primarily focus on evaluating direct protective efficacy, i.e., vaccine efficacy in preventing the disease, with further accumulation of safety data. Results of phase III studies are used to apply for licensure of a vaccine.[2,3] Once a vaccine is licensed, various studies are done to monitor and evaluate the effectiveness and safety of the vaccine in routine usage, generically referred to as phase IV studies.[2,3]

The estimation of vaccine efficacy is a vital step in the process of vaccine development and approval. It is the direct effect of a vaccine measured in prelicensure randomized clinical trials where vaccination is allocated under optimal conditions.[3,4] From the public health point of view, knowing the vaccine efficacy allows for the estimation of the effective fraction of people that need to be immunized, beyond which no epidemic outbreak can happen, which is also known as the herd immunity threshold.[3] Overestimation of efficacy comes with the danger of not reaching the herd immunity threshold at the end of the vaccination campaign for a particular disease.[5] There might be a wastage of resources and an eventual failure in preventing the disease despite achieving expected coverage. Underestimating efficacy can increase both the costs and duration of a vaccination campaign, and in extreme cases, it can lead to roadblocks in planning, procurement of funding, and implementation owing to considerations of practical feasibility.[5] Demonstrating the burden of the disease prevented by the vaccine is a critical step in the development of the vaccine, its uptake by the policy makers, program managers and community in any country. Hence, it is essential that all aspects are taken into consideration while estimating the vaccine efficacy including setting up the robust surveillance system to pick all the cases, especially in the high burden disease areas, using standard case definition of the diseases, case ascertainment in the field, and methodological rigor to ensure that reliable estimates are produced. This chapter delves into the methodological aspects of estimating the vaccine efficacy in the clinical trials, vaccine effectiveness, the difference between the two, and the challenges and measures to resolve those.

UNDERSTANDING VACCINE EFFICACY

Vaccine efficacy is the percentage reduction in the incidence of the vaccine-preventable disease due to the vaccination.[4] It is essentially the direct effect of a vaccine in reduction of the disease incidence measured in randomized clinical trials, where vaccination is allocated under optimal research conditions before licensure.[4] It can be estimated as one minus a particular measure of relative risk.[2] Several measures of efficacy can be defined according to the risk considered such as efficacy for susceptibility to disease, clinical illness, colonization, progression, pathogenicity, infectiousness, indirect effects, population-level effects, etc.[3] Accordingly, there are various types of vaccine efficacy depending upon the outcome of interest. These are described here and summarized in **Table 1**.

Vaccine Efficacy for Susceptibility to Infection

It measures how well a vaccine protects against an infection to the vaccine-preventable disease. To estimate this, all the suspected infections (symptomatic and asymptomatic) meeting the standard case definition are included in the study and tested for the occurrence of the causative organism. In such cases, vaccine efficacy against infection due to the given pathogen is estimated.

Vaccine Efficacy for Susceptibility to Disease

It measures how well a vaccine protects against a clinical disease. With most infectious agents, the major interest is in preventing clinical illness. Usually, while evaluating vaccines against infectious agents such as measles, influenza, or pertussis, it is often ascertained by observing individuals clinically, in which case asymptomatic infections are not included. This may be

TABLE 1: Types of vaccine efficacy.

Types	Description	Example
Vaccine efficacy for susceptibility to infections (VE_S)	• Measure of protectiveness of vaccination against the infection • Denotes how well a vaccinated individual is protected against getting infected by the respective infectious agent	• COVID-19 pandemic vaccine efficacy against infection was lower than against the disease[5,6] • While evaluating the effects of vaccines against infectious agents such as measles, pertussis, or influenza, asymptomatic cases are not included and usually vaccine efficacy for susceptibility to disease (VE_{SP}) is calculated
Vaccine efficacy for susceptibility to disease (VE_{SP})	• Measures how well a vaccine protects against a disease • Evaluated by observing individuals clinically for the symptoms, in which case asymptomatic infections are not included and may be followed by a biological test to confirm the infectious agent under study	*COVID-19*: In a study to assess the safety and efficacy of BNT162b2 mRNA COVID-19 vaccine, persons 16 years of age or older were randomly assigned in a 1:1 ratio to receive two doses, 21 days apart, of either placebo or the vaccine candidate. It showed 95.0% vaccine efficacy [95% confidence interval (CI), 90.3–97.6] as there were 8 cases of COVID-19 among 21,720 with BNT162b2 injection and 162 cases among those 21,728 assigned to placebo[7]
Vaccine efficacy against colonization (VEcol)	• Measures the efficacy of vaccines in preventing colonization of the infectious agent • Colonized individuals are generally asymptomatic but play an important role in transmission to other susceptible individuals who in their turn might develop severe disease • In the case of infectious agents which colonize the throat and nose passages without causing overt disease, the efficacy of a vaccine against colonization is estimated	The 2013 study by Auranen et al. presents a framework for estimating vaccine efficacy against colonization by *Streptococcus pneumoniae*[8]

Continued

Continued

Types	Description	Example
Vaccine efficacy for progression or pathogenicity (VE_P)	• Measures the efficacy of vaccination in preventing a postinfection outcome • Measures of interest can be the effect of prophylactic vaccination on the rate or probability of progression to diseases on being infected, severe disease, or reduction in the duration of being infected	In a systematic review and meta-analysis, the combined efficacy of full vaccination was 44.5% (95% CI 27.8–57.4) for preventing asymptomatic infections, 76.5% (69.8–81.7) for preventing symptomatic infections, 95.4% (95% credible interval 88.0–98.7) for preventing hospitalization, 90.8% (85.5–95.1) for preventing severe infection, and 85.8% (68.7–94.6) for preventing death. The combined efficacy of full vaccination was 44.5% (95% CI 27.8–57.4) for preventing asymptomatic infections, 76.5% (69.8–81.7) for preventing symptomatic infections, 95.4% (95% credible interval 88.0–98.7) for preventing hospitalization, 90.8% (85.5–95.1) for preventing severe infection, and 85.8% (68.7–94.6) for preventing death[9]
Vaccine efficacy for infectiousness (VE_I)	• Measures the reduction in the ability of a vaccinated infected person to transmit the infectious agents to others compared to an unvaccinated infected person • It might be because of a reduction in the infectiousness of the disease or a reduction in the duration of the infectious period of the disease in the vaccinated person	A study from Belgian contact tracing data for high-risk exposure contacts between 26/01/2021 and 14/12/2021 estimated VE_I estimates for BNT162b2 and ChAdOx1 as 71% (CI 68–74) and 53% (CI 49–57), respectively[10]
Total vaccine efficacy (VE_T)	The combined protective effect of both individuals (infected and susceptible) coming in contact with being vaccinated, as opposed to neither of them being vaccinated	In the Belgian study conducted to estimate vaccine efficacy against transmission of SARS-CoV-2-infection by variants of concern, VE_T estimates were higher for mRNA-vaccines, over 90%, compared to viral vector vaccines Ad26COV2.S and ChAdOx, showing 66% and 80%, respectively for alpha after 0–50 days of vaccination[10]

followed by a biological test to confirm the infectious agent under study to confirm the causative organism. In such cases, vaccine efficacy for susceptibility to disease (VE_{SP}) is calculated, which denotes the vaccine efficacy against disease due to the given pathogen. Many a time, we use both VE_S and VE_{SP} simultaneously in the randomized control trials.

Vaccine Efficacy against Colonization (VEcol)

It is important in infectious agents such as pneumococcal, meningococcal, and *Haemophilus influenza* type b bacteria, which colonize the throat and nose passages without causing overt disease. Colonized individuals are generally asymptomatic but play an important role in transmission to other susceptible individuals who, in turn, might develop severe disease.

Vaccine Efficacy for Progression or Pathogenicity (VE_P)

It measures the efficacy of vaccination in preventing a postinfection outcome. Here, the measure of interest can be the effect of prophylactic vaccination on the rate or probability of progression to diseases/severity. It could be a measure of the effect of vaccination on the probability of severe disease or reduction in the duration of being infected.

Vaccine efficacy for susceptibility to infection (VE_S), VE_{SP}, and VE_P are measures of the direct protective effects of vaccination. The important difference is that VE_S and VE_{SP} evaluate outcomes in participants who are susceptible to infection, whereas VE_P estimates outcomes in participants who are already infected; hence, denominators to estimate the risk are different.

Vaccine Efficacy for Infectiousness

It measures the reduction in the ability of a vaccinated infected person to transmit the infectious agents to others compared to an unvaccinated infected person. It might be because of a reduction in the infectiousness of the disease or a reduction in the duration of the infectious period of the disease in the vaccinated person.

Total Vaccine Efficacy (VE_T)

The combined effect of the scenario with both individuals coming in contact being vaccinated as opposed to neither vaccinated is termed total vaccine efficacy (VE_T). Vaccine efficacy for infectiousness (VE_I) and VE_T are of immense public health significance because a vaccine that reduces infectiousness has wide public health implications with respect to a communicable disease in the community.

In most of the controlled clinical trials, the "outcome of interest" is usually disease, and the vaccine efficacy is measured based on how many people who got vaccinated developed the outcome, compared to how many people who got the placebo or were unimmunized also developed the same outcome. Once the study is complete, the numbers of diseased people in each group are compared to calculate the relative risk of getting the disease depending on whether the subjects received the vaccine. From this, we estimate the efficacy—a measure of how much the vaccine lowered the risk of contracting the disease. If a vaccine has high efficacy, fewer people in the group that received the vaccine would contract the disease than the people in the group that were unimmunized. For example, let us imagine a vaccine with a proven efficacy of 80%. This means that out of the people in the vaccine trial, those who received the vaccine were at an 80% lower risk of developing the disease than the group who received the placebo. This is calculated by comparing the number of cases of disease in the vaccinated group versus the placebo group. Hence, an efficacy of 80% does not mean that 20% of the vaccinated group will become ill. Vaccine efficacy depends on several factors, such as the type of vaccine, age at which it is administered, number of doses of the vaccine administered, gap between administration of two doses, administration of booster doses, route of administration, potency of vaccines as well as technique of administration.[4] Many variations of the above, such as the ideal age of administration, number of doses, the gap between doses, need for boosters, and route of administration, are tested during the different phases of vaccine trials, to ultimately arrive at a version of the vaccine with the highest possible efficacy.[4]

METHODOLOGICAL APPROACHES TO ESTIMATE VACCINE EFFICACY

As information on exposure to infection is difficult to collect, studies estimate vaccine efficacy for susceptibility to get the disease simply from the incidence of people who become clinically ill (as per case definition) among the vaccinated compared to unvaccinated groups.[3] In estimating the direct protective effects of vaccination, three necessary conditions for valid inference are given by Greenwood and Yule (1915),[11] which are as follows:

1. The people must be alike in all material respects. Relevant covariates can include sociodemographic factors such as age and gender, prior disease history, previous history of vaccination, and preexisting immune levels such as antibody titer.
2. The effective exposure to the disease must be identical in the case of vaccinated and unvaccinated individuals.
3. The criteria of the fact of vaccination and the fact of the disease having occurred must be independent.

The efficacy of a vaccine is usually assessed by prelicensure randomized clinical trials (phase III clinical trials) where vaccination is allocated under optimal conditions and the disease occurrence between the vaccinated and nonvaccinated groups are compared. Double-blinded randomized controlled trials, which further equalize the chances of exposure among vaccinated and unvaccinated, ensure that these criteria are met so that any differences in the risk in the two groups are likely be due to the biological effects of the vaccine. In most of the randomized controlled clinical trials, the "outcome of interest" is usually disease, and the vaccine efficacy is measured based on how many people who got vaccinated developed the outcome, compared to how many people who got the placebo or were unimmunized also developed the same outcome. Once the study is complete, the numbers of diseased people in each group are compared to calculate the relative risk of getting the disease depending on whether the subjects received the vaccine. From this, we estimate the efficacy—a measure of how much the vaccine lowered the risk of contracting the disease. Assuming an "idealized" clinical trial where:

Number of randomized individuals in the unvaccinated (control) group = Nu

Number of randomized individuals in the vaccinated group = Nv

Number of cases of disease developed among unvaccinated (control) population = Cu

Number of cases of disease developed among vaccinated population = Cv

Risk/incidence of the disease among unvaccinated (control) group, Ru = Cu/Nu

Risk/incidence of the disease among vaccinated population, Rv = Cv/Nv

Relative Risk = Rv/Ru

The vaccine efficacy (VE) is calculated as:

VE = (Risk/incidence of the disease among the unvaccinated – Risk/incidence of the disease among the vaccinated)/Risk/incidence of disease among the unvaccinated × 100%

VE = (Ru – Rv)/Ru × 100%

Or, VE = (1 – Relative risk) × 100%

(The obtained value is multiplied by 100 to express the vaccine efficacy in percentage)

The measure of risk can be the incidence rate, hazard rate, or attack rate, which are not related to the measure of exposure. It can also be a form of disease transmission probability, which is dependent on exposure to infection. The estimate of this efficacy is obtained from the relative risk in the vaccinated individuals compared to the unvaccinated individuals, as shown by the formula above. If a vaccine has high efficacy, fewer people in the group that received the vaccine would contract the disease than the people in the group that were unimmunized.

***Example 1*:** Estimation of vaccine efficacy of rotavirus vaccine in a randomized control trial.[7]

A study was conducted to evaluate the vaccine efficacy of three doses of oral rotavirus vaccine 116E against severe rotavirus gastroenteritis among infants in India. It was a randomized double-blind placebo-controlled trial, and the primary outcome of the study was severe hospitalized rotavirus gastroenteritis. Three doses of ROTAVAC®/placebo were given with childhood vaccines at 6–7 weeks, ≥10 weeks, and ≥14 weeks following inclusion and exclusion criteria. Families were contacted weekly at home by trained field workers to ascertain efficacy outcomes. Trained field workers collected information on the characteristics of gastroenteritis episodes for each day. A stool sample was collectedfor each episode of gastroenteritis and was examined for rotavirus with a commercial enzyme immunoassay to detect rotavirus. Efficacy estimates for the first year of life included events that occurredtill 1 year of age. Among the 4,354 vaccinated children, 57 developed severe gastroenteritis, whereas 65 out of 2,187 children receiving a placebo developed the same outcome.

	Severe gastroenteritis		
Exposure	**Present**	**Absent**	**Total**
Vaccinated	57	4297	4354
Unvaccinated	65	2122	2187
Total	122	6419	6541

Vaccine efficacy is calculated as:

VE = (Risk/incidence of the disease among the unvaccinated – Risk/incidence of the disease amongvaccinated)/ Risk/incidence of disease among the unvaccinated × 100%

VE = (Ru – Rv)/Ru × 100% or (1 – relative risk) × 100% Ru = 65/2,187 = 2.9%

Rv = 57/4,354 = 1.3%

= 1 – 1.3/2.9 = 1 – 0.45 = 55%

Hence, vaccine efficacy was calculated as 55%.

UNDERSTANDING VACCINE EFFECTIVENESS

The effectiveness of a vaccine is the real-world performance of a vaccine.[4] It is assessed after the vaccine is licensed and introduced in the healthcare delivery system.[4] A vaccine effectiveness of 80% would mean that in a vaccinated population, 80% fewer people would contract the disease on meeting the disease agent.[4] Effectiveness in the real world can differ from the efficacy measured in a trial, because of the much bigger and more variable population getting vaccinated in uncontrolled conditions, difference in geographic parameters, introduction of vaccine in sub populations not included or under-represented in the original trials (e.g., children and pregnant women), suboptimal consideration of the cold-chain necessary for optimal effectiveness of the vaccine, incompleteness of the vaccination schedule, incorrect time spacing between the vaccine doses administered, emergence of new variants of the infectious agent, varying techniques of administration due to uneven training, and many other factors.[4] Widespread vaccination can also have indirect effects due to changes in the collective level of immunity in the population, the herd immunity.[3] The indirect effect of vaccination at the population level in unvaccinated and vaccinated groups might not be the same. The former is called indirect vaccination effectiveness, whereas the latter is total vaccination effectiveness.[3] The overall effectiveness of a vaccination strategy within a particular population is the weighted average of the outcomes in these vaccinated and unvaccinated people.[3]

Methodological Approaches to Measure Vaccine Effectiveness

Once the vaccine is licensed, we need to investigate the vaccine effectiveness in real-world settings. In that scenario, it is unethical to conduct randomized controlled trials with no vaccine to be given to the control group. Hence, we resort to conducting observational studies, such as cohort and case-control studies, to determine the vaccine effectiveness in wider population groups, in whom the effectiveness may differ from the efficacy observed in clinical trials due to reasons as discussed earlier.

Cohort Study Design to Estimate the Vaccine Effectiveness

In a cohort study, two groups of similar individuals with and without exposure to a vaccine are followed for a certain period (often, it is the time they have probability to get the clinical disease). Vaccine effectiveness (VE1) is calculated as:

$$\textit{Vaccine effectiveness (VE1)} = [(IRu - IRv)/IRu)] \times 100\%$$

where,

IRu = Incidence rate of disease among unvaccinated

IRv = Incidence rate of disease among vaccinated

Example 2: Estimation of vaccine effectiveness of influenza vaccine in a cohort study.

To estimate the vaccine effectiveness of the influenza vaccine, the disease of interest is influenza. Let usassume that a random sample of 50 vaccinated (exposed) and 50 unvaccinated (unexposed) individualswas taken from a population in which the outcome of interest, i.e., the presence of influenza, is ascertainedby a positive diagnostic test. The following results were observed:

	Influenza		
Exposure	**Present**	**Absent**	**Total**
Vaccinated	2	48	50
Unvaccinated	8	42	50
Total	10	90	100

VE1 = [(IRu – IRv)/IRu] × 100%

IRu = 8/50 = 0.16; Irv = 2/50 = 0.04; VE1 = [(0.16 – 0.04)/0.16] × 100 = 75%

Here, the unexposed group carried a 4-fold (=16%/4%) increase in the risk of infection comparedwith the vaccinated group. In other words, vaccination decreased the risk of infection by 75%, which is the estimated effectiveness.

Case-control Study Design to Estimate the Vaccine Effectiveness

In a case-control study, which is retrospective, we compare the odds of disease among the vaccinated and nonvaccinated groups. Vaccine effectiveness (VE1) is calculated as:

VE1 = [(Oddsu – Oddsv)/Oddsu)] × 100% or

VE1 = (1 – OR) × 100%

where,

Oddsu = Odds of disease among unvaccinated

Oddsv = Odds of disease among vaccinated

OR = Odds ratio is the odds of disease among the vaccinated compared to the odds of disease among the unvaccinated.

Example 3: Estimation of effectiveness of rotavirus vaccine in a case-control study.
In a study to estimate the effectiveness of a vaccine to rotavirus-associated gastroenteritis, random sample of 50 test-positive rotavirus children and 50 test-negative rotavirus children were selected. The history of the study participants for being vaccinated was as follows:

Exposure	Rotavirus-associated gastroenteritis		Total
	Present	Absent	
Vaccinated	8	23	31
Unvaccinated	32	17	49
Total	40	40	80

The odds ratio (OR) is calculated as = (8/23)/(32/17) = 8 × 17/23 × 32 = 136/736 = 0.18
= 0.18 (for the exposure of vaccination among the patients having rotavirus-associated gastroenteritis)
Here, the effectiveness of vaccine against the disease is estimated to be (1 – 0.18) × 100 = 81%.

Estimating Herd Immunity

The population-level effectiveness of a vaccination evaluating indirect, direct, and overall herd effect has population as its unit of inference and requires several communities to be included in the study to account for potential variability. It facilitates comparison between different levels of vaccination coverage, as well as varying allocation within different age groups, or otherwise defined subgroups. It is generally estimated when there is a phase-wise introduction of the vaccine in the country.

Consider an example of two districts (district A and district B) in a state. Vaccination was launched in a phase-wise manner and district A is covered first. Hence, district A has a proportion of the population vaccinated and some unvaccinated population as well. District B has an unimmunized population. The direct effects of vaccination on the population can be assessed within district A that receives the vaccine, and indirect effects can be assessed by comparing the effects with district B, as described here and given in **Figure 1**.

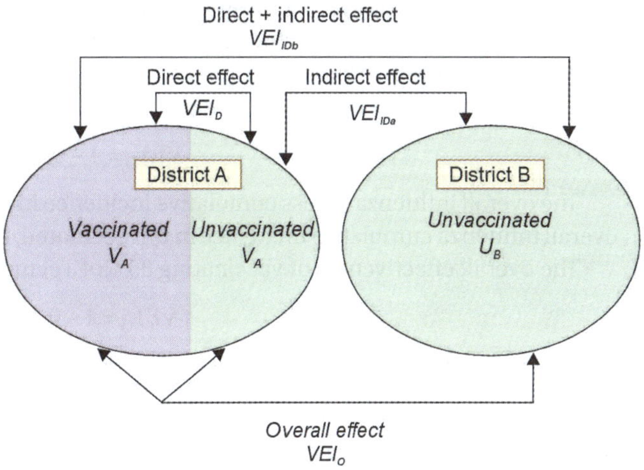

FIG. 1: Types of effects of a vaccination program in a state with phase-wise introduction of vaccine in districts A and B.
Source: With permission from Hanquet G, et al. 2013.[12]

Direct effect is a percentage reduction in the incidence of the disease in district A due to vaccination.

$$VE1_D = 1 - RV_A/RU_A$$

where,

$VE1_D$ = Vaccine effectiveness direct

RV_A is the risk/incidence of disease among vaccinated (VA) in the district A.

RU_A is the risk/incidence of disease among unvaccinated (U_A) in the district A.

Indirect effect of the vaccination in district A is then studied by comparing the disease incidence in unvaccinated (RU_A) people of population in district A to the disease incidence among unvaccinated (RU_B) people of population in district B. It is estimated as:

$$VEI_{IDa} = 1 - RU_A/RU_B$$

where,

VEI_{IDa} = Vaccine effectiveness indirect (a)

RU_A is the risk/incidence of disease among unvaccinated (U_A) in the district A RU_B is the risk/incidence of disease among unvaccinated (U_B) in the district B.

Direct plus indirect effects of the vaccination in district A are studied by comparing the disease incidence in vaccinated (RV_A) population in district A to the disease incidence among unvaccinated (RU_B) people of population in district B. It is estimated as:

$$VEI_{IDb} = 1 - RV_A/RU_B$$

where,
VEI_{IDb} = Vaccine effectiveness indirect (b)
RU_A is the risk/incidence of disease among vaccinated (V_A) in the district A

RU_B is the risk/incidence of disease among unvaccinated (U_B) in the district B.

Overall or combined effect of vaccination (total herd effect) in the state is the overall percentage reduction in the districts due to the vaccination. The average disease incidence (Ravg) in the total population (vaccinated and unvaccinated) in district A is compared with the disease incidence (RU_B) in the unvaccinated population in district B. The overall effectiveness of the vaccine or population-level effect of the vaccine compares the average outcomes in the vaccinated communities with those of the unvaccinated communities **(Fig. 1)**.

$$VE1_O = 1 - Ravg/RU_B$$

where,
$VE1_O$ = Vaccine effectiveness overall
Ravg = Average incidence rate of disease in district A

RU_B is the risk/incidence of disease among the unvaccinated (U_B) in district B.

Exercise 4: Direct and overall vaccine effectiveness.

A study by Monto et al. (1969) estimated the direct vaccine effectiveness ($VE1_D$) and the overall effect($VE1_O$) of an influenza vaccination program. Before the epidemic of 1968, they vaccinated 85% ofthe school-age children in Tecumseh, Michigan, against a Hong Kong influenza strain. A 10-week epidemic from November 17, 1968, to January 26, 1969, occurred, following which the weekly mean influenza illness rates in vaccinated and unvaccinated children were 0.072 and 0.090, respectively.

Direct vaccine effectiveness is estimated as:

$$VE1_D = 1 - 0.072/0.090 = 0.20\ (20\%)$$

The overall influenza illness cumulative incidence in Tecumseh for the epidemic period was 0.14, andthe adjusted overall influenza cumulative incidence in unvaccinated, neighboring Adrian, Michigan, was 0.42 for the same period. The overall effectiveness of vaccinating 85% of Tecumseh's school children was estimated to be:

$$VE1_O = 1 - 0.14/0.42 = 0.67 \text{ or } 67\%.$$

It is higher than its previously estimated efficacy of 20%.

VACCINE EFFICACY VERSUS VACCINE EFFECTIVENESS

The major difference between vaccine efficacy and vaccine effectiveness is given in **Table 2**. In most of the scenarios, estimated vaccine efficacy is higher than vaccine effectiveness, as vaccine efficacy is estimated in the controlled environment and constant monitoring and supervision of the vaccine storage with regard to cold chain maintenance and administration is followed. However, in certain conditions such as vaccination against infectious diseases such as pneumococcal pneumonia

TABLE 2: Differences between vaccine efficacy and vaccine effectiveness.

Parameters	Vaccine efficacy	Vaccine effectiveness
Study design	Phase III vaccine trial	Cohort and case control
Goal	Licensure of vaccine, estimates protection conferred to a healthy individual	Conduct of study in real-world settings, results that are meaningful to policymakers
Vaccine storage and administration	Strictly followed with constant monitoring	Storage and administration as per the routine immunization program in the national health system
Age administered and intervals between doses	Specific age groups enrolled, and dosing intervals are strictly followed	Recommended age for administration and intervals between doses as per the national immunization schedule of the country
Persons to be vaccinated	*Strict*: With specific exclusion in trials (screening out some disease conditions) as per the approved study protocol	Not selective. Instructions followed as per the national immunization guidelines of the country

and *Heamophilus influnzae* type b, vaccine effectiveness might be higher than vaccine due to additional benefit of reduction in the colonization of the organism in the nasopharynx resulting in lower transmission and infection rates among the vaccinated group compared to the unvaccinated group.[3]

LIMITATIONS

Transmission patterns can differ among communities. This variability could have an impact on the effects of vaccination among various communities.[3] A lack of consideration of various transmission patterns might influence the magnitude of the indirect effects of vaccination. At times, the effectiveness can be more than the efficacy because of its indirect effects, which are difficult to study during clinical trials owing to its limited participation and controlled setting.[3] Also, measuring the vaccine effectiveness at different stages of an epidemic's progression can lead to significant variations in the estimation of efficacy.[5]

CONCLUSION

To conclude, phase III clinical trials are done to assess the efficacy of vaccines prior to licensure of the vaccine. In today's time, when various vaccines are being developed on an accelerated timeline, especially in the midst of epidemics and pandemics, it is important to know how to assess vaccine efficacy in absolute and relative terms. It is also important to understand the difference between this calculated efficacy from the eventual effectiveness of the vaccine in the population, and how this can be assessed postlicensure of a vaccine. In addition, it is vital to be able to interpret the efficacy and effectiveness findings of a vaccine and correctly understand its public health implications.

REFERENCES

1. World Health Organization. (2024). Vaccines and immunization. [online] Available from https://www.who.int/health-topics/vaccines-and-immunization#tab=tab_1 [Last accessed March, 2025].
2. Plotkin SA, Orenstein WA, Offit PA, Edwards KM (Eds). Plotkin's Vaccines, 7th edition. Elsevier; 2017.
3. Halloran ME, Longini IM, Struchiner CJ. Statistics for Biology and Health Design and Analysis of Vaccine Studies. New York: Springer; 2010.
4. World Health Organization. (2024). Vaccine efficacy, effectiveness and protection. [online] Available from www.who.int/news-room/feature-stories/detail/vaccine-efficacy-effectiveness-and-protection [Last accessed March, 2025].
5. Scala A, Cavallo P. Measuring the efficacy of a vaccine during an epidemic. PLoS One. 2023;18(9):e0290652.
6. Al Kaabi N, Zhang Y, Xia S, Yang Y, Al Qahtani MM, Abdulrazzaq N, et al. Effect of 2 Inactivated SARS-CoV-2 Vaccines on Symptomatic COVID-19 Infection in Adults: A Randomized Clinical Trial. JAMA. 2021;326(1):35-45.
7. Polack FP, Thomas SJ, Kitchin N, Absalon J, Gurtman A, Lockhart S, et al. Safety and Efficacy of the BNT162b2 mRNA Covid-19 Vaccine. New Engl J Med. 2020;383(27):2603-15.
8. Auranen K, Rinta-Kokko H, Halloran ME. Estimating Strain-Specific and Overall Efficacy of Polyvalent Vaccines Against Recurrent Pathogens from a Cross-sectional Study. Biometrics. 2013;69(1):235-44.
9. Yang ZR, Jiang YW, Li FX, Liu D, Lin TF, Zhao ZY, et al. Efficacy of SARS-CoV-2 vaccines and the dose–response relationship with three major antibodies: A systematic review and meta-analysis of randomised controlled trials. Lancet Microbe. 2023;4(4):e236-46.
10. Braeye T, Catteau L, Brondeel R, van Loenhout JAF, Proesmans K, Cornelissen L, et al. Vaccine effectiveness against onward transmission of SARS-CoV2-infection by variant of concern and time since vaccination, Belgian contact tracing, 2021. Vaccine. 2022;40(22):3027-37.
11. Greenwood M, Yule GU. The Statistics of Anti-typhoid and Anti-cholera Inoculations, and the Interpretation of such Statistics in General. J R Soc Med. 1915;8:113-94.
12. Hanquet G, Valenciano M, Simondon F, Moren A. Vaccine effects and impact of vaccination programmes in post licensure studies. Vaccine. 2013;31:5634-42.

CHAPTER 9

Modeling and Vaccine Evaluation

Ankit Sheth

INTRODUCTION

Modeling in vaccinology refers to the use of mathematical and statistical techniques to simulate the behavior of vaccines and diseases within populations. These models are vital tools for understanding and predicting the complex dynamics of infectious diseases and the impact of vaccination strategies.[1] These models help researchers and policymakers to predict how vaccines will perform in real-world settings, assess how many people need to be vaccinated to achieve desired outcomes, and evaluate the potential effects of vaccination on overall disease burden. The importance of modeling in vaccinology lies in its ability to inform public health decisions, immunization strategies, and policymaking. Models simplify complex situations by combining data from various sources.

- *Predicting vaccine efficacy*: Models can simulate various scenarios to predict how effective a vaccine will be in preventing disease. This includes accounting for factors like varying levels of vaccine coverage, differences in vaccine efficacy among different populations, and potential mutations in pathogens.
- *Coverage needs*: Models help to determine the proportion of the population that needs to be vaccinated to achieve herd immunity. By analyzing patterns of disease transmission and vaccination coverage, models provide estimates of the necessary vaccination rates to control or eliminate a disease.
- *Impact assessment*: Models can estimate the potential impact of vaccination programs on public health. This includes predicting reductions in disease incidence, hospitalizations, and mortality rates, as well as evaluating the cost-effectiveness of vaccination campaigns.
- *Policy and planning*: In essence, models in vaccinology assist in making informed decisions about vaccination strategies, resource allocation, and public health interventions.[2] They can also be used to forecast and plan for potential outbreaks or emerging threats.

HISTORICAL PERSPECTIVE

Early Beginnings

- *18th–19th century:* The concept of modeling in public health dates to the work of pioneers like John Snow, who used mapping to understand cholera outbreaks in London. However, early models were rudimentary compared to modern standards.
- The development of more sophisticated mathematical models began with the work of Sir Ronald A Fisher and other statisticians who applied their methods to epidemiology. These models were used to understand the spread of diseases and the effects of vaccination.

Key Milestones in Vaccine Modeling

Kermack and McKendrick Model[3] (1926–1927)

Kermack and McKendrick introduced the susceptible-infected-recovered (SIR) model and derived an equation to determine the final size of an epidemic. This model was instrumental in studying infectious disease spread and the effects of vaccination on population health. The model divided the population into compartments based on disease status. They highlighted that a critical threshold for population density is necessary for large epidemics to occur; if the population density is below this threshold, large outbreaks are unlikely.[4] This is the earliest and most influential model in infectious disease epidemiology.

Measles Modeling (1970s)

During the 1970s, significant advancements in modeling were made in response to measles outbreaks. Researchers used mathematical models to evaluate the impact of vaccination on measles transmission, helping to guide immunization programs. These models demonstrated that high vaccination coverage could lead to herd immunity and the eventual elimination of measles.

HIV/AIDS Epidemic and Modeling (1980s)

The emergence of the human immunodeficiency virus/acquired immunodeficiency syndrome (HIV/AIDS) epidemic in the 1980s led to a surge in modeling efforts to understand the disease's spread and evaluate the potential impact of various interventions, including vaccines. These models were instrumental in highlighting the importance of targeted vaccination strategies and identifying high-risk populations.

Polio Eradication Efforts (2000s)

In the early 2000s, modeling played a crucial role in the global polio eradication initiative. Models were used to assess the feasibility of eradicating polio, predict the outcomes of different vaccination strategies, and guide resource allocation. This period marked a significant shift toward more sophisticated models that incorporated a wide range of epidemiological, demographic, and behavioral factors. The rise of agent-based models (ABMs) represented a significant leap forward. ABMs simulate individual interactions and behaviors, providing a more granular view of disease spread and vaccination effects. These models have been used to study the impact of vaccination strategies on diseases such as influenza and coronavirus disease 2019 (COVID-19).

Recent Advances: COVID-19 Pandemic

The COVID-19 pandemic has underscored the importance of modeling in vaccinology like never before. Since the onset of the pandemic, models have been used extensively to predict the spread of severe acute respiratory syndrome coronavirus 2 (SARS-CoV-2), evaluate the effectiveness of different vaccines, and inform vaccination rollout strategies. Advanced modeling techniques, such as ABMs and machine learning (ML), have been employed to account for the complexity and uncertainty associated with the virus and its variants. The integration of real-time data and ML techniques into vaccine modeling has enhanced the ability to predict and respond to emerging infectious diseases. The COVID-19 pandemic showcased the critical role of modeling in guiding public health responses and vaccine development efforts.

TYPES OF MODELS USED IN VACCINE IMPACT ASSESSMENT

In vaccine impact assessment, *compartmental models* are fundamental tools that help researchers and policymakers understand the dynamics of infectious diseases and the potential effects of vaccination strategies. These models categorize the population into distinct compartments, each representing a specific state related to the disease. By tracking the flow of individuals between these compartments, they provide insights into how diseases spread and how vaccines can alter these dynamics.

Susceptible-infected-recovered Model

The SIR model is one of the simplest and most widely used compartmental models. It divides the population into three compartments:

1. *Susceptible (S):* Individuals who are not yet infected but are at risk of contracting the disease.
2. *Infectious (I):* Individuals who are infected and capable of transmitting the disease to susceptible individuals.
3. *Recovered (R):* Individuals who have recovered from the disease and are assumed to have immunity, thus cannot be infected again.

Transition rates: The transitions between these compartments are governed by two parameters: (1) the transmission rate (β) and (2) the recovery rate (γ). Individuals move from the susceptible compartment to the infectious compartment at a rate proportional to the number of contacts between susceptible and infectious individuals. This is often modeled using the transmission rate (β) and the number of contacts. The rate of moving from infectious to recovered is defined by the recovery rate (γ).

The SIR model is particularly useful for diseases that confer long-term immunity after infection, such as measles or chickenpox.

The model is described by the following differential equations:

$$dS/dt = -\beta SI/N$$
$$dI/dt = \beta SI/N - \gamma I$$
$$dR/dt = \gamma I$$

Here, N is the total population, and β and γ are the transmission and recovery rates, respectively.

Applications in Vaccinology

- By introducing a vaccination compartment (V) where individuals transition from susceptible to vaccinated, the SIR model can be extended to assess the impact of vaccination programs. This allows the model to simulate the reduction in the number of susceptible individuals and, consequently, the decrease in the disease's spread. This helps estimate how vaccination affects disease prevalence and herd immunity.
- The model is used to calculate the basic reproduction number (Ro) and assess the required vaccination coverage to achieve herd immunity.

Susceptible-exposed-infectious-recovered Model

The susceptible-exposed-infectious-recovered (SEIR) model adds an additional compartment to the SIR model to account for individuals who are exposed to the disease but not yet infectious. This is particularly useful for diseases with an incubation period where individuals are not immediately infectious after exposure. The compartments are:

- *Susceptible (S):* Individuals who are not infected and can contract the disease.
- *Exposed (E):* Individuals who have been exposed to the disease but are not yet infectious. This compartment accounts for the incubation period.
- *Infectious (I):* Individuals who are infected and capable of transmitting the disease to susceptible individuals.
- *Recovered (R):* Individuals who have recovered from the disease and are assumed to have immunity.

Transition rates: Individuals move from susceptible to exposed at a rate determined by the transmission rate (β). They then progress from exposed to infectious at a rate defined by the inverse of the incubation period. Finally, they recover at a rate defined by the recovery rate (γ).

The SEIR model is described by:

$$dS/dt = -\beta SI/N$$
$$dE/dt = \beta SI/N - \sigma E$$
$$dI/dt = \sigma E - \gamma I$$
$$dR/dt = \gamma I$$

Here, σ is the rate at which exposed individuals become infectious, and β and γ are the transmission and recovery rates, respectively.

Applications in Vaccinology

- The SEIR model is especially useful for diseases with a significant incubation period, such as influenza and COVID-19. It provides a more accurate representation of disease dynamics and helps in planning vaccination strategies that account for delayed infection.
- Like the SIR model, the SEIR model can be extended to include vaccination, allowing for the evaluation of how vaccines affect each stage of the disease progression and overall transmission dynamics.

Deterministic versus Stochastic Models

Deterministic Models

Deterministic models operate on the principle that given a set of initial conditions and parameters, the outcome is predictable and consistent. These models use fixed mathematical equations to describe how different variables interact over time.

Characteristics

- *Predictability:* Given the same initial conditions and parameters, deterministic models always produce the same results. There is no randomness in the system.
- *Simplicity:* These models often involve simpler equations and are easier to analyze. They can provide clear insights into the average behavior of a system.
- *Equations:* The behavior of the system is described by differential equations or algebraic equations, such as those in the SIR or SEIR models.

Applications in Vaccinology

- Deterministic models are used to understand the average behaviors of disease spread and the impact of vaccination strategies. They are particularly useful for studying large populations where individual variability has a minimal effect on overall outcomes.
- These models help estimate the level of vaccination coverage needed to achieve herd immunity by solving equations that describe the transmission dynamics and vaccination impacts.

Limitations

- *Lack of variability:* Deterministic models do not account for the inherent variability and randomness, such as differences in individual behaviors or random events.
- *Assumptions:* They often rely on simplifying assumptions that may not capture the complexities of actual disease dynamics.

Stochastic Models

Stochastic models incorporate randomness and variability into the system. Instead of providing a single, fixed outcome, these models account for the inherent uncertainty and unpredictability in the system.

Characteristics

- *Randomness:* Stochastic models include random variables and processes, which means that the same initial conditions can lead to different outcomes in different simulations.
- *Complexity:* These models are often more complex and computationally intensive, as they require simulating numerous possible outcomes to understand the range of possible behaviors.
- *Equations:* The behaviors of the system are described using probabilistic methods, such as stochastic differential equations.

Applications in Vaccinology

- Stochastic models are useful for simulating disease outbreaks and assessing the impact of vaccination

strategies in real-world scenarios where random events and individual variations play a significant role.
- They account for variability in individual behaviors, contact patterns, and transmission rates, providing a more nuanced understanding of disease dynamics.

Limitations

- *Computational intensity:* Stochastic models can be computationally demanding and require extensive simulations to obtain reliable results.
- *Interpretation:* The outcomes are probabilistic, making it more challenging to interpret results and draw definitive conclusions.

Agent-based Models

Agent-based models simulate individual entities, or "agents," that interact with each other and their environment according to specified rules. Each agent represents a distinct unit, such as a person, and can have its own characteristics and behaviors.

Characteristics

- *Individual simulation:* ABMs model each agent separately, allowing for a detailed representation of interactions and behaviors within a population.
- *Rule-based interaction:* Agents follow specific rules or behaviors that dictate their interactions with other agents and their environment. These rules can change over time or be influenced by the state of the system.
- *Emergent behavior:* The collective behavior of the system emerges from the interactions of individual agents. This allows ABMs to capture complex patterns and dynamics that are difficult to model with simpler approaches.

Applications in Vaccinology

- ABMs can simulate how individuals in a population respond to vaccination campaigns, including variations in vaccine uptake, social interactions, and compliance with health guidelines.
- They provide insights into how individual behaviors and social networks affect disease spread and vaccination impact. For example, ABMs can model how people with different levels of vaccine acceptance might influence overall vaccination coverage and disease dynamics.
- ABMs allow researchers to test different vaccination strategies and public health policies in a virtual environment before implementing them in the real world.

Limitations

- *Complexity and computation:* ABMs can be computationally intensive, especially for large populations or detailed simulations. They require careful calibration and validation to ensure accuracy.
- *Data requirements:* Accurate modeling requires detailed data on individual behaviors, interactions, and network structures, which may not always be available.
- *Stochastic and deterministic models* provide different perspectives on disease dynamics and vaccine impact, with stochastic models capturing the variability and randomness inherent in real-world systems, and deterministic models offering clear, predictable insights based on fixed parameters. *ABMs* add another layer of detail by simulating individual entities and their interactions, allowing for a nuanced understanding of complex systems. Each approach has its strengths and limitations, and often, a combination of these models is used to provide a comprehensive view of vaccine impact and disease dynamics.

Dynamic versus Static Models

Dynamic Models

Dynamic models account for changes over time. They incorporate temporal variations and allow for the study of how a system evolves and responds to different factors, such as vaccination programs, changes in disease transmission, or shifts in population demographics.

Characteristics

- *Time dependence:* Dynamic models explicitly include time as a variable, meaning that they describe how the state of the system changes over time. This allows for the analysis of temporal dynamics such as outbreaks, disease progression, and the impact of interventions.
- *Differential equations:* These models often use differential equations to represent the rates at which individuals move between different states (e.g., susceptible, infected, and recovered) over time. For example, in the SIR model, differential equations describe how the number of susceptible, infectious, and recovered individuals change with time.
- *Feedback mechanisms:* Dynamic models can incorporate feedback mechanisms where changes in one part of the system affect other parts. For instance, increasing vaccination coverage might reduce disease incidence, which in turn reduces transmission rates.

Applications in Vaccinology

- Dynamic models are used to predict the course of epidemics and the impact of vaccination programs

over time. They can simulate how different vaccination rates or strategies might influence disease spread and overall public health.
- These models help to evaluate the effectiveness of various public health interventions by showing how changes in vaccination policies or disease control measures to affect disease dynamics over time.
- Dynamic models can estimate how vaccination coverage needs to change over time to maintain herd immunity and prevent outbreaks.

Examples:
- *SIR and SEIR models:* These models dynamically track the progression of diseases and the effects of vaccination over time, allowing researchers to simulate how epidemics evolve and assess the impact of vaccination strategies.
- *Agent-based models:* When used in a dynamic context, these models simulate how individuals interact over time, incorporating changes in behavior and vaccination uptake to observe long-term effects on disease dynamics.

Static Models

Static models do not account for changes over time. They provide a snapshot of the system at a particular point in time and assume that the parameters and states remain constant. These models are useful for understanding equilibrium or steady-state conditions rather than temporal dynamics.

Characteristics

- *Time independence:* Static models assume that the system does not change with time. They provide a static view of the system, focusing on the relationships between variables at a specific moment.
- *Algebraic equations:* These models typically use algebraic equations to describe the relationships between different variables without considering how these relationships evolve over time.
- *Equilibrium analysis:* Static models are often used to analyze equilibrium conditions, where the rates of change are balanced, and the system is in a steady state.

Applications in Vaccinology

- Static models can be used to estimate the necessary vaccination coverage to achieve herd immunity before an epidemic occurs, based on a snapshot of current population dynamics and disease transmission rates.
- These models help to assess the cost-effectiveness of vaccination programs by evaluating outcomes such as disease incidence and healthcare costs under various static scenarios.
- Static models can analyze different hypothetical scenarios and their immediate impact without considering how these scenarios might change over time.

Examples:
- Static models are used to calculate the basic reproduction number (R0), which represents the average number of secondary infections produced by a single infectious individual in a fully susceptible population. This calculation helps to determine the level of vaccination needed to prevent outbreaks.
- These models are useful in cross-sectional studies where data is collected at a single point in time to understand the prevalence of disease and vaccination coverage.

Usually, the best model for an outbreak is developed only after the outbreak has happened, as it relies on real-world data from the event.[5,6]

APPLICATIONS OF MODELING IN VACCINE IMPACT ASSESSMENT

Predicting Vaccine Efficacy

To predict the effectiveness of new vaccines before they deployed widely, models use data from clinical trials, such as vaccine efficacy rates and adverse effects, to simulate how the vaccine will perform in larger populations.
- *Compartmental models:* Such as SIR or SEIR models, simulate disease dynamics and incorporate vaccine efficacy to predict reductions in disease incidence.
- *Stochastic models:* These include randomness to account for variability in vaccine responses and disease transmission.
- *Agent-based models:* Simulate individual interactions and behaviors, allowing for detailed predictions of vaccine impact based on real-world scenarios.
    - Different levels of vaccine coverage and efficacy are tested to predict the overall impact on disease spread and public health outcomes.
    - Include estimated reductions in disease cases, potential changes in transmission rates, and projected healthcare cost savings.

Applications

- Inform decisions about broader deployment based on trial results
- Provide insights into how effective the vaccine will be under various real-world conditions.

Determining Herd Immunity Thresholds

To calculate the proportion of the population that needs to be vaccinated to achieve herd immunity and prevent disease spread. Models use:

- *Basic reproduction number (R0): R_0* is the average number of people that a single infected person will infect in a completely susceptible population (i.e., a population where no one has immunity to the disease).
- *Herd immunity threshold (p) calculation: p* represents the proportion of the population that needs to be immune (typically through vaccination) to stop the spread of the disease. The formula to calculate this threshold is:

$$p = [1 - \{1\}/\{R_0\}]$$

Where, p = herd immunity threshold and R_0 = basic reproduction number.

Higher R_0 values indicate more contagious diseases, requiring a higher proportion of the population to be immune to achieve herd immunity.

- *Dynamic models:* Adjust for varying transmission rates, population mobility, and other factors.
- Models incorporate vaccine efficacy to determine the effective coverage needed to achieve herd immunity, accounting for partial vaccine protection.

Applications

- Guide vaccination campaigns to ensure adequate coverage
- Help in planning responses to outbreaks and assessing the effectiveness of vaccination programs

Resource Allocation

To determine the optimal distribution of vaccines in different regions, especially during shortages or emergencies.

- Models estimate vaccine needs based on population size, disease prevalence, and transmission dynamics.
- *Geographic distribution*:
  - Analyze disease spread and vaccination coverage across different regions to prioritize areas with higher disease risk or lower vaccine coverage
  - Evaluate the most cost-effective distribution strategies, considering factors such as logistics, population density, and healthcare infrastructure
- Simulate different allocation strategies to determine their impact on disease reduction and resource utilization.

Applications

- Guide vaccine distribution during outbreaks or pandemics
- Ensure that vaccines are allocated to underserved or high-risk populations effectively

Policy Development

To assist policymakers in designing and evaluating vaccination strategies and public health policies.

- Models simulate the impact of various vaccination strategies, such as phased rollouts, targeted vaccination of high-risk groups, and combination with other public health measures.
- *Impact assessment*:
  - Evaluate the economic and health outcomes of different policies
  - Assess how different strategies impact disease incidence, mortality rates, and overall public health
- Models help to identify the most effective strategies for achieving public health goals and inform decisions on vaccination schedules, coverage levels, and additional interventions.

Applications

- Develop and refine vaccination strategies based on predicted outcomes
- Provide evidence-based recommendations for vaccine mandates, funding, and public health initiatives

DATA REQUIREMENTS AND CHALLENGES

Accurate modeling in vaccine impact assessment relies on high-quality data across various domains. The data requirements and the challenges associated with collecting this data are as follows:

Data Inputs for Models

Epidemiological Data

Types of Data

- *Disease incidence and prevalence:* Information on the number of new and existing cases of the disease in different populations and regions.
- *Transmission rates:* Data on how frequently the disease spreads from one person to another, often represented by parameters like the basic reproduction number (R0).
- *Disease progression:* Information on the stages of disease (e.g., incubation period and infectious period) and how these vary across different populations.

Sources

- *Surveillance systems:* Public health databases and disease monitoring systems provide ongoing data on incidence and prevalence.

- *Historical data:* Past records and epidemiological studies offer insights into disease patterns and trends.

Vaccine Efficacy

Types of Data

- *Clinical trial results:* Data on how effective the vaccine is in preventing disease under controlled conditions, including efficacy rates and duration of protection.
- *Effectiveness:* Information on vaccine performance in general population settings, accounting for variations in adherence and exposure.

Sources

- *Clinical trials:* Phase I-III trials provide data on vaccine safety and efficacy.
- Ongoing studies and data collection post-approval offer insights into real-world effectiveness.

Population Demographics

Types of Data

- *Age distribution:* Information on the age structure of the population, as disease susceptibility and vaccine efficacy can vary with age.
- *Population density:* Data on how many people live in a given area, which affects disease transmission and vaccine distribution strategies.
- *Risk factors:* Data on factors such as comorbidities and socioeconomic status that influence disease risk and vaccine effectiveness.

Sources

- *Census data:* National and local population surveys provide demographic details.
- *Health surveys:* Data from health and lifestyle surveys offer information on risk factors and health behaviors.

Social Behavior Patterns

Types of Data

- *Vaccination coverage:* Information on the proportion of the population that has received the vaccine.
- *Behavioral patterns:* Data on social interactions, mobility, and contact patterns, which influence disease spread and vaccine uptake.
- *Compliance and attitudes:* Insights into public attitudes toward vaccination and compliance with health guidelines.

Sources

- *Surveys and polls:* Conducted to gauge public opinion and vaccination behaviors.
- *Contact tracing studies:* Provide data on interaction patterns and how they affect disease transmission.

Challenges in Data Collection

Data Availability

Challenges

- *Inconsistent reporting:* Variability in data reporting standards and practices across regions can lead to gaps or inconsistencies in available data.
- *Limited access:* Some regions or populations may lack comprehensive data collection systems, making it difficult to gather necessary information.

Solutions

- Implementing standardized data collection protocols can improve consistency.
- Encouraging collaboration and data sharing among organizations can enhance data availability.

Data Quality

Challenges

- *Accuracy issues:* Errors in data collection, reporting, or recording can compromise the quality of the data.
- *Incomplete data:* Missing data or incomplete records can lead to inaccuracies in model predictions.

Solutions

- Regularly validating data through cross-checks and quality control measures.
- Enhancing data collection methods and technologies to ensure accuracy and completeness.

Data Representativeness

Challenges

- *Sampling bias:* Data may not accurately represent the entire population if certain groups are underrepresented or if the sample is not randomly selected.
- *Cultural and regional differences:* Variations in disease dynamics, vaccine efficacy, and social behaviors across different regions can affect the generalizability of the data.

Solutions

- Ensuring that data collection encompasses a diverse range of population groups and regions
- Developing models that account for regional and cultural differences to improve relevance and accuracy

Data Integration

Challenges

- Combining data from different sources (e.g., clinical trials and surveillance systems) can be challenging due to differences in data formats and definitions.

- Keeping data up to date is crucial for accurate modeling, but timely updates can be difficult to manage.

Solutions

- Using data integration techniques and frameworks to standardize and merge data from various sources
- Implementing systems for continuous data collection and updating to maintain the relevance of the data

CASE STUDIES IN VACCINE MODELING

Eradication of Smallpox

The global eradication of smallpox, certified in 1980 by the World Health Organization (WHO), is a significant milestone in public health. This success was made possible by a global vaccination campaign that relied heavily on modeling to guide its strategies.

Modeling Techniques

- *Compartmental models (SIR models):* The SIR models were used to understand the dynamics of smallpox transmission. These models helped to estimate the basic reproduction number (R0) of smallpox and predict the spread of the disease under different scenarios.
- *Ring vaccination strategy:* Models demonstrated that a targeted approach, such as ring vaccination (vaccinating contacts and contacts of an infected person), could be more efficient than mass vaccination. This strategy minimized the number of vaccinations needed by focusing on high-risk groups and proved highly effective in containing outbreaks.

Strengths and Limitations of Modeling Techniques

- *Strengths:* The models used for smallpox eradication were relatively simple but effective in guiding decision making. They allowed for the rapid adjustment of strategies based on real-time data and demonstrated that targeted interventions could achieve high impact with limited resources.
- *Limitations:* The models required accurate data on case identification and transmission patterns. In regions with poor surveillance or reporting, the models' predictions could be less reliable. Also, SIR models did not account for spatial heterogeneity or population movements, which could affect transmission dynamics.

Control of Polio

Polio control and eradication efforts have been ongoing since the Global Polio Eradication Initiative (GPEI) was launched in 1988. Vaccine modeling has been essential in identifying the best strategies for interrupting transmission, especially in areas with persistent outbreaks.

Modeling Techniques

- *Agent-based models:* These models simulate the actions and interactions of individuals or agents to assess the impact of different vaccination strategies on polio transmission. ABMs have been particularly useful in understanding the complex dynamics in areas with varied population density, movement, and vaccine coverage.
- *Dynamic transmission models:* These models incorporate various factors, including immunity levels, birth rates, and seasonality, to predict polio spread and assess the impact of vaccination campaigns. They have been used to evaluate the effectiveness of oral polio vaccines (OPVs) versus inactivated polio vaccines (IPVs) in different settings.

Strengths and Limitations of Modeling Techniques

- *Strengths:* Agent-based and dynamic transmission models can capture complex population dynamics and provide more granular predictions, which is crucial for tailoring interventions in different regions. These models have helped to optimize vaccine allocation and scheduling of supplementary immunization activities (SIAs).
- *Limitations:* The complexity of these models requires substantial computational resources and detailed data, which may not always be available. Uncertainties in parameter estimates, such as vaccine efficacy and population immunity, can affect model outputs. Additionally, models might not fully account for unforeseen factors like political instability or public resistance to vaccination.

Global Strategy for COVID-19 Vaccination

The COVID-19 pandemic required an unprecedented global vaccination effort. Modeling played a vital role in guiding vaccine development, allocation, and distribution strategies. Early in the pandemic, models were used to predict the spread of the virus, estimate the impact of nonpharmaceutical interventions (NPIs), and evaluate vaccination strategies.

Modeling Techniques

- *Compartmental models (SEIR models):* Susceptible-exposed-infectious-recovered models were used to simulate COVID-19 transmission dynamics. These models included additional compartments (such as exposed) to reflect the latent period of the virus and were crucial in predicting the impact of different vaccination rates on epidemic curves.

- *Stochastic models:* These models incorporate randomness and are used to account for the variability in COVID-19 transmission. Stochastic models helped to assess the probability of different outcomes under varying levels of vaccination and public health measures, providing a range of possible scenarios rather than a single deterministic outcome.
- *Optimization models:* These models were used to optimize vaccine distribution and allocation strategies to maximize public health benefits, considering factors such as vaccine availability, logistics, and population prioritization (e.g., healthcare workers, elderly).

Strengths and Limitations of Modeling Techniques

- *Strengths:* SEIR and stochastic models provided valuable insights into the potential course of the pandemic and the impact of vaccination under different scenarios. They informed public health decisions on the timing and intensity of interventions and helped prioritize high-risk groups for vaccination. Optimization models facilitated efficient resource allocation and logistics planning.
- *Limitations:* The rapidly evolving nature of COVID-19, including the emergence of new variants and changing public behavior, presented challenges for modeling. Early models often had to be revised as more data became available, highlighting the need for flexibility and adaptive modeling approaches. The accuracy of predictions was also limited by uncertainties in key parameters, such as transmission rates, vaccine efficacy against variants, and duration of immunity.

The following lessons are learned from these case studies:

- *Adaptability and flexibility*: The success of vaccine modeling in these case studies highlights the importance of adaptable and flexible models that can be updated as new data and understanding emerge. In rapidly evolving situations, such as the COVID-19 pandemic, models need to be able to incorporate new information quickly.
- *Data quality and availability*: High-quality, timely data are critical for accurate modeling. The smallpox eradication campaign benefited from robust surveillance systems, while polio control efforts have sometimes been hindered by data gaps. COVID-19 models have similarly been affected by variations in data quality and reporting.
- *Targeted strategies*: Models have shown that targeted vaccination strategies, such as ring vaccination for smallpox and prioritization of high-risk groups for COVID-19, can be highly effective as compared to mass interventions. However, these strategies require accurate case identification and effective contact tracing.
- *Limitations of predictive accuracy*: While models can provide valuable insights, they are not infallible and should be used in conjunction with other decision-making tools. Uncertainties in model parameters and assumptions can lead to inaccuracies, underscoring the importance of interpreting model outputs with caution.
- *Importance of global coordination*: For diseases that require global action, like polio and COVID-19, models have underscored the need for coordinated international efforts and data sharing. The global strategy for smallpox eradication also demonstrated the value of a unified approach to vaccination campaigns.

MODELING VACCINE IMPACT IN LOW-RESOURCE SETTINGS

Modeling vaccine impact in low-resource settings involves adapting models to address specific challenges, such as limited healthcare infrastructure, varied vaccine delivery methods, and varied public health behavior. Here is a detailed exploration of how models can be adjusted for these settings:

Adapting Models for Limited Healthcare Infrastructure

Challenges

- Inadequate or incomplete data on disease incidence, vaccine coverage, and population demographics can hinder accurate modeling.
- Weak healthcare infrastructure may affect vaccine distribution, administration, and monitoring, influencing the effectiveness of vaccination programs.

Adaptations

- Use simpler models or hybrid approaches that require less detailed data but still provide valuable insights. For instance, compartmental models such as SIR or SEIR can be adjusted to focus on core parameters.
- Employ statistical techniques or use proxy data to estimate missing information. For example, use survey data to infer vaccine coverage rates or disease prevalence where direct data is lacking.
- Simulate various scenarios to understand the impact of infrastructure limitations on vaccine distribution and effectiveness. This helps to identify critical areas where interventions are needed.

For example:
GAVI Alliance: Models have been adapted to account for limited data and infrastructure in low-resource settings to guide vaccine introductions and optimize impact.

Accommodating Varying Vaccine Delivery Methods

Challenges

- Variability in vaccine delivery methods, such as mobile clinics, outreach programs, or fixed sites, can affect the reach and effectiveness of vaccination campaigns.
- Maintaining vaccine efficacy in regions with limited cold chain facilities can be challenging, impacting vaccine effectiveness.

Adaptations

- Incorporate different vaccine delivery methods into the models to assess their impact. For example, models can simulate the effectiveness of outreach programs versus fixed-site clinics in reaching remote populations.
- Include variables related to cold chain management in the models, such as storage conditions and transportation reliability, to estimate their impact on vaccine efficacy and coverage.
- Adjust models to account for variable vaccination schedules and campaign timing based on local logistics and resource availability.

For example:
Polio eradication campaigns: Models have been used to evaluate the effectiveness of different delivery strategies, including mass vaccination campaigns and targeted outreach in hard-to-reach areas.

Addressing Variability in Public Health Behavior

Challenges

- *Vaccine hesitancy:* Public attitudes toward vaccination may vary, affecting vaccine uptake and coverage.
- *Cultural and social factors:* Local customs, beliefs, and social structures can influence vaccine acceptance and administration.

Adaptations

- Include data on public attitudes, vaccine hesitancy, and cultural factors in the models. This helps in understanding how these factors might influence vaccine uptake and disease spread.
- Simulate the impact of tailored communication strategies and community engagement initiatives to improve vaccine acceptance and coverage.

For example:
HIV/AIDS programs: Models have been adapted to account for social and behavioral factors affecting healthcare utilization and vaccine uptake in different communities.

ETHICAL CONSIDERATIONS IN VACCINE MODELING

Modeling plays a crucial role in guiding public health decisions, but it also raises several ethical considerations, especially when decisions have significant impacts on public health.

Equity and Access

Models can influence decisions about vaccine allocation, which can affect equitable access to vaccines. There is a risk that models may prioritize certain populations over others, potentially exacerbating existing health disparities.

- *Inclusive data*: Ensure that models use data representative of diverse populations, including marginalized and underserved groups. This helps to make equitable recommendations and prevent biases.
- *Equitable allocation*: Use models to evaluate and promote fair vaccine distribution strategies, such as prioritizing high-risk groups or regions with limited access to healthcare. This helps ensure that vulnerable populations receive adequate protection.
- *Transparency*: Clearly communicate the criteria and assumptions used in models to stakeholders and the public, fostering trust and understanding about how decisions are made.

Example:
COVID-19 vaccination campaigns: Ethical frameworks and models were used to prioritize vaccine distribution to healthcare workers, high-risk individuals, and underserved communities to ensure equitable access.

Informed Consent and Public Engagement

Decisions based on models can affect public health interventions and policies, and it is crucial that affected populations are informed about how these decisions are made.

- *Public communication*: Engage with the public to explain the role of models in decision making and how model predictions influence public health policies.

This includes being transparent about uncertainties and limitations.
- *Stakeholder involvement*: Involve community representatives and stakeholders in the modeling process to ensure that diverse perspectives are considered and that policies reflect the needs and values of different groups.

Example:
Vaccination prioritization: In the early stages of vaccine rollouts, engaging with community leaders and the public to explain prioritization criteria helped to manage expectations and increase acceptance.

Model Assumptions and Uncertainties

Models rely on assumptions and can have inherent uncertainties. Decisions based on these models can have significant consequences, and it is important to address how these uncertainties are managed and communicated.
- *Transparent reporting*: Clearly communicate the assumptions, limitations, and uncertainties of models to policymakers and the public. This helps to ensure that decisions are made with a clear understanding of potential risks and limitations.
- *Adaptive strategies*: Implement adaptive strategies that allow for adjustments based on new data and emerging evidence. This helps to address uncertainties and improve decision making over time.

Example:
Smallpox eradication: Early models had to be updated as new data became available, highlighting the importance of flexibility and transparency in modeling assumptions.

Public Health versus Individual Rights

Public health models often aim to protect the broader community, which can sometimes conflict with individual rights, such as autonomy and privacy.
- *Proportionality*: Ensure that public health measures recommended by models are proportionate to the risk and benefit, balancing collective health benefits with individual rights.
- *Privacy*: Respect privacy when collecting and using data for modeling purposes. Implement robust data protection measures to safeguard individual information.

Example:
COVID-19 lockdowns and mandates: Decisions based on models led to public health measures that impacted individual freedoms. Ethical considerations included balancing the benefits of controlling the pandemic with respect for personal liberties.

Ethical Use of Model Predictions

Models can be misinterpreted or misused to justify decisions that may not align with ethical principles or public health goals.
- *Ethical oversight*: Establish ethical review processes to oversee the use and interpretation of models, ensuring that decisions are aligned with ethical standards and public health objectives.
- *Accountability*: Hold decision makers accountable for how model predictions are used, ensuring that they are applied responsibly and ethically.

Example:
Resource allocation: In situations of vaccine shortages, models can guide allocation decisions. Ethical oversight is needed to ensure that allocation prioritizes fairness and maximizes public health benefits.

Ethical considerations in vaccine modeling are critical for ensuring that public health decisions are made with fairness, transparency, and respect for individual rights. Addressing issues of equity, informed consent, model assumptions, and the balance between public health and individual rights helps to guide ethical decision making and fosters trust in public health interventions.

FUTURE DIRECTIONS IN VACCINE MODELING

Advancements in Technology

Advancements in computational power and data science are significantly enhancing vaccine modeling capabilities, making it possible to achieve more accurate, detailed, and timely insights into vaccine effectiveness and disease dynamics.

Increased Computational Power

High-performance Computing

- *Complex simulations*: High-performance computing (HPC) resources, including powerful supercomputers and clusters, allow for the execution of complex models that simulate detailed interactions within large populations. This includes capturing the nuances of disease spread, vaccine impact, and the effects of various intervention strategies.
- *Speed and efficiency*: HPC accelerates the processing of large datasets and complex algorithms, which improves the speed of simulations and the ability to run multiple scenarios or sensitivity analyses quickly. This is critical for real-time decision making and rapid response to emerging public health threats.

Cloud Computing

- *Scalability and flexibility*: Cloud-based platforms provide on-demand access to scalable computing resources. Researchers can expand or contract their computational capabilities based on the needs of their models, without investing in physical infrastructure. This flexibility supports large-scale data analysis and complex simulations.

- *Collaboration and accessibility*: Cloud computing facilitates collaboration among researchers and public health officials by providing centralized access to models and data. This enhances the ability to share insights and coordinate responses across different locations and organizations.

Graphics Processing Units

Parallel processing: Graphics processing units (GPUs) are designed for parallel processing and are particularly effective at handling large-scale computations. They are used to accelerate the training of ML models and run complex simulations, reducing the time required for data processing and analysis.

Example: During the COVID-19 pandemic, HPC and cloud computing were extensively used to model virus transmission and vaccine impact, enabling quick updates and scenario analyses as new data emerged.

Advancements in Data Science

Big Data Integration

Diverse data sources: Modern data science techniques enable the integration of diverse datasets, including electronic health records, real-time surveillance data, social media, and demographic information. This comprehensive approach enhances the accuracy and relevance of models by incorporating a wide range of variables and trends.

Real-time analytics: Advanced analytics tools allow for the real-time processing of data, enabling models to be continuously updated with the latest information. This dynamic capability supports timely decision making and adaptive responses to changing conditions.

Machine Learning and Artificial Intelligence

- Machine learning algorithms can identify patterns and trends within large datasets that may not be apparent through traditional statistical methods. This improves the accuracy of predictions regarding disease spread, vaccine efficacy, and public health interventions.
- Artificial intelligence (AI) can help to develop adaptive models that adjust predictions and strategies based on new data and evolving trends. This enhances the ability to respond to emerging challenges and refine vaccination strategies.

Advanced statistical methods: Advanced statistical methods and tools, such as Bayesian inference and ensemble methods, enhance model accuracy by providing sophisticated approaches to parameter estimation and uncertainty quantification.

Example:
Flu vaccine development: Data science techniques, including ML, are used to analyze influenza strain data, predict vaccine effectiveness, and optimize vaccine formulation based on genetic variations and historical data.

Integration of Genomic and Omics Data

Genomic Data

- *Tracking variants*: Incorporating genomic data allows models to track viral mutations and assess their impact on vaccine effectiveness. This helps in adapting vaccines to new strains and understanding how genetic variations affect vaccine response.
- *Personalized approaches*: Genomic data can be used to develop personalized vaccination strategies; tailoring vaccines based on individual genetic profiles to improve efficacy and minimize adverse effects.

Omics Data

Systems biology insights: Omics technologies (e.g., proteomics and metabolomics) provide insights into the molecular mechanisms of immune responses. Integrating this data into models helps in understanding how vaccines interact with the immune system and optimizing vaccine design.

Example:
Personalized vaccines: Research integrating omics data with vaccine models aims to develop personalized vaccine approaches, enhancing effectiveness by considering individual genetic and biological factors.

Integrating Artificial Intelligence in Vaccine Modeling

Artificial intelligence and ML are increasingly playing pivotal roles in enhancing vaccine modeling through improved accuracy and predictive power.

Enhanced Predictive Accuracy

Pattern Recognition

- AI and ML algorithms excel at recognizing complex patterns in large datasets that traditional statistical methods might miss. This helps in understanding intricate disease dynamics and vaccine responses by uncovering subtle correlations and trends.
- Machine learning models, such as neural networks and ensemble methods, can refine predictions based

on historical data and emerging patterns. This leads to more precise forecasts of disease spread, vaccine efficacy, and the impact of vaccination strategies.

Adaptive Learning

- AI-driven models can continuously learn and adapt from new data. As real-time information becomes available, these models update their predictions, improving their accuracy over time and allowing for rapid adjustments in public health strategies.
- AI models can simulate various scenarios and outcomes more effectively by learning from past data and adjusting predictions based on new variables or changing conditions.

Example: During the COVID-19 pandemic, ML models were used to predict infection rates, assess the impact of public health measures, and evaluate vaccine effectiveness. These models adapted to new data on virus variants and vaccination coverage, providing valuable insights for policymakers.

Personalized Vaccine Strategies

Individual Risk Assessment

- AI can integrate diverse data sources, such as genetic information, health records, and lifestyle factors, to assess individual risk profiles. This allows for the development of personalized vaccination strategies tailored to an individual's specific health risks and conditions.
- Machine learning algorithms can predict how individuals with different risk factors might respond to vaccines. This includes forecasting potential adverse reactions and optimizing vaccine dosages or schedules based on individual characteristics.

Tailored Vaccination Plans

- By analyzing individual health data, AI can recommend personalized vaccination plans. For instance, it can suggest different vaccine types or schedules based on genetic predispositions or preexisting health conditions.
- Personalized approaches aim to increase vaccine efficacy by addressing specific risk factors and optimizing the vaccine's impact on different population segments. This can lead to better health outcomes and more efficient use of resources.

CONCLUSION

Summary of Key Points

Modeling is a fundamental tool in the field of vaccinology, playing a critical role in assessing and predicting the impact of vaccines.

Predicting Vaccine Efficacy and Impact

Simulation of Disease Dynamics

- *Forecasting outcomes:* Models simulate how diseases spread and how vaccines will perform under various scenarios. By projecting these outcomes, they provide estimates of vaccine efficacy and how different vaccination strategies might influence disease prevalence.
- *Understanding interventions:* Models help to evaluate the potential impact of different interventions, such as mass vaccination campaigns or targeted vaccination strategies. They predict how these interventions will alter disease dynamics and reduce incidence.

Example:
COVID-19 pandemic: During the pandemic, models were used to predict how different vaccination rates and strategies would affect infection rates, hospitalizations, and deaths. This informed decisions on vaccine rollout and public health measures.

Determining Herd Immunity Thresholds

Coverage Needs

- *Herd immunity:* Models calculate the proportion of the population that needs to be vaccinated to achieve herd immunity. This is essential for preventing disease outbreaks and protecting vulnerable individuals who cannot be vaccinated themselves.
- *Dynamic adjustments:* They also help to adjust these thresholds based on emerging data, such as the introduction of new variants or changes in vaccine efficacy.

Example:
Measles control: Models have been used to determine the vaccination coverage needed to maintain herd immunity against measles, guiding public health efforts to prevent outbreaks and ensure community protection.

Optimizing Resource Allocation

Efficient Use of Vaccines

- *Strategic deployment:* Models help to determine how to allocate limited vaccine supplies most effectively. This includes deciding which populations to prioritize, such as high-risk groups or areas with high transmission rates.
- *Cost-effectiveness:* They also assist in evaluating the cost-effectiveness of different vaccination strategies, ensuring that resources are used efficiently to maximize public health benefits.

Example:
Polio eradication: During the global polio eradication efforts, models were used to prioritize vaccination efforts

in regions with the highest risk of outbreaks, ensuring that resources were allocated to where they would have the most impact.

Guiding Policy Development

Informed Decision-making

- *Simulating scenarios:* Models allow policymakers to simulate various vaccination strategies and their potential outcomes. This helps in evaluating the effectiveness of different approaches and making informed decisions about public health policies.
- *Scenario analysis:* They provide insights into the potential consequences of policy decisions, such as changes in vaccination schedules or the introduction of new vaccines.

Example:
Vaccination mandates: Models have been used to assess the impact of vaccination mandates in schools or workplaces, guiding policies that aim to increase vaccination coverage and protect public health.

Addressing Ethical and Equity Considerations

Fair Distribution

- *Equity analysis:* Models can assess the equity of vaccine distribution strategies, ensuring that vaccines are accessible to all segments of the population, including underserved and marginalized groups.
- *Ethical guidelines:* They help in developing ethical guidelines for vaccine distribution, balancing public health benefits with individual rights and ensuring fair access.

Example:
COVID-19 vaccine equity: During the COVID-19 pandemic, models were used to evaluate the impact of different distribution strategies on vaccine equity, helping to address disparities and ensure fair access to vaccines across different communities.

Modeling is indispensable for understanding and predicting the impact of vaccines. It provides essential insights into vaccine efficacy, herd immunity thresholds, resource allocation, and policy development. By simulating disease dynamics and vaccination strategies, models help to guide public health decisions, optimize vaccine deployment, and ensure equitable access. As we face new and evolving public health challenges, the continued refinement and application of modeling will remain crucial in advancing vaccine strategies and protecting global health.

Call for Continued Research and Development

The need for ongoing research and development in vaccine modeling is crucial to ensure that models remain accurate, relevant, and effective as new vaccines and diseases emerge.

Adapting to Emerging Diseases

- *Rapid response*: Emerging infectious diseases, such as novel pathogens or variants, require the development of new models to predict their spread and assess potential vaccines. Research must focus on creating adaptable modeling frameworks that can quickly incorporate data on new diseases and provide timely predictions.
- *Early warning systems*: Models need to integrate real-time surveillance data to identify potential outbreaks and assess the effectiveness of emerging vaccines. This requires ongoing refinement of models to include new disease characteristics and transmission patterns.

Incorporating Advances in Vaccine Technology

- *New technologies*: The development of new vaccine technologies, such as mRNA vaccines and vector-based vaccines, requires updates to modeling approaches. Research should focus on integrating data specific to these new technologies to evaluate their effectiveness and optimize their use.
- *Personalized vaccines*: Advances in personalized medicine, including vaccines tailored to individual genetic profiles, necessitate the development of models that can predict individual responses and adjust vaccination strategies accordingly.

Enhancing Model Accuracy and Reliability

- *Advanced techniques*: Ongoing research should explore new algorithms and ML techniques to improve the accuracy and predictive power of models. This includes enhancing the ability to process and analyze large, complex datasets and refining statistical methods used in modeling.
- *Uncertainty handling*: Research must focus on better methods for quantifying and addressing uncertainties in models, providing more reliable predictions and helping policymakers make informed decisions.

Integrating Diverse Data Sources

- *Data integration*: Models need to incorporate a wide range of data sources, including electronic health records, genomic data, and real-time surveillance information. Research should focus on developing methods for integrating these data types into models to enhance their accuracy and relevance.

- *AI and ML*: Continued exploration of AI and ML can enhance models by identifying patterns and trends that traditional methods miss, providing more accurate predictions and insights.

Addressing Ethical and Equity Issues

- *Equitable access*: Research must address how models can better incorporate equity considerations to ensure fair vaccine distribution. This includes analyzing the impact of different distribution strategies on underserved and marginalized populations.
- *Ethical frameworks*: Developing ethical guidelines and frameworks for vaccine modeling ensures that models are used responsibly and that public health interventions uphold principles of equity and justice.

Enhancing Public Health Preparedness

Models should be continuously updated and refined to plan for potential future scenarios, including the emergence of new diseases and changes in vaccine technologies. This proactive approach enhances public health preparedness and response capabilities.

Ongoing research and development are essential to refine vaccine modeling and ensure its relevance in the face of new vaccines and emerging diseases. By focusing on adapting to new pathogens, incorporating advances in vaccine technology, enhancing model accuracy, integrating diverse data sources, addressing equity issues, and improving public health preparedness, researchers can ensure that vaccine models continue to provide valuable insights and guide effective public health interventions.

REFERENCES

1. LSHTM. Modelling and Economic Evaluation of Vaccines. [online] Available from https://www.lshtm.ac.uk/research/centres/centre-mathematical-modelling-infectious-diseases/vaccines [Last accessed March, 2025].
2. Dembek ZF, Chekol T, Wu A. Best practice assessment of disease modelling for infectious disease outbreaks. Epidemiol Infect. 2018;146(10):1207-15.
3. Kermack WO, McKendrick AG. A Contribution to the Mathematical Theory of Epidemics. Proceedings of The Royal Society A: Mathematical, Physical and Engineering Sciences. 1927;115(772):700-21.
4. Bacaër N. McKendrick and Kermack on epidemic modelling (1926–1927). In: A Short History of Mathematical Population Dynamics. London: Springer; 2011.
5. Shoman H, Karafillakis E, Rawaf S. The link between the West African Ebola outbreak and health systems in Guinea, Liberia and Sierra Leone: a systematic review. Global Health. 2017;13(1):1.
6. Sharareh N, S Sabounchi N, Sayama H, MacDonald R. The Ebola Crisis and the Corresponding Public Behavior: A System Dynamics Approach. PLoS Curr. 2016;8:ecurrents.outbreaks.23badd982187 0a002fa86bef6893c01d.

CHAPTER 10

Frontiers in Vaccine Technology: mRNA Vaccines

Abhishek Padhi, Praggya Mishra, Krupal J Joshi, Ashwini Agarwal

INTRODUCTION

Messenger RNA (mRNA) vaccines have emerged as a revolutionary technology in immunization, significantly impacting public health by providing an effective response to the COVID-19 pandemic. Unlike traditional vaccines, which often utilize inactivated or attenuated forms of pathogens, mRNA vaccines leverage a synthetic strand of mRNA to instruct cells to produce a target antigen, typically a viral protein that triggers an immune response. This approach offers several advantages, including faster development times, ease of modification in response to emerging viral variants, and a robust safety profile due to the absence of live virus components.[1]

The development of mRNA vaccine technology can be traced back to the early 1990s when researchers first explored the potential of mRNA as a therapeutic tool. However, early efforts were hampered by challenges such as the instability of mRNA molecules and their susceptibility to degradation by ribonucleases present in the body. These hurdles made it difficult to achieve efficient delivery and sustained expression of the target antigens, which are crucial for inducing a strong immune response.[1]

Significant advancements were made in the late 2010s with the development of lipid nanoparticles (LNPs) as delivery vehicles, which protect mRNA from enzymatic degradation and facilitate its uptake by cells. This breakthrough enabled the stabilization and effective delivery of mRNA, setting the stage for the successful deployment of mRNA vaccines during the COVID-19 pandemic.[2]

The COVID-19 pandemic highlighted the potential of mRNA vaccines to revolutionize vaccine development and deployment. The rapid development and emergency use authorization of the Pfizer-BioNTech (BNT162b2) and Moderna (mRNA-1273) vaccines within a year of the virus's emergence demonstrated the technology's speed and adaptability. Unlike traditional vaccine development, which often takes years, mRNA vaccines can be designed quickly once the genetic sequence of the target virus is known. This capability is particularly valuable in responding to emerging infectious diseases and variants, allowing for swift modifications to the vaccine composition without the need for extensive retooling of manufacturing processes.[2]

The mechanism of action for mRNA vaccines is based on delivering a piece of genetic code that instructs cells to produce a specific antigen. Once inside the body, the mRNA is taken up by cells, typically antigen-presenting cells (APCs), which use the host cell machinery to translate the mRNA into the encoded protein. This protein is then processed and displayed on the cell surface, where it is recognized by the immune system, prompting the activation of both humoral and cellular immune responses. This process not only generates antibodies against the pathogen but also activates T cells, providing a comprehensive immune defense that includes memory components to ensure long-lasting protection.[1]

Despite the remarkable success of mRNA vaccines against COVID-19, challenges remain, particularly regarding their storage and distribution. The inherent instability of mRNA requires storage at ultra-low temperatures, which poses logistical challenges, especially in low-resource settings. However, ongoing research aims to improve the thermal stability of mRNA vaccines, potentially allowing for storage at standard refrigeration temperatures, which would greatly enhance their accessibility and ease of distribution globally.[1,2]

In conclusion, mRNA vaccines represent a paradigm shift in vaccine technology, offering rapid development, adaptability, and a favorable safety profile. As research continues to address the remaining challenges, such as stability and delivery, mRNA vaccines are poised to play a central role in future pandemic preparedness and in expanding the range of diseases that can be effectively targeted by vaccination strategies.

MECHANISM OF ACTION

The mechanism of mRNA vaccines revolves around the delivery of synthetic mRNA into host cells, where it serves as a template for producing a specific antigen that triggers an immune response. This process is distinct from traditional vaccines, which often rely on using whole pathogens (live attenuated or inactivated) or protein subunits to stimulate immunity. mRNA vaccines provide a safer and more versatile approach by leveraging the body's cellular machinery to produce the desired antigen internally, thereby initiating a natural immune process.[1,2]

Step-by-step Mechanism

1. *Introduction and uptake*: Upon administration via intramuscular injection, the mRNA vaccine, encapsulated in LNPs, enters the body. LNPs are crucial as they protect the mRNA from enzymatic degradation in the extracellular environment and facilitate its uptake by cells, particularly APCs such as dendritic cells and macrophages. The LNPs fuse with the cell membrane, allowing the encapsulated mRNA to enter the cytoplasm of the host cell.
2. *Translation and protein synthesis*: Once inside the cytoplasm, the host cell's ribosomes read the mRNA sequence and translate it into a protein. This protein is typically a spike protein from a virus, such as the SARS-CoV-2 spike protein used in COVID-19 vaccines.[3] The synthetic mRNA is designed to resemble naturally occurring mRNA, including modifications to the cap and poly-A tail, which stabilize the mRNA and enhance its translation efficiency. This process bypasses the nucleus, so the mRNA does not integrate into the host genome, ensuring safety and mitigating concerns over potential genomic alterations.[4]
3. *Immune system activation*: The newly synthesized viral protein (antigen) is then processed by the cell and presented on its surface via major histocompatibility complex (MHC) molecules. APCs present these antigens on MHC class I or II molecules, depending on the pathway. MHC class I presentation primarily activates cytotoxic T cells (CD8+ T cells), which can destroy infected cells, while MHC class II presentation activates helper T cells (CD4+ T cells) and induces B-cell maturation. This dual pathway stimulation ensures a robust cellular and humoral immune response.[4]
4. *Antibody production and memory cell formation*: The antigen presentation stimulates B cells to differentiate into plasma cells that produce antibodies specific to the viral protein. These antibodies can neutralize the virus by binding to it and preventing its entry into host cells. Simultaneously, helper T cells release cytokines that further enhance the immune response by promoting the differentiation of more B cells and cytotoxic T cells. Importantly, the immune system also forms memory B and T cells that remain in the body long term, providing durable immunity and a rapid response if the body is exposed to the actual pathogen in the future.[4,5]
5. *Advantages of mRNA-based mechanisms*: This approach mimics a natural infection more closely than traditional vaccines, as the antigen is produced inside the host cells, similar to a viral infection. This intracellular antigen production is vital for activating cytotoxic T lymphocytes, which are essential for clearing infected cells and providing long-term immunity. The flexibility of mRNA vaccines also allows for the rapid adjustment of the encoded antigen, which is particularly beneficial in responding to emerging variants of viruses such as SARS-CoV-2.[2]
6. *Immune system modulation and safety considerations*: Unlike traditional vaccines that use inactivated pathogens or subunit proteins, mRNA vaccines do not pose a risk of causing disease, as they do not use live components. Furthermore, mRNA vaccines are nonreplicating and do not alter the host's DNA, as the mRNA does not enter the nucleus. This ensures a high safety profile while still achieving strong immunogenicity. However, ongoing studies aim to refine the vaccine formulations to minimize any potential adverse effects and optimize the immune responses generated.[4]
7. *Challenges and future directions*: While the fundamental mechanism of mRNA vaccines provides several advantages, challenges remain, particularly concerning the stability and storage requirements of mRNA. mRNA is inherently unstable and requires cold-chain logistics, typically ultra-cold temperatures, to maintain its integrity. Research is underway to improve the thermal stability of mRNA vaccines, enabling more accessible global distribution, especially in low-resource settings.

ADVANTAGES OVER TRADITIONAL VACCINES

Messenger RNA vaccines offer several distinct advantages over conventional vaccine platforms. Firstly, they do not require the use of live pathogens or inactivated viruses, which significantly reduces the risks associated with infection and contamination during the manufacturing process. This safety feature is a major benefit as it eliminates the possibility of the vaccine causing disease in the recipient, a concern that sometimes arises with live-attenuated vaccines.

Secondly, mRNA vaccines can be designed and produced much more rapidly than traditional vaccines.

The production process for mRNA vaccines involves synthesizing a strand of mRNA that encodes a specific antigen, which can be achieved relatively quickly once the genetic sequence of the pathogen is known. This rapid development capability is especially crucial in responding to emerging infectious diseases, as demonstrated by the COVID-19 pandemic. The mRNA vaccines developed by Pfizer-BioNTech and Moderna were authorized for emergency use within a year of the virus's emergence, showcasing the technology's speed and flexibility in addressing public health crises.[6]

Moreover, mRNA vaccines can be easily modified to address viral mutations or new strains. This adaptability is particularly valuable in the context of rapidly evolving pathogens, such as influenza or coronaviruses, where frequent changes in the virus can render existing vaccines less effective. The ability to quickly update the vaccine composition without the need for developing new production processes allows for a more responsive and dynamic approach to vaccination campaigns.[7]

Another advantage is that mRNA vaccines do not require adjuvants, which are substances added to some vaccines to enhance the immune response. The mRNA in these vaccines naturally stimulates the immune system, reducing the need for additional components that could potentially cause adverse reactions. This simplicity in formulation further contributes to the overall safety and efficacy profile of mRNA vaccines.[7]

Finally, the production of mRNA vaccines does not rely on cell cultures or eggs, which are common substrates for traditional vaccine production. This difference not only streamlines the manufacturing process but also avoids issues related to allergies and cross-contamination. The use of a cell-free production system also simplifies scaling up manufacturing, making it easier to meet global demand in a pandemic setting.[7,8]

These advantages collectively position mRNA vaccines as a revolutionary technology in the field of immunization, offering a safer, faster, and more adaptable solution to preventing infectious diseases. As research and development continue to improve mRNA technology, it is likely that these vaccines will play an increasingly prominent role in global vaccination strategies.[7,8]

RECENT TECHNOLOGICAL ADVANCES

Recent advances in mRNA technology have significantly enhanced the stability, delivery, and immunogenicity of mRNA vaccines, which have been pivotal to their successful deployment. A key innovation in this area has been the development of LNPs as a primary delivery system. LNPs protect the mRNA from degradation by enzymes in the extracellular environment and facilitate its uptake by cells, ensuring that the mRNA reaches the cytoplasm intact. This approach has been critical in improving the stability of mRNA vaccines and ensuring their efficient delivery into host cells, a necessary step for effective antigen presentation and immune activation.[9]

Lipid nanoparticles consist of a mixture of lipids that form a protective shell around the mRNA, shielding it from nucleases that would otherwise degrade the RNA before it reaches the target cells. This delivery system also enhances the endosomal escape of mRNA once it is taken up by the cells, allowing the mRNA to reach the ribosomes in the cytoplasm, where it is translated into the target protein antigen. The optimization of LNP formulations, including the ratio of lipids and the type of lipids used, has led to more effective delivery and reduced reactogenicity, further enhancing the safety profile of mRNA vaccines.[7,8]

In addition to LNPs, advances in self-amplifying RNA (saRNA) technologies have also been a focus of recent research. saRNA differs from conventional mRNA in that it not only encodes the antigen but also includes sequences that enable the RNA to replicate itself once inside the host cell. This replication mechanism allows a single strand of saRNA to produce many copies of itself, amplifying the production of the target antigen within the cell. As a result, saRNA can elicit a stronger immune response with lower doses compared to traditional mRNA vaccines.[8,10]

The use of saRNA can also reduce the amount of RNA required for vaccination, which is particularly advantageous in scaling up vaccine production and reducing costs. Furthermore, the ability to amplify RNA within cells helps generate a more robust and durable immune response, enhancing both the magnitude and duration of immunity. Research into optimizing saRNA constructs and delivery methods is ongoing, with a focus on maximizing the immunogenicity while minimizing potential side effects.[3]

These technological advancements, including LNPs and saRNA, represent significant steps forward in the field of mRNA vaccines. By improving the delivery and stability of mRNA, as well as enhancing the immune response, these innovations have expanded the potential applications of mRNA technology beyond infectious diseases to include cancer immunotherapy and other therapeutic areas.[11]

CHALLENGES AND LIMITATIONS

Despite their significant advantages and promise, mRNA vaccines face several challenges that need to be addressed to fully realize their potential. One of the primary challenges is the stability of mRNA molecules. mRNA is inherently unstable and prone to rapid degradation by ribonucleases in the environment and within the body. To preserve the integrity of the mRNA, these vaccines require storage at extremely low temperatures, typically between –80° and –20°C. This stringent cold chain requirement poses significant logistical challenges, especially in low-resource settings where access to ultra-cold storage facilities is limited. Efforts are currently underway to develop thermostable formulations that could be stored at higher temperatures, which would simplify distribution and expand access to these vaccines globally.[3]

Another limitation of mRNA vaccines is the ongoing evaluation of their long-term safety. While the safety profiles of mRNA vaccines such as those developed for COVID-19 (Pfizer-BioNTech and Moderna) have been generally favorable, with millions of doses administered worldwide, there are still concerns about rare but serious adverse effects. Reports of autoimmune responses, such as myocarditis (inflammation of the heart muscle), particularly in younger populations, have emerged. These incidents are rare and often resolve with appropriate treatment, but they highlight the need for continuous monitoring and research to understand the underlying mechanisms and long-term effects of mRNA vaccines fully.[11]

Additionally, the production and scalability of mRNA vaccines require access to specialized equipment and raw materials, such as LNPs for delivery and nucleotides for mRNA synthesis. This dependency can create bottlenecks in production, particularly during global surges in demand, as seen during the COVID-19 pandemic. Furthermore, intellectual property rights and manufacturing capacities are predominantly held by companies in high-income countries, which can limit the ability of low- and middle-income countries to produce these vaccines independently. Addressing these supply chain and equity issues is critical for ensuring broad and equitable access to mRNA vaccines worldwide.[11]

Moreover, the current generation of mRNA vaccines may need further optimization to enhance their immunogenicity across different populations and against various pathogens. This includes developing strategies to ensure robust and long-lasting immune responses, which may require booster doses or additional modifications to the mRNA sequence or delivery mechanisms. As the technology continues to evolve, ongoing research will be essential to refine these vaccines to maximize their effectiveness and safety across diverse global populations.[3]

In conclusion, while mRNA vaccines have demonstrated their revolutionary potential in rapidly addressing infectious diseases such as COVID-19, several challenges and limitations remain. Overcoming these hurdles will require concerted efforts in scientific research, logistical planning, and global cooperation to ensure that mRNA vaccines can be effectively and equitably deployed worldwide.

FUTURE DIRECTIONS

Looking to the future, mRNA vaccine technology is poised to extend its impact far beyond the realm of infectious diseases, with promising applications in cancer immunotherapy. In this context, mRNA can be engineered to produce tumor-specific antigens that trigger a targeted immune response against cancer cells. This approach leverages the body's own immune system to recognize and destroy cancerous cells, offering a personalized treatment strategy that could revolutionize cancer therapy. The adaptability of mRNA technology, which allows for rapid development and customization, is particularly valuable in creating vaccines tailored to the unique mutations present in individual tumors.[12]

Moreover, the inherent flexibility of mRNA technology positions it as an essential tool in pandemic preparedness and response. The COVID-19 pandemic has demonstrated the technology's capacity for rapid adaptation, enabling swift updates to vaccine formulations in response to emerging variants of concern. This capability is not only crucial for addressing current public health emergencies but also for preemptively developing vaccines against potential future pathogens. The platform's ability to be quickly modified and scaled up ensures that mRNA vaccines can be at the forefront of global efforts to mitigate the impact of pandemics.[5]

In addition to expanding the scope of mRNA vaccines, there is a growing emphasis on the global distribution and manufacturing of these vaccines. A critical aspect of this expansion is the establishment of mRNA vaccine production facilities in low- and middle-income countries. Such efforts aim to democratize access to this cutting-edge technology and reduce dependency on manufacturing hubs in high-income countries. The World Health Organization (WHO) and various private sector entities are actively working to build and support these facilities, addressing supply chain challenges and promoting geopolitical equity in vaccine distribution.[13]

The establishment of local manufacturing capabilities is expected to enhance regional pandemic preparedness, ensuring that vaccines can be produced and distributed rapidly in response to outbreaks. This approach also helps to mitigate the risks associated with global supply chain disruptions, which were evident during the early stages of the COVID-19 pandemic. By decentralizing production and fostering self-sufficiency in vaccine manufacturing, low- and middle-income countries can play a more active role in global health security.[13]

In parallel with these efforts, ongoing research is focused on overcoming the current limitations of mRNA vaccines, such as their need for ultra-cold storage and transport. Innovations aimed at improving the stability and thermal tolerance of mRNA vaccines could further broaden their accessibility, particularly in regions with limited cold chain infrastructure. Additionally, advancements in delivery systems and formulations will continue to enhance the efficacy and safety of mRNA vaccines, potentially reducing the need for booster doses and improving long-term immunity.[12,5]

In conclusion, the future of mRNA vaccine technology is bright, with potential applications extending beyond infectious diseases to areas such as cancer immunotherapy. The global expansion of manufacturing capabilities, coupled with continued research and innovation, will ensure that mRNA vaccines remain a pivotal tool in public health, capable of responding to both current and future challenges.

CONCLUSION

Messenger RNA vaccines signify a transformative leap in vaccine technology, providing a rapid, adaptable, and potentially safer alternative to conventional vaccines. The COVID-19 pandemic showcased the speed and effectiveness with which mRNA vaccines could be developed and deployed, highlighting their role in modern immunization strategies. Unlike traditional vaccines that often involve lengthy development times and complex production processes, mRNA vaccines offer a streamlined approach that can be quickly adjusted to target new pathogens and variants, making them invaluable tools for future pandemic preparedness and response.

Despite their many advantages, mRNA vaccines still face several challenges, including stability issues that necessitate ultra-cold storage and ongoing concerns about long-term safety and rare adverse effects. Addressing these challenges requires sustained investment in research and development to improve vaccine formulations, enhance delivery systems, and expand global manufacturing capabilities. Such efforts are crucial to ensuring that mRNA vaccines can be produced and distributed equitably worldwide, particularly in low- and middle-income countries where access to advanced healthcare technology is often limited.

Moreover, the potential applications of mRNA vaccines extend beyond infectious diseases. The technology's flexibility allows for its use in other areas, such as cancer immunotherapy, where mRNA can be tailored to produce tumor-specific antigens, opening new avenues for personalized medicine. As research continues to advance, the scope of mRNA vaccine technology will likely broaden, offering new solutions for a wide range of medical challenges.

In summary, mRNA vaccines have revolutionized the field of immunization by providing a versatile and powerful tool against both existing and emerging diseases. Continued innovation and global collaboration will be key to overcoming the current limitations of this technology and fully realizing its potential in protecting global health.

REFERENCES

1. Kairuz D, Samudh N, Ely A, Arbuthnot P, Bloom K. Advancing mRNA technologies for therapies and vaccines: An African context. Front Immunol. 2022;13:1018961.
2. Wilson B, Geetha KM. Lipid nanoparticles in the development of mRNA vaccines for COVID-19. J Drug Deliv Sci Technol. 2022;74:103553.
3. Parry PI, Lefringhausen A, Turni C, Neil CJ, Cosford R, Hudson NJ, et al. Spikeopathy: COVID-19 spike protein is pathogenic, from both virus and vaccine mRNA. Biomedicines. 2023;11(8):2287.
4. Alberts B, Johnson A, Lewis J, Raff M, Roberts K, Walter P. T cells and MHC proteins. In: Molecular Biology of the Cell. 4th ed. Garland Science; 2002.
5. Alberts B, Johnson A, Lewis J, Raff M, Roberts K, Walter P. B cells and antibodies. In: Molecular Biology of the Cell. 4th ed. Garland Science; 2002.
6. Al Fayez N, Nassar MS, Alshehri AA, Alnefaie MK, Almughem FA, Alshehri BY, et al. Recent advancement in mRNA vaccine development and applications. Pharmaceutics. 2023;15(7): 1972.
7. Chaudhary N, Weissman D, Whitehead KA. mRNA vaccines for infectious diseases: principles, delivery and clinical translation. Nat Rev Drug Discov. 2021;20(11):817-38.
8. Rosa SS, Prazeres DM, Azevedo AM, Marques MP. mRNA vaccines manufacturing: Challenges and bottlenecks. Vaccine. 2021;39(16): 2190-200.
9. Pardi N, Hogan MJ, Porter FW, Weissman D. mRNA vaccines—a new era in vaccinology. Nat Rev Drug Discov. 2018;17(4):261-79.
10. Blakney AK, Ip S, Geall AJ. An update on self-amplifying mRNA vaccine development. Vaccines. 2021;9(2):97.
11. Eftekhari Z, Zohrabi H, Oghalaie A, Ebrahimi T, Shariati FS, Behdani M, et al. Advancements and challenges in mRNA and ribonucleoprotein-based therapies: From delivery systems to clinical applications. Mol Ther Nucleic Acids. 2024;35(3):102313.
12. Shi Y, Shi M, Wang Y, You J. Progress and prospects of mRNA-based drugs in pre-clinical and clinical applications. Signal Transduct Target Ther. 2024;9(1):322.
13. World Health Organization. Establishment of a COVID-19 mRNA vaccine technology transfer hub to scale up global manufacturing. Geneva: WHO; 2021.

CHAPTER 11

Therapeutic Vaccines: Expanding the New Horizon

Vani Jayaraman, Radha A, Annarao Kulkarni

INTRODUCTION

Prophylactic vaccines prevent disease by introducing an antigen into a healthy individual, which triggers immunity for a specific disease. Advancements in technology and a deeper understanding of the human immune system have led to the development of therapeutic vaccines. A therapeutic vaccine helps to strengthen the immune system to preexisting illnesses such as cancer, precancerous lesions, autoimmune disorders (ADs), and chronic infections.

Thus, a therapeutic vaccine is designed to induce an immune response that treats disease progression in a patient already suffering from a disease or infected with an organism.

The difference between prophylactic and therapeutic vaccines lies in their application: Prophylactic vaccines are administered to healthy individuals while therapeutic vaccines are given as postexposure treatments and are generally well tolerated by patients.[1] Therapeutic vaccines intend to promote lasting antitumor memory, eliminate minimal residual disease, induce tumor regression, and minimize adverse reactions.[2]

The three types of therapeutic vaccines are:

1. Molecular-based vaccine (peptide/protein-based vaccine, DNA/RNA-based vaccine)
2. Vector-based vaccine (natural or genetically engineered bacteria, yeast, and fungi as carriers)
3. Cell-based vaccine (dendritic cell or genetically modified cell vaccine)[3]

The different types of therapeutic vaccines are depicted in **Figure 1**.

Vaccines can also be categorized, according to the disease into tumor-targeted vaccines, infectious disease-targeted vaccines, and chronic disease-targeted vaccines.

THERAPEUTIC CANCER VACCINE

The concept of cancer immunotherapy was first proposed by Dr William Coley in 1890. He discovered that patients with cancer would spontaneously regress from

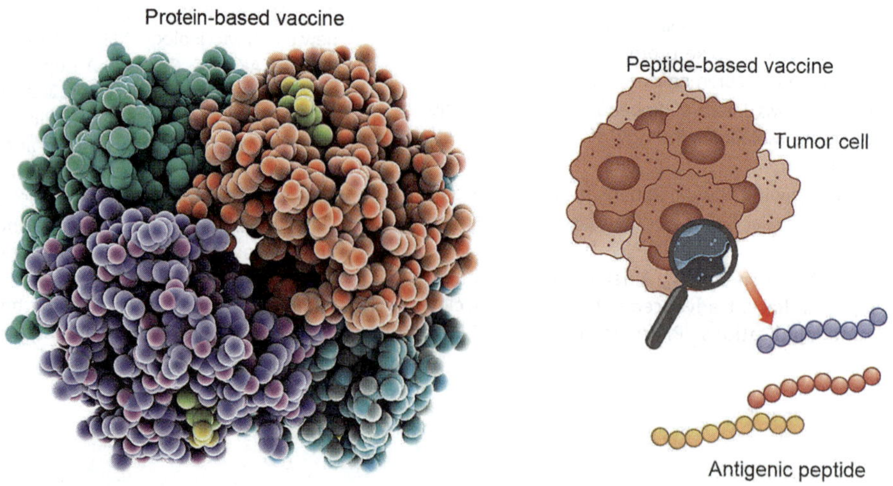

FIG. 1: *Continued*

Continued

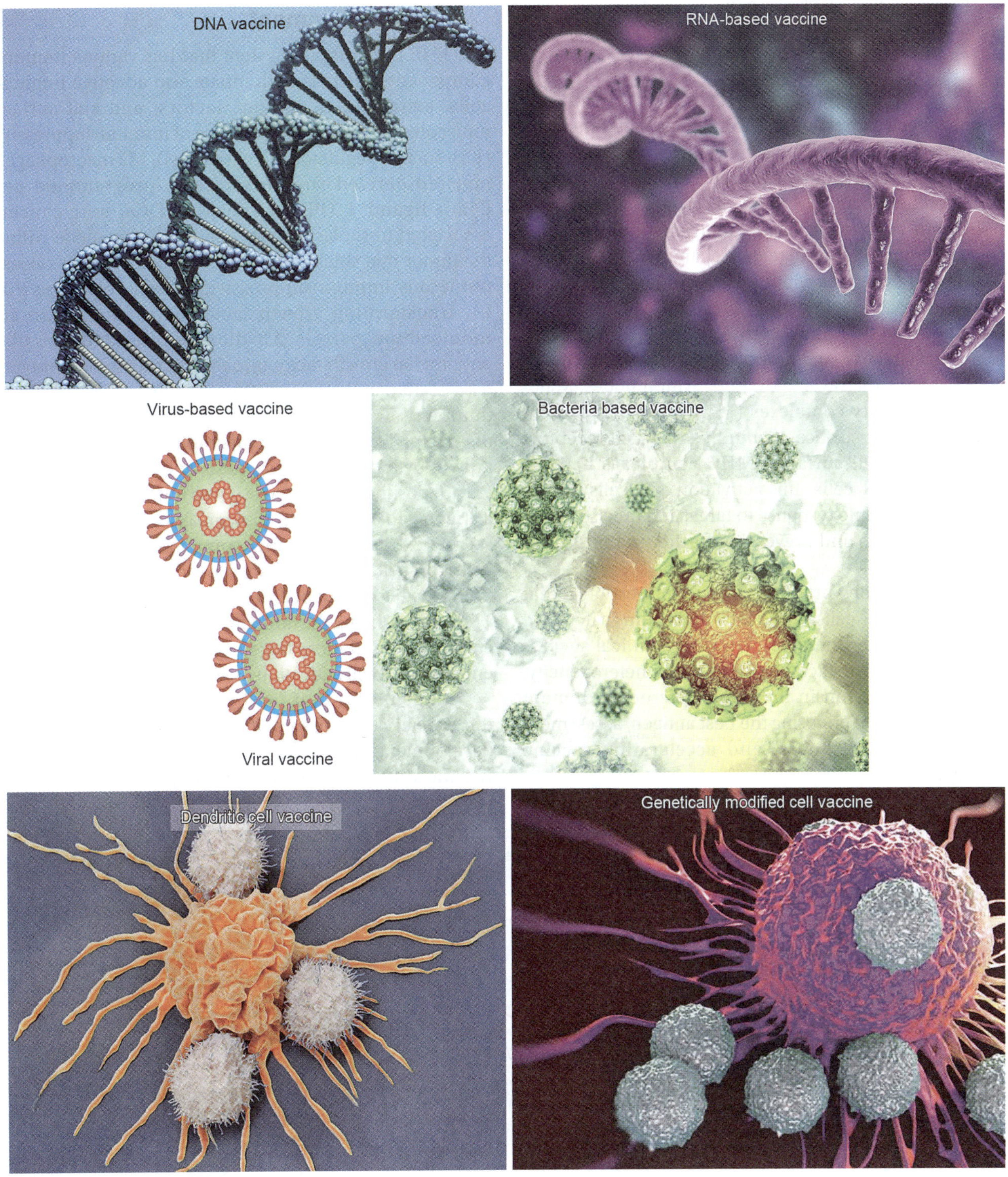

FIG. 1: Categories of therapeutic vaccine.

their illness when bacterial products were administered to them.[4] Immunological control of tumor growth and theory of immunosurveillance were proposed in 1950s and 1967, respectively. Further studies proposed that adaptive immunity was crucial for tumor regression and control. In 1991, melanoma antigen-1 (MAGE-1), the first tumor-associated antigen (TAA) was identified and the studies proved that immune system responds to tumor antigens. Since then, TAA-based cancer vaccine studies have been conducted. **Figure 2** illustrates the therapeutic cancer vaccine development and its key milestones.

Mechanism of Therapeutic Cancer Vaccines

The cancer cell expresses unique antigens that differ from healthy cells; a therapeutic vaccine utilizes the presence of these antigens and trains the immune system to recognize and target the cancer cells. Once the tumor antigens enter the body in various forms, the adjuvants in the vaccine activate immune system to release chemokines (CCL2 and CXCL1) and cytokines which recruit antigen-presenting cells (APCs) at the injection site. The APCs, such as dendritic cell (DC) phagocytose, express and process them intracellularly, and process the antigens effectively. The activated DCs travel to draining lymph nodes. Major histocompatibility complexes (MHCs) on DCs present antigens on their surface. By binding to T-cell receptors (TCR) on the cell surfaces, MHC complexes activate antigen-specific T cells. This activation of T-cells initiate an adaptive immune response to target and precise killing of the tumor cells and preventing further tumor growth **(Fig. 2)**.[5]

Cancer vaccines produce an immune response that can kill the tumor cells specifically and is thus safer than the current cancer therapies. However, clinical success rate is modest due to factors such as tumor heterogeneity, immune suppression in the tumor microenvironment (TME), difficulty in choosing the best antigen, assessment of the immune response, and accelerating vaccine production.

Immune Suppression in Tumor Microenvironment

The TME is a complex system that has various immune components, such as both innate and adaptive immune cells, extracellular immune factors, and cell surface molecules. However, the presence of immunosuppressive cells, such as regulatory T cells (Tregs), M2 macrophages, myeloid-derived suppressor cells, programmed cell death ligand 1 (PD-L1)-positive DCs, and cancer-associated fibroblasts creates an inhibitory niche within the tumor that shields immune attack. These cells release numerous immunosuppressive signals, including PD-L1, transforming growth factor-beta, interleukin-10, indoleamine pyrrole 2,3 dioxygenase, and vascular endothelial growth factor into the microenvironment and act directly or indirectly on effector T cells to dampen tumor immunity. Tregs inhibit the activation and proliferation of effector T cells, and M2 macrophages promote tumor growth by inducing angiogenesis and tissue remodeling. PD-L1-positive DCs suppress T-cell function by presenting antigens to them, and cancer-associated fibroblasts secrete extracellular matrix components that physically restrict T-cell infiltration into the tumor **(Fig. 3)**.

Strategies developed to overcome the suppression of TME are depleting the immunosuppressive cells, immune checkpoint inhibition, targeting the tumor structure, and enhancing T-cell activation or survival signaling.

Antigen, adjuvant, and platform for delivery are the crucial components of therapeutic cancer vaccine development. Each plays a distinct role in determining the vaccine's effectiveness and specificity.

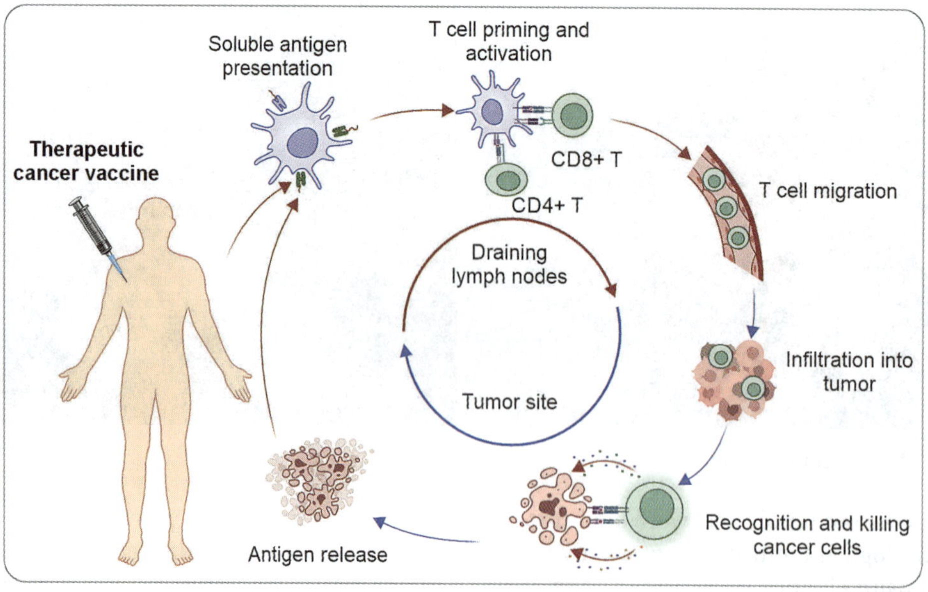

FIG. 2: Mechanism of action of therapeutic vaccine.

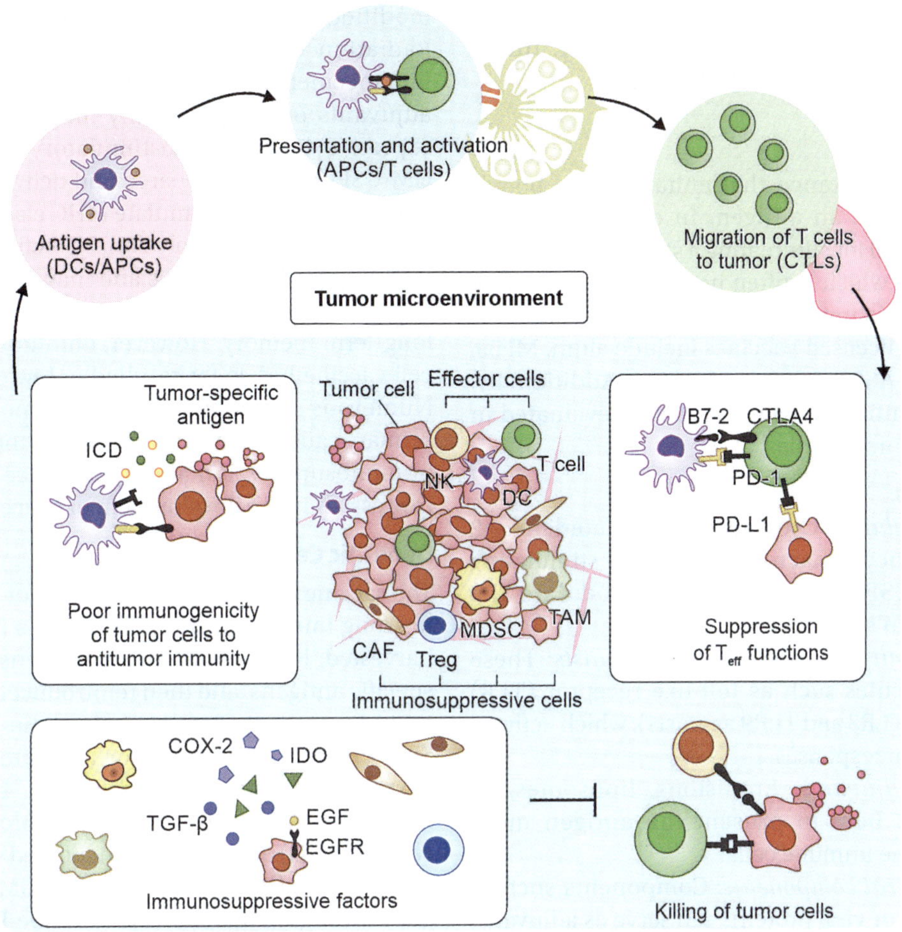

FIG. 3: Immune cells in immunosuppressive tumor microenvironment (TME).

(APC: antigen-presenting cell; CAF: cancer associated fibroblasts; DC: dendritic cell; EGF: epidermal growth factor; EGFR; epidermal growth factor receptor MDSC: myeloid-derived suppressor cell; NK: natural killer; TGF-β: transforming growth factor beta; Treg: regulatory T cells)

Antigen

The antigen is a specific molecule which upon recognition triggers an immune response. Based on the expression frequency, tumor antigens are broadly categorized into TAA and tumor-specific antigen (TSA):

- *Tumor-associated antigens:* These are normal proteins that are overexpressed in cancer cells. For example, carcinoembryonic antigen (CEA) and HER2/neu, cancer testis antigens (MAGE1 and MAGE3), viral antigens [*E6* and *E7* genes of human papillomavirus (HPV)], differentiation antigens (Gp100), tyrosinase, Epstein–Barr virus nuclear antigen 1 (EBNA 1) expressed by Burkitt's lymphoma, and nasopharyngeal carcinoma cells.
- *TSAs:* Also known as neoantigens, these are the class of antigens that develop from somatic mutations specific to tumors. Neoantigens, in contrast to TAAs, are specific to the tumor. The danger of autoimmunity is decreased by this specificity. They are more likely to be identified by the immune system as alien and are not subjected to central tolerance, a process in which the thymus teaches the immune system to distinguish between self and non-self. They are immunogenic. Their unique properties have made them a center of interest in the development of personalized cancer immunotherapies.

  Examples for TSAs are mutated oncogene products (mRas) and T-cell receptor idiotype in lymphoid malignancies.

One of the major obstacles for vaccine research was the identification of potent neoantigen. Nevertheless, scientific developments such as sequencing the entire cancer genome, creation of an algorithm for predicting epitopes, and the expansion of available immunotherapy options such as immune checkpoint inhibitors (ICIs), radiotherapy, have hastened the development of personalized tumor therapy. Neoantigen-specific T-cell-based therapy has demonstrated promise in preclinical and early clinical research.[6]

An antigen is chosen for the development of a therapeutic vaccine based on its immunogenicity, tumor specificity, and its expression in the tumor.

Adjuvant

An adjuvant is a substance that enhances the body's immune response to an antigen. In cancer vaccines, adjuvants are crucial for stimulating a strong and effective immune reaction, which is often necessary to overcome the immune evasion strategies of cancer cells. Some of the adjuvants used in licensed vaccines include alum, MF59, CpG 1018, AS01, AS02, AS03, and AS04.[7] Additionally, several high-potential adjuvants are being evaluated in preclinical and clinical studies.

Types of adjuvants:

- *Immune modulators:* Cytokines such as interleukin-2 (IL-2), granulocyte macrophage-colony stimulating factor (GM-CSF), and interferons modulate the immune system's activity.
- *Pattern recognition receptor (PRR) agonists:* These include molecules such as toll-like receptor (TLR) agonists (e.g., TLR3 and TLR9 agonists), which activate innate immune responses.
- *Particulate adjuvants:* Emulsions, liposomes, or nanoparticles help to present the antigen more effectively to the immune cells.
- *Bacterial or viral components:* Components such as bacterial DNA or viral proteins can serve as adjuvants by mimicking infection, thereby stimulating an immune response.

Adjuvants enhance antigen presentation, stimulation of inflammatory responses, and prolonged antigen exposure.

Platform for Delivery

The delivery platform refers to the method used to introduce the vaccine into the body. The choice of platform affects how the antigen is processed and presented to the immune system, influencing the overall efficacy of the vaccine. An extracellular protein is processed along the class II MHC pathway and will predominantly elicit a CD4+ response, whereas an intracellular protein is processed along the class I pathway and will predominantly elicit a CD8+ response, which is the preferred response for cancer vaccine.

Various types of delivery platforms are described here.

Whole Cell Cancer Vaccine

Whole cell cancer vaccine has been investigated from past 20 years and are the earliest vaccines to be explored for cancer vaccination. Tumor cells, either from the patient (autologous) or from a tumor cell line (allogeneic), are modified to express immune-stimulating molecules. Radiation or lysis renders the tumor cells dormant. Enhancement of immunogenicity is achieved by adding adjuvants or by genetically modifying tumor cells to express cytokines or costimulatory substances such as GM-CSF. They are prepared and delivered with all tumor antigen peptides to stimulate MHC class I and class II DCs to produce a strong polyclonal T-cell immune response. It stimulates CD4+ T cells and may also encourage CD8+ T cells to produce a more potent antitumor effect and long-term memory. However, immunization with whole-cell vaccine has so far resulted in low efficacy outcomes. Numerous investigations have demonstrated that the primary causes of the low efficacy are the tumor's inherent immunosuppression and the absence of tumor antigen expression in the development of cancer.[8]

Dendritic Cell Vaccine

The vaccine uses DCs, which are potent APCs, to stimulate a strong immune response. Patient's dendritic cells are harvested, loaded with tumor antigens or other disease-specific antigens, and then reintroduced into the patient's body to activate T cells against the target cells, e.g., Sipuleucel-T (Provenge) for asymptomatic metastatic castrate-resistant prostate cancer. It is prepared by harvesting APCs from peripheral blood mononuclear cells (PBMCs) of the patient, incubated with prostatic acid phosphatase (PAP), and merged to GM-CSF. The patient goes through leukapheresis to refine PBMCs, then they are processed in the laboratory where PAP is merged and reinfused to the patient. The requirement of leukaphereses and cell culture processing of PBMCs is one of the pitfalls of DC platform. Different approaches of antigen loading include pulsing of DCs with tumor antigens or lysate, by producing DC-tumor cell hybridoma or pulse DCs with dexasones obtained from autologous DCs.[9-12] The immunogenicity can be enhanced by genetically modifying DCs to express the genes for GM-CSF or other cytokines. The presentation of the DCs can be achieved by genetic approaches such as plasmid or viral vectors which will favor stimulation of MHC class I response. When compared to naturally circulating DCs which have the benefit of effortless separation from blood stream and very efficient in producing to the T cells, monocyte-derived DCs require prolonged time of ex-vivo culturing. In melanoma patients, the primary plasmacytoid DC-based vaccine has shown to be effective.[13,14] In the treatment of metastatic cancer, autologous primary myeloid DC-based vaccine has shown to be effective. Several factors, including decreased TAA expression on tumor cells, overexpression of checkpoint proteins, suboptimal avidity of TAA-specific T lymphocytes, and lack of suitable adjuvants necessary for inducing

TLR-mediated DC maturation, contributed to some of the DC vaccine failures observed in the clinical trials.[15-17] ICIs and the DC vaccination could be used together increase clinical efficacy.[18,19] Neoantigens are recommended as an antigen source for DC vaccine development since they have less immunological tolerance and are less toxic than TAAs.

Peptide-based Vaccine

Peptide-based vaccines are subunit vaccines that utilize specific peptides from TAAs to induce immune response. It is administered along with an adjuvant or immunomodulator to enhance the immunogenicity. However, drawbacks of these peptides are less immunogenicity, difficulty in epitope selection, and mutation of the chosen epitopes. To overcome these challenges, mutipeptide vaccines targeted against multiple TAA epitopes were developed for melanoma and glioblastoma (GBM) patients, demonstrating good clinical outcomes.[20] The gp100 peptide and CAP1-6D are examples of modified vaccines to enhance immunogenicity. In comparison with the minimal peptide vaccine, synthetic long peptide vaccines have higher affinity to the MHC molecules and have shown good immunogenicity.[21] E6 and E7 long peptide vaccine against HPV 16 confirmed stimulation of both CD4+ and CD8+ T-cell response. Personalized peptide vaccination (PPV) in which, based on the host's preexisting immunity, HLA-matched peptides are chosen and delivered.

Phase I and II trials of PPVs in various cancers such as prostate cancer, lung cancer, bladder cancer, and others demonstrated antigen-specific response and good clinical outcomes. Gliovac is a personalized peptide vaccine designed to treat GBM, an aggressive type of brain cancer. It uses a combination of tumor-associated peptides from the patient's tumor and from allogeneic sources (tumors from other patients) to stimulate a strong immune response. In phase II trials, Gliovac proved to prolong survival in patients with recurrent GBM.

Protein-based Vaccine

They are simpler to make and do not rely on the patient's MHC specificity. There are two kinds of protein-based vaccines being evaluated.

1. *Anti-idiotypes vaccines:* It consists of antibodies which target the idiotype of another antibody. These patient-tailored autologous antibodies mimic the three-dimensional structure of an antigen. Idiotype proteins are generated via a variety of methods, such as hybridoma technology, and the polymerase chain reaction (PCR) technique. Then, proteins are coupled to an immunogen, such as keyhole limpet hemocyanin (KLH) and an adjuvant, such as GM-CSF, to increase immunogenicity. The vaccine has been evaluated in patients with B-cell lymphoma and myelomas. Early studies revealed significant CD4+ response when combined with aggressive debulking surgery and chemotherapy. However, subsequent studies did not prolong the survival rate in patients.[22]
2. *Heat shock protein (HSP)-based vaccine:* HSPs are generated when tumor cells are mildly heated. It stimulates predominant CD8+ response after binding to tumor cells.[23] They are harmless and immunogenic. Nevertheless, in phase III trial, the vaccine did not reveal the expected results in melanoma patients. In melanoma and non–small cell lung carcinoma (NSCLC), the MAGE-3 as an antigen with adjuvant is being investigated. A large phase III study is underway to assess its efficacy.

DNA Vaccine

DNA vaccines are easy to produce and carry in-built adjuvant and concentrated form of TAAs, and they must undergo additional steps of transcription and translation before cross-presentation by DCs when compared to RNA and peptide vaccines. When a high dose of vaccine is administered via the intramuscular (IM) route along with electroporation, it stimulates CD4+ and CD8+ responses. DNA vaccine encoding chemokines or costimulatory molecules will enhance the immunogenicity.[24,25] However, DNA vaccines did not show encouraging results in cancer. Some of the techniques used to enhance the responses were innovation of better adjuvant, vectors, and enhanced delivery systems. For cancers such as lymphoma, cervical cancer, prostatic carcinoma, melanomas, liver cancer and breast cancer, DNA vaccines have been investigated.

RNA Vaccine

RNA vaccines are easy to produce and carry in-built adjuvants. These vaccines do not require transcription such as DNA vaccines. Vaccines are injected directly into the lymph node and as lipoplex nanoparticle intravenously. The messenger ribonucleic acid (mRNA) vaccine, consisting of 10 personalized antigens, revealed remarkable antitumor response when it was injected intranodally in melanoma patients. The RNA lipoplex vaccine encoding 4 antigens stimulated good T-cell response with partial clinical responses when it is given along with anti-PD-1 therapy for patients with anti-PD-1 resistance before the combination therapy. The mRNA neoantigen cancer vaccine BNT122 is being evaluated in a randomized phase II trial as a first-line treatment along with pembrolizumab in patients with untreated melanoma.[26]

Vector-based Vaccine

Recombinant viruses and bacteria can be used as vector to deliver antigens, and they can induce remarkable antitumor immune responses. The preclinical studies showed positive results, whereas clinical trials revealed unacceptable results with stand-alone cancer vaccines. The T-VEC, an oncolytic herpes simplex 1 virus coupled with GM-CSF, along with standard neoadjuvant therapy in phase II trial in patients with triple-negative breast cancer, showed promising results.[27]

When Busch and Fehleisen et al.[28] discovered that an infection with *Streptococcus pyogenes* might cause a tumor to shrink, *Salmonella strains* are attracted to the TME to absorb metabolic nutrients, while *Bacillus* is very active, primarily in hypoxic TME.[29,30] In conclusion, microorganisms provide several benefits as possible delivery systems for anticancer therapy. They proliferate in a hypoxic TME, travel into the tumor's remote regions, and are drawn to the tumor to absorb nutrients. These properties make them a promising candidate for anticancer therapy.

Novel Antigen Platform Delivery

Currently, nano-drug delivery technologies are being developed to improve the cancer vaccine's precision targeting and DCs' ability of antigen uptake. It consists of lipid nanoparticle technology (LNPs), bacteria-derived outer membrane vesicles, exosomes, and amphiphilic vaccines. A lipo-polyplex vector, which has a bilayer structure with polymer- and phospholipid-encapsulated mRNA constituting the inner core and outer core, respectively, is one method, while a customized DC-mimicking nano-vaccine is another.

Immune Checkpoint Inhibitor

One of the challenges faced by the therapeutic vaccine is immunosuppression of the tumor environment, which guard the tumor cells from host immune system. Immune checkpoint inhibition is a fascinating strategy to overcome the immunosuppression in TME and enhance the antitumor immune response.

Immune checkpoint inhibitors such as anti-CTLA-4, anti-PD1, and anti-PDL1 are revolutionizing cancer therapeutics. Tumor cells evade immune response by stimulating immune checkpoint pathways, thereby suppressing antitumor immune response. ICIs block these signaling pathways and promote immune-mediated tumor lysis. Therefore, a combination of therapeutic vaccine along with ICIs is emerging methods to increase response rate and survival of cancer patients.

US FDA-approved ICIs are pembrolizumab, atezolizumab, cemiplimab, nivolumab, ipilimumab and avelumab for melanoma, non-small cell lung cancer, head and neck squamous cell cancer, renal cell carcinoma, and others.

Current Scenario

List of FDA-approved therapeutic vaccines:[31,32]

- Sipuleucel-T (Provenge, commercialized by Dendreon, Inc.), a DC-based vaccine, is the first FDA-approved cancer vaccine, for the treatment of metastatic castration-resistant prostate cancer. In Dores et al., 2019 study, Provenge given to treat the male patients suffering from advanced prostate cancer shown to prolong the survival.
- Bacillus Calmette-Guérin (TheraCys) is a live-attenuated vaccine which makes use of *Mycobacterium bovis* strain for bladder invasive cancer.
- Talimogene Laherparepvec (T-VEC or Imlygic) is a vaccine for advanced oncolytic melanoma.

A list of therapeutic vaccines which are undergoing clinical trial is mentioned in **Table 1**.[5]

TABLE 1: Ongoing clinical trials of therapeutic cancer vaccine.

Clinical trials	Target antigen	Indication	Combination therapy	Administration route	Start year
mRNA cancer vaccine					
NCT05933577 (phase 3)	Neoantigen mRNA	High-risk melanoma	Pembrolizumab	Intramuscular injection	2023
NCT05886439 (phase 1b/2a)	Neoantigen mRNA	Incurable lung cancer	Pembrolizumab or durvalumab	Not mentioned	2023
NCT05198752 (phase 1)	Neoantigen mRNA	Multiple solid tumors		Subcutaneous injection	2022
NCT04486378 (phase 2)	Neoantigen mRNA	Resected stage II (high risk) and stage III colorectal cancer	Pembrolizumab	Intravenous injection	2020
NCT03815058 (phase 2)	Neoantigen mRNA	Advanced melanoma	Pembrolizumab	Intravenous injection	2019

Continued

Continued

Clinical trials	Target antigen	Indication	Combination therapy	Administration route	Start year
NCT02036956 (phase 1/2)	Neoantigen mRNA	Multiple solid tumors		Intramuscular injection	2018
NCT03639714 (phase 1/2)	Neoantigen mRNA	NSCLC, gastroesophageal adenocarcinoma, and urothelial carcinoma	Nivolumab ipilimumab	Intramuscular injection	2018
NCT04382898	KLK-2, KLK-3, PAP, HOXB13, and NKX3.1	Prostate cancer	Cemiplimab	Intravenous injection	2020
DNA vaccine					
NCT03988283 (phase 1)	Neoantigen DNA	Recurrent brain tumor		Intramuscular injection + electroporation	2023
NCT05743595 (phase 1)	Neoantigen DNA	Glioblastoma	Retifanlimab	Intramuscular injection + electroporation	2023
NCT04251117 (phase 1/2a)	Neoantigen DNA	Advanced hepatocellular carcinoma	Pembrolizumab	CELLECTRA 2000 EP device	2020
NCT03122106 (phase 1)	Neoantigen DNA	Resected pancreatic/ cancer		Intravenous injection	2018
NCT03548467 (phase 1/2a)	Neoantigen DNA	Melanoma, NSCLC/RCC, UC, SCCHN		Intravenous injection	2018
NCT05350501 (phase 2)	Oncomimics peptides, UCP2	Colorectal cancer	Nivolumab	Not mentioned	2023
NCT05286060 (phase 2)	HPV16/18 E6/E7	HPV9-positive head and neck cancer	Pembrolizumab	Intramuscular injection + electroporation	2022
NCT05455658 (phase 2)	MDM2, YB1, SOX2, CDC25B, CD105 Plasmid	Early stage TNBC		Intradermal injection	2022
NCT03655756 (early phase 1)	Emm55 streptococcal antigen plasmid	Unresectable melanoma		Intertumoral injection	2018
NCT05269381 (phase 1)	Neoantigen peptides	Advanced solid tumors	Pembrolizumab	Intravenous injection	2022
NCT05010200 (phase 1)	Personalized multipeptides	Prostate cancer		Intracutaneous injection	2022
Peptide vaccine					
NCT03645148 (phase 1)	Neoantigen peptides	Advanced pancreatic cancer	Radiofrequency ablation	Subcutaneous injection	2018
NCT05937295 (phase 1)	Montanide ISA 51 VG	Fibrolamellar hepato-cellular carcinoma	Atezolizumab	Subcutaneous injection	2023
NCT05283109 (phase 1b)	Not mentioned	Glioblastoma	Radiation therapy and temozolomide	Not mentioned	2023
NCT05609994 (phase 1)	IDH1 peptide	Recurrent IDH1 mutant lower-grade glioma	Vorasidenib	Intracutaneous injection	2023
NCT04206254 (phase 2/3)	Heat shock protein gp96-peptide	Liver cancer		Subcutaneous injection	2019
NCT03879694 (phase 1)	Surviving long peptide	Metastatic neuroendocrine tumor	Octreotide acetate	Subcutaneous injection	2019

(NSCLC: non–small cell lung carcinoma; RCC: renal cell carcinoma; SCCHN: squamous cell carcinomas of the head and neck; TNBC: triple-negative breast cancer)

THERAPEUTIC VACCINES AGAINST AUTOIMMUNE DISEASES

Autoimmune disorders result from the immune system erroneously attacking the body's own healthy cells and tissues, causing persistent inflammation, tissue injury, and impaired organ function. Existing treatments primarily rely on broad immunosuppression, leaving patients vulnerable to infections and necessitating lifelong treatments. To address these unmet needs, therapeutic vaccine development aims to restore immune equilibrium by inducing immune tolerance to autoantigens, offering a potential avenue for a cure rather than mere symptom management.[33]

Personalized medicine, particularly in the context of neoantigen-based vaccines, is being researched. The vaccines are tailored to an individual's specific autoimmune pathology, aiming to induce tolerance to autoantigens.[34] Plasmid DNA[35] and mRNA[36] vaccines have garnered high interest as a multiutility platform suitable for prevention and therapy, from personalized medicine.

Autoantibodies are predictable biomarkers of Ads and can also act as vaccine targets such as type 1 diabetes (anti-Gad antibodies), rheumatoid arthritis (RA) [HLA-DR4 allele, anticitrullinated protein antibodies (ACPAs)], multiple sclerosis (MS) (genetic markers, vitamin D deficiency, and MRI scans), celiac disease (HLA-DQ2 or HLA-DQ8 alleles), systemic lupus erythematosus (SLE) [antinuclear antibodies (ANAs)], Graves' disease, and Hashimoto's thyroiditis [thyroid peroxidase antibodies (TPOAb) and thyroglobulin antibodies (TgAb)].[37]

The next wave of truly transformative therapeutics should aspire to provide a cure by selectively suppressing pathogenic autoantigen-specific immune responses while leaving the rest of the immune system intact to control infectious diseases and malignancies. Three main areas of active research in immune tolerance are:

1. Tolerogenic vaccines aiming at robust, lasting autoantigen-specific immune tolerance.
2. T-cell therapies using Tregs to establish active dominant immune tolerance to delete pathogenic immune cells.
3. IL-2 therapies aiming at expanding immunosuppressive Tregs in vivo.[38]

THERAPEUTIC VACCINES IN INDIVIDUAL AUTOIMMUNE DISORDERS

Multiple Sclerosis

In multiple sclerosis, the patient's own immune cells attack self-antigens in the central nervous system (CNS), namely the myelin sheath that protects nerve cells of the brain and spinal cord. Several phase I/II trials have demonstrated the safety and feasibility of therapeutic vaccination strategies for MS. However, a magic bullet precisely targeted to an invader is yet to be available as a solution because of the high patient-to-patient variability in antigen reactivity. MOG, MBP, PLP peptides, apitopes (ATX-MS-1467), mannosylated liposomes containing MBP peptides, TCR peptide vaccination, MBP-encoding DNA vaccine, tol DC pulsed with myelin-derived peptides are some of the various approaches that have entered the research for the treatment of multiple sclerosis and are at various phases (I and II).[39]

THERAPEUTIC VACCINES AGAINST NONCOMMUNICABLE DISEASE (OTHER NONCOMMUNICABLE DISEASE)

Efforts are underway to develop noncommunicable disease (NCD) vaccines to address not only cancer and autoimmune diseases but also hypertension, tobacco addiction, atherosclerosis, obesity, asthma, and Crohn's disease, among others.[40]

THERAPEUTIC VACCINES AGAINST INFECTIOUS DISEASES

Prophylactic vaccines against hepatitis B virus (HBV) and HPV have achieved great success. However, some viruses can cause persistent infection in some humans, e.g., individuals at high risk for HPV infection. HPV has developed various approaches to escape immune surveillance, such as the low expression of viral proteins and the inhibition of antiviral immunity by suppressing APC function and the expression of MHC I molecules. The concept of therapeutic vaccines is based on the constant or unique expression of specific antigens, such as HPV viral E6 and E7, tumor neoantigens, and HBsAg, in established diseases.[41]

Hepatitis B

The main reason for HBV persistence after treatment with multiple drugs is dysfunctional HBV-specific T and B cells, with characteristics of low frequency, functional defects, and exhaustion. Therapeutic vaccination aims to reconstitute the systemic immune system and elicit or augment existing HBV-specific B- and T-cell responses, representing a rational strategy to overcome immune tolerance and cure chronically HBV-infected patients.[42]

Human Immunodeficiency Virus

The main hurdles in developing an effective human immunodeficiency virus (HIV) vaccine include the high variability of HIV, genetic diversity, and a lack of understanding about immune protection. Among the many HIV vaccine candidates, RV-144 was the only vaccine that was tested in a clinical trial and achieved 31.2% efficacy in Thailand. DNA, peptide, protein, viral, mRNA, and DC vaccines have been tested in clinical trials. Protein, peptide, and DNA-based vaccines aim to induce cellular immunity and humoral immunity to viral proteins, but these vaccines have yet to provide effective treatment.[43]

UNMET NEEDS AND CHALLENGES IN THE DEVELOPMENT OF THERAPEUTIC VACCINES

There is a strong focus on unmet needs such as vaccine against cancer, infectious disease, and chronic noncommunicable disease. The challenges faced in the development of therapeutic vaccines are complex pathogens [e.g., HIV, malaria, and tuberculosis (TB)], tumor heterogeneity, immune suppression in TME in cancer, immune dysfunction in chronic disease, and the design of novel adjuvants.

When compared to conventional cancer treatments, therapeutic cancer vaccines offer a focused and less harmful option. Therapeutic cancer vaccines may play a key role in comprehensive cancer therapy regimens with the potential to improve patient survival rates and quality of life.

CONCLUSION

In contrast to the current drugs or monoclonal antibody, the therapeutic vaccine has the advantage of high specificity, no drug resistance, less adverse effects, and long-lasting effects.

REFERENCES

1. Li T, Qian C, Gu Y, Zhang J, Li S, Xia N. Current progress in the development of prophylactic and therapeutic vaccines. Sci China Life Sci. 2023;66:679-710.
2. Saxena M, van der Burg SH, Melief CJM, Bhardwaj N. Therapeutic cancer vaccines. Nat Rev Cancer. 2021;21:360-78.
3. Shahnazari M, Samadi P, Pourjafar M, Jalali A. Therapeutic vaccines for colorectal cancer: the progress and future prospect. Int Immunopharmacol. 2020;88:106944.
4. Nauts HC. Bacteria and cancer: antagonisms and benefits. Cancer Surv. 1989;8(4):713-23.
5. Fan T, Zhang M, Yang J, Zhu Z, Cao W, Dong C. Therapeutic cancer vaccines: advancements, challenges, and prospects. Signal Transduct Target Ther. 2023;8(1):450.
6. Phuengkham H, Ren L, Shin IW, Lim YT. Nanoengineered immune niches for reprogramming the immunosuppressive tumor microenvironment and enhancing cancer immunotherapy. Adv Mater. 2019;31:1803322.
7. Wirth TC, Kühnel F. Neoantigen Targeting-Dawn of a New Era in Cancer Immunotherapy? Front Immunol. 2017;8:1848.
8. Pulendran B, Arunachalam PS, O'Hagan DT. Emerging concepts in the science of vaccine adjuvants. Nat Rev Drug Discov. 2021;20(6):454-75.
9. Sondak VK, Sosman JA. Results of clinical trials with an allogeneic melanoma tumour cell lysate vaccine: melacine. Semin Cancer Biol. 2003;13(6):409-15.
10. Vermorken J, Claessen A, van Tinteren H, Gall HE, Ezinga R, Meijer S, et al. Active specific immunotherapy for stage II and stage III human colon cancer: a randomised trial. Lancet. 1999;353(9150):345-50.
11. Wallack MK, Sivanandham M, Balch CM, Urist MM, Bland KI, Murray D, et al. Surgical adjuvant active specific immunotherapy for patients with stage III melanoma: the final analysis of data from a phase III, randomized, double-blind, multicenter vaccinia melanoma oncolysate trial. J Am Coll Surg. 1998;187(1):69-79.
12. Boczkowski D, Nair SK, Snyder D, Gilboa E. Dendritic cells pulsed with RNA are potent antigen-presenting cells in vitro and in vivo. J Exp Med. 1996;184(2):465-72.
13. Najafi S, Mortezaee K. Advances in dendritic cell vaccination therapy of cancer. Biomed Pharmacother. 2023;164:114954
14. Tel J, Aarntzen EH, Baba T, Schreibelt G, Schulte BM, Benitez-Ribas D, et al. Natural human plasmacytoid dendritic cells induce antigen-specific T-cell responses in melanoma patients. Cancer Res. 2013;73(3):1063-75.
15. Schreibelt G, Bol KF, Westdorp H, Wimmers F, Aarntzen EH, Duiveman-de Boer T, et al. Effective clinical responses in metastatic melanoma patients after vaccination with primary myeloid dendritic cells. Clin Cancer Res. 2016:22(9):2155-66.
16. Jang GY, Kim YS, Lee SE, Lee JW, Han HD, Kang TH, et al. Improvement of DC-based vaccines using adjuvant TLR4-binding 60S acidic ribosomal protein P2 and immune checkpoint inhibitors. Cancer Immunol Immunother. 2021;70(4):1075-88.
17. Mastelic-Gavillet B, Balint K, Boudousquie C, Gannon PO, Kandalaft LE. Personalized dendritic cell vaccines—recent breakthroughs and encouraging clinical results. Front Immunol. 2019;10:766.
18. Grenier JM, Yeung ST, Khanna KM. Combination immunotherapy: taking cancer vaccines to the next level. Front Immunol. 2018;9:610.
19. Hirayama M, Nishimura Y. The present status and future prospects of peptide-based cancer vaccines. Int Immunol. 2016;28(7):319-28.
20. Zhao J, Chen Y, Ding ZY, Liu JY. Safety and efficacy of therapeutic cancer vaccines alone or in combination with immune checkpoint inhibitors in cancer treatment. Front Pharmacol. 2019:10:1184.
21. Slingluff CL, Petroni GR, Chianese-Bullock KA, Smolkin ME, Hibbitts S, Murphy C, et al. Immunologic and clinical outcomes of a randomized phase II trial of two multi-peptide vaccines for melanoma in the adjuvant setting. Clin Cancer Res. 2007;13(21):6386-95.
22. Melief CJ, van der Burg SH. Immunotherapy of established (pre) malignant disease by synthetic long peptide vaccines. Nat Rev Cancer. 2008;8(5):351-60.
23. Kenter GG, Welters MJ, Valentijn AR, Lowik MJ, Berends-van der Meer DM, Vloon AP, et al. Vaccination against HPV-16 oncoproteins for vulvar intraepithelial neoplasia. N Engl J Med. 2009;361(19):1838-47.

24. Butts C, Murray N, Maksymiuk A, Goss G, Marshall E, Soulières D, et al. R andomized phase IIB trial of BLP25 liposome vaccine in stage IIIB and IV non-small-cell lung cancer. J Clin Oncol. 2005;23(27):6674-81.
25. Tamura Y, Peng P, Liu K, Daou M, Srivastava PK. Immunotherapy of tumors with autologous tumor-derived heat shock protein preparations. Science. 1997;278(5335):117-20.
26. Gilewski TA, Ragupathi G, Dickler M, Powell S, Bhuta S, Panageas K, et al. Immunization of high-risk breast cancer patients with clustered sTn-KLH conjugate plus the immunologic adjuvant QS-21. Clin Cancer Res. 2007;13(10):2977-85.
27. American Association of Cancer Research. (2020). Personalized Cancer Vaccine Plus Atezolizumab Shows Clinical Activity in Patients with Advanced Solid Tumors. [online] Available from https://www.aacr.org/about-the-aacr/newsroom/news-releases/personalized-cancer-vaccine-plus-atezolizumab-shows-clinical-activity-in-patients-with-advanced-solid-tumors/ [Last accessed March, 2025].
28. Soliman H, Hogue D, Han H, Mooney B, Costa R, Lee MC, et al. Oncolytic T-VEC virotherapy plus neoadjuvant chemotherapy in nonmetastatic triple-negative breast cancer: a phase 2 trial. Nat Med. 2023;29:450-7.
29. Oelschlaeger TA. Bacteria as tumor therapeutics? Bioeng Bugs. 2010;1(2):146-7.
30. Derré L, Cesson V, Lucca I, Cerantola Y, Valerio M, Fritschi U, et al. Intravesical Bacillus Calmette Guerin Combined with a Cancer Vaccine Increases Local T-Cell Responses in Non-muscle-Invasive Bladder Cancer Patients. Clin Cancer Res. 2017;23:717-25.
31. Zheng JH, Nguyen VH, Jiang SN, Park SH, Tan W, Hong SH, et al. Two-step enhanced cancer immunotherapy with engineered Salmonella typhimurium secreting heterologous flagellin. Sci Transl Med. 2017;9:eaak9537.
32. Hargrave A, Mustafa AS, Hanif A, Tunio J, Hanif S. Recent Advances in Cancer Immunotherapy with a Focus on FDA-Approved Vaccines and Neoantigen-Based Vaccines. Vaccines. 2023;11(11):1633-3.
33. Kim A, Xie F, Abed OA, Moon JJ. Vaccines for immune tolerance against autoimmune disease. Adv Drug Deliv Rev. 2023;203:115140.
34. Prajeeth CK, Dittrich-Breiholz O, Talbot SR, Robert PA, Huehn J, Stangel M. IFN-γ Producing Th1 Cells Induce Different Transcriptional Profiles in Microglia and Astrocytes. Front Cell Neurosci. 2018;12:352.
35. Voysey M, Clemens SAC, Madhi SA, Weckx LY, Folegatti PM, Aley PK, et al. Safety and efficacy of the ChAdOx1 nCoV-19 vaccine (AZD1222) against SARS-CoV-2: An interim analysis of four randomised controlled trials in Brazil, South Africa, and the UK. Lancet 2021;397:99-111.
36. Pardi N, Hogan MJ, Porter FW, Weissman D. mRNA vaccines—A new era in vaccinology. Nat Rev Drug Discov. 2018;17:261-79.
37. Niazi SK. Anti-Idiotypic mRNA Vaccine to Treat Autoimmune Disorders. Vaccines (Basel). 2023 Dec 21;12(1):9.
38. Moorman CD, Sohn SJ, Phee H. Emerging therapeutics for immune tolerance: Tolerogenic vaccines, T cell therapy, and IL-2 therapy. Front Immunol. 2021;12:657768.
39. Willekens B, Cools N. Beyond the Magic Bullet: Current Progress of Therapeutic Vaccination in Multiple Sclerosis. CNS Drugs. 2018;32(5):401-10.
40. Darrow JJ, Kesselheim AS. A new wave of vaccines for non-communicable diseases. Food Drug Law J. 2015;70(2):243-58.
41. Tian Y, Hu D, Li Y, Yang L. Development of therapeutic vaccines for the treatment of diseases. Mol Biomed. 2022;3:40.
42. Boni C, Fisicaro P, Valdatta C, Amadei B, Di Vincenzo P, Giuberti T, et al. Characterization of hepatitis B virus (HBV)-specific T-cell dysfunction in chronic HBV infection. J Virol. 2007;81(8):4215-25.
43. Tian Y, Hu D, Li Y, Yang L. Development of therapeutic vaccines for the treatment of diseases. Mol Biomed. 2022;3:40.

CHAPTER 12

Vaccination and Disease Control

Krupal J Joshi, Bhautik Modi

INTRODUCTION

From at least the 15th century, people in different parts of the world attempt to prevent illness by intentionally exposing healthy people. In the year 1796, Dr Edward Jenner created the world's first successful vaccine. The term Vaccine was coined which derives from the Latin word 'Vacca' for cow. Following this, the era of vaccination begins and researchers started targeting different disease which can be prevented by vaccines.

Vaccine-preventable diseases (VPDs) are significant public health issue in India. In India, the Universal Immunization Program (UIP) provides free immunization against around 12 vaccine-preventable diseases, including 11 nationally and 3 sub-nationally, aiming to reduce childhood mortality and morbidity.

Any adverse medical event after vaccination should be reported as an AEFI, regardless of whether it is directly caused by the vaccine.

This chapter outlines the current scenario of different VPDs and vaccine coverage, comprehensive strategies employed in India to eliminate VPDs, supported by evidence and best practices along with a brief on adverse medical event after vaccination.

CURRENT SCENARIO OF VACCINE-PREVENTABLE DISEASES AND VACCINE COVERAGE

Tuberculosis

Tuberculosis (TB), caused by bacteria *Mycobacterium tuberculosis*, is a major health issue in developing countries and is closely linked to poverty, making its control a matter of justice and human rights. TB control strategies are struggling, particularly where TB and human immunodeficiency virus (HIV)/acquired immunodeficiency syndrome (AIDS) intersect, and drug-resistant strains are worsening the crisis. The Bacillus Calmette–Guérin (BCG) vaccine protects against severe forms of TB in children but does not prevent primary infection or reactivation of latent infection. In 2023, around 87% of children had received the BCG vaccine in their first year of life.[1]

Diphtheria

The number of cases and deaths due to diphtheria has reduced significantly due to vaccination, but it remains a major health concern for children in countries with low routine immunization coverage. In diphtheria-endemic regions, cases usually appear sporadically. The disease is fatal in 5–10% of cases, especially among young children.[3]

As the diphtheria vaccine is a bacterial toxoid, it is an inactivated toxin from the bacteria but still capable of triggering immunity. It is usually administered in combination with other vaccines, such as tetanus, pertussis, Hib, and Hep-B. For adults and adolescents, a lower-concentration combination of diphtheria and tetanus toxoids (Td vaccine) is often used.

The **Figures 1 and 2** shows the prevalence of diphtheria globally and in India corresponding to the coverage of the diphtheria, tetanus, and pertussis (DPT) vaccine first dose and third dose. It has been observed that in the last 4 years, the number of diphtheria cases has increased globally.

Measles

Measles is a highly contagious viral disease which leads to high fever and rash and can result in complications such as encephalitis, blindness, or death. In the year 2023, around 83% of children had received at least one dose of a measles vaccine by 2 years of age, and around 74% had received at least two doses of the vaccine. Additionally, 190 member states had included two doses of the measles-containing vaccine in their national immunization schedules.

Measles anywhere is a threat everywhere. Measles poses a global threat, no matter where it occurs. Due to its highly contagious nature, measles can quickly spread

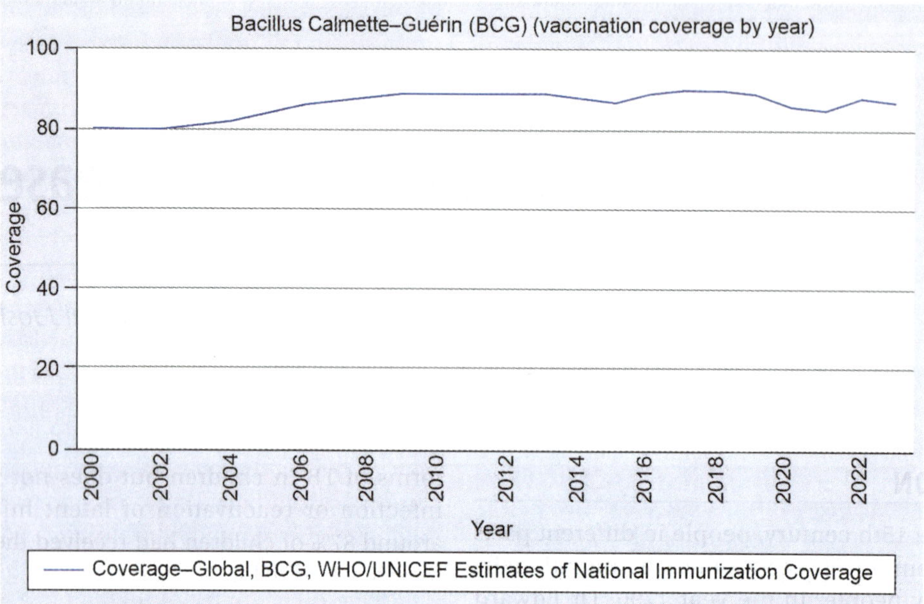

FIG. 1: Global coverage of BCG vaccine.[2]

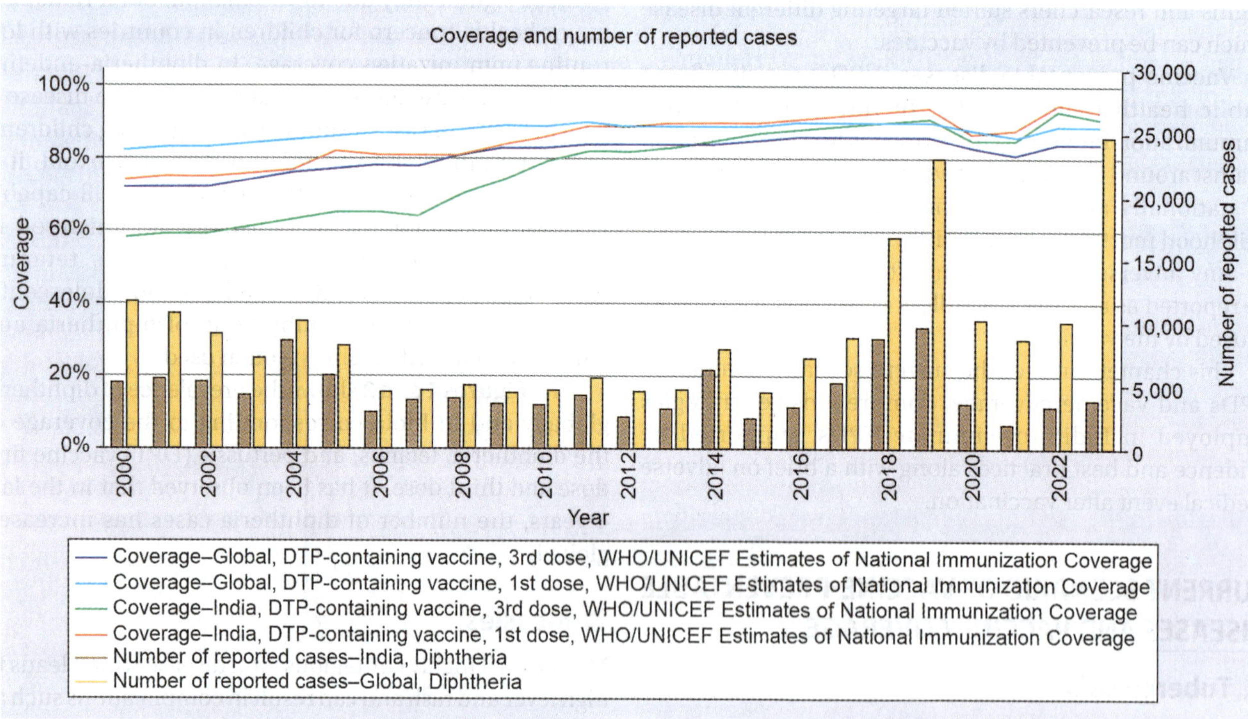

FIG. 2: Number of reported cases of diphtheria globally and in India with coverage of the diphtheria, tetanus, and pertussis (DPT) vaccine first dose and third dose.[2]

across borders. The graph illustrates the global and Indian prevalence of measles in relation to the coverage rates of both doses of the measles vaccine. It is been observed that global cases of measles have decreased as the coverage of vaccines increases. Unvaccinated individuals are at risk of contracting measles while traveling abroad and can easily transmit the virus to others upon their return.

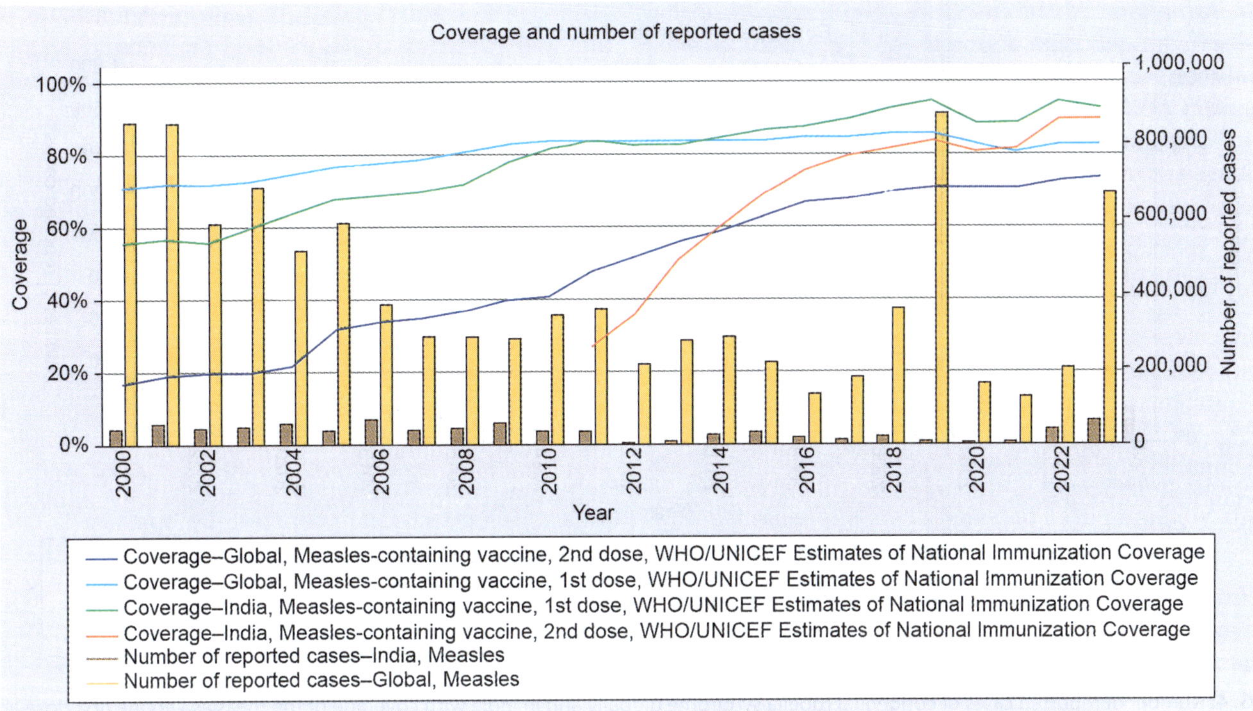

FIG. 3: Number of reported cases of measles globally and in India with coverage of the measles vaccine first dose and second dose.[2]

Figure 3 depicts that; between 2000 and 2022, vaccination efforts have averted an estimated 57 million deaths. In 2022 alone, the disease claimed over 1,36,000 lives.

Rubella

Rubella is a viral disease, mild in children, but infection in early pregnancy can lead to congenital rubella syndrome, causing defects in eyes, ears, heart, and brain. In the year 2023, the rubella vaccine has been introduced in 175 member states, with coverage estimated at 71%.

Congenital rubella syndrome is used as an indirect indicator of the disease burden of rubella in the community. India has introduced the rubella antigen in the national immunization schedule in the form of two doses of measles-rubella (MR) vaccine after a successful MR campaign in 2016–2017. The trend of congenital rubella syndrome increased in the last 5 years **(Fig. 4)**.

Haemophilus Influenza Type B

Haemophilus influenza type B (Hib) is causing meningitis and pneumonia in children. In the year 2023, the Hib vaccine is covered in 193 member states, with global coverage for three doses estimated at 77% **(Fig. 5)**. However, coverage varies significantly by region, the European Region achieving an estimated 94%, while the Western Pacific Region lags at just 33%.[4]

Hepatitis B

It is a viral infection that mainly affects the liver. In the year 2023, 190 member states had introduced the hepatitis B vaccine, achieving an estimated global coverage of 83% for three doses **(Fig. 6)**. This coverage peaks at 79% in Western Pacific Region, while the African Region has a much lower rate of just 17%.[4]

Polio

Polio, or poliomyelitis, is a highly infectious viral disease that is caused by the poliovirus. Most infections are asymptomatic or mild, with symptoms such as fever, fatigue, headache, and sore throat. In severe cases, it can cause permanent paralysis, typically in the legs. If the respiratory muscles are affected, it can be life-threatening. Globally, an estimated 83% of infants received three doses of the polio vaccine in the year 2023. Of the three strains of wild poliovirus, type 2 was eradicated in 1999, and type 3 was eradicated in 2020 **(Fig. 7)**. Despite significant progress, polio remains endemic in Afghanistan and Pakistan.[5] All countries having weak public health and immunization systems remain at risk of polio importation from these countries. Polio has been eliminated from most countries, including India and China, by maintaining a high level of coverage of the polio vaccine.

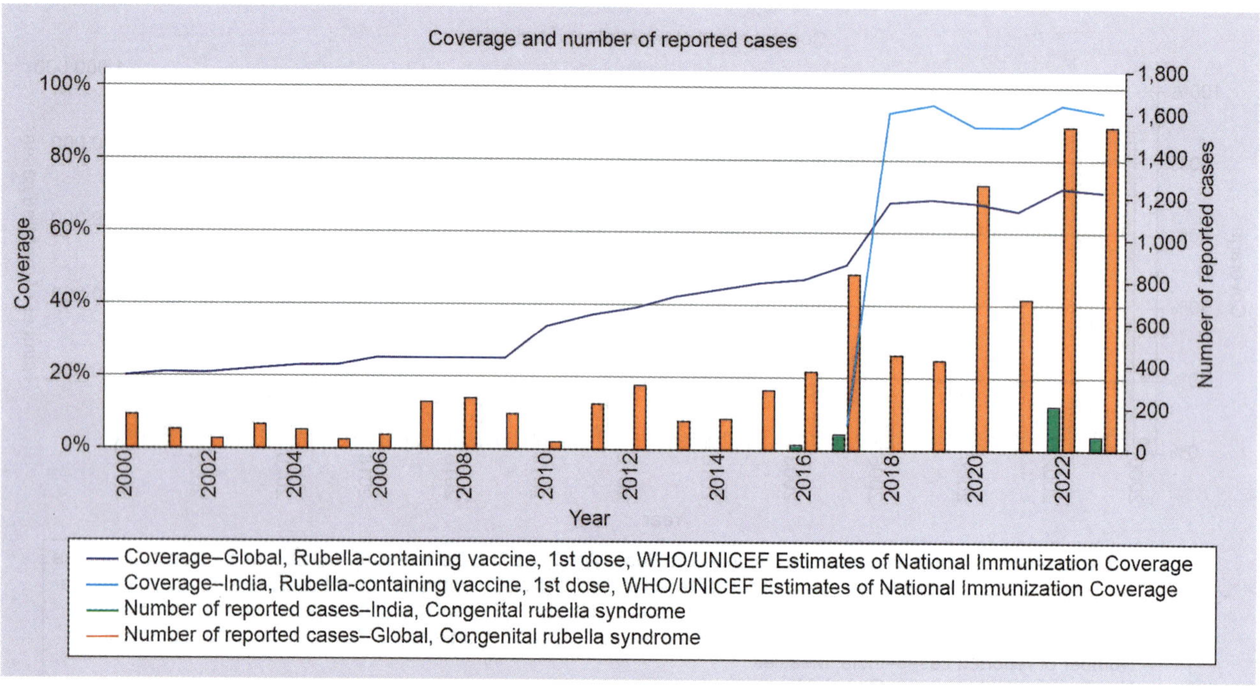

FIG. 4: Number of reported cases of congenital rubella syndrome globally and in India with coverage of the measles vaccine first dose and second dose.[2]

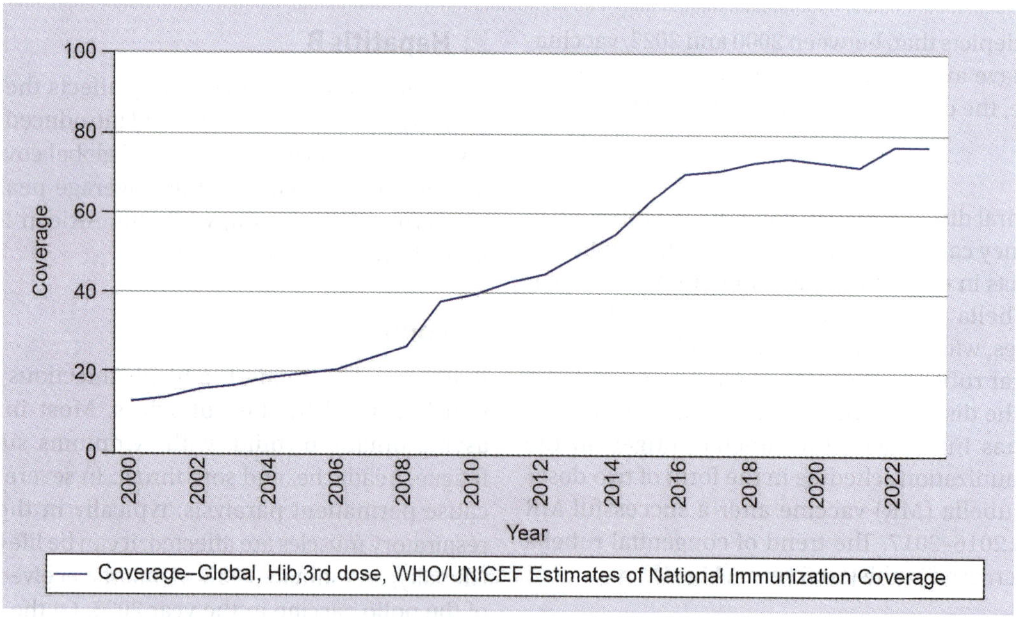

FIG. 5: Global coverage of *Haemophilus influenza* type B (Hib) vaccine third dose.[2]

Rotavirus

It is the leading cause of severe diarrheal disease in young children. **Figure 8** shows that; in the year 2023, the rotavirus vaccine is included in 123 countries, with global coverage of around at 55%.[6]

Tetanus

Tetanus is caused by *Clostridium tetani,* a bacterium that thrives in low-oxygen environments. The spores of this bacterium are ubiquitous and found in the environment regardless of location. Once in the body, *C. tetani* produces

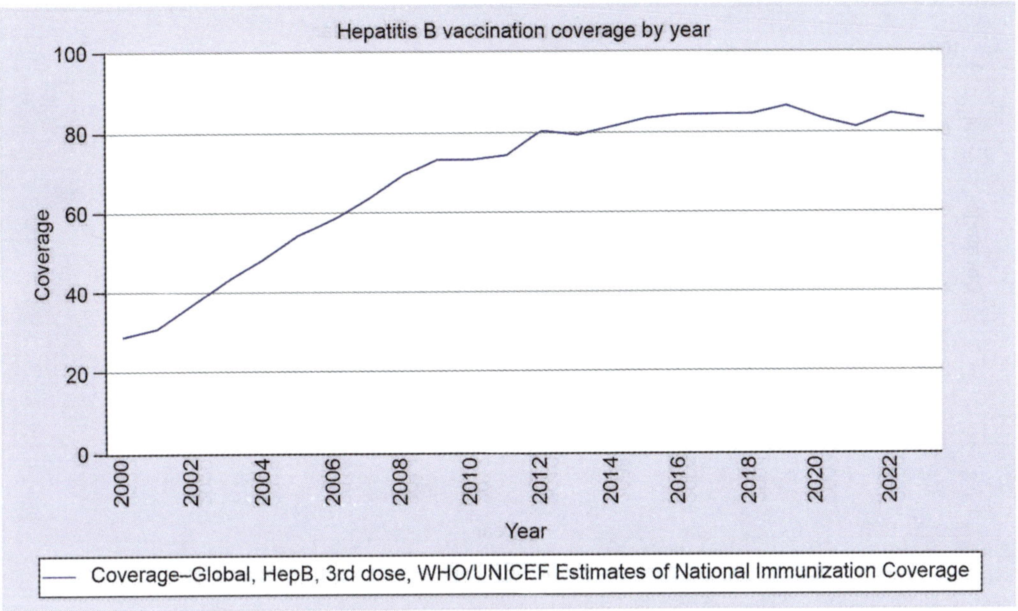

FIG. 6: Global coverage of hepatitis B (Hep B) vaccine third dose.[2]

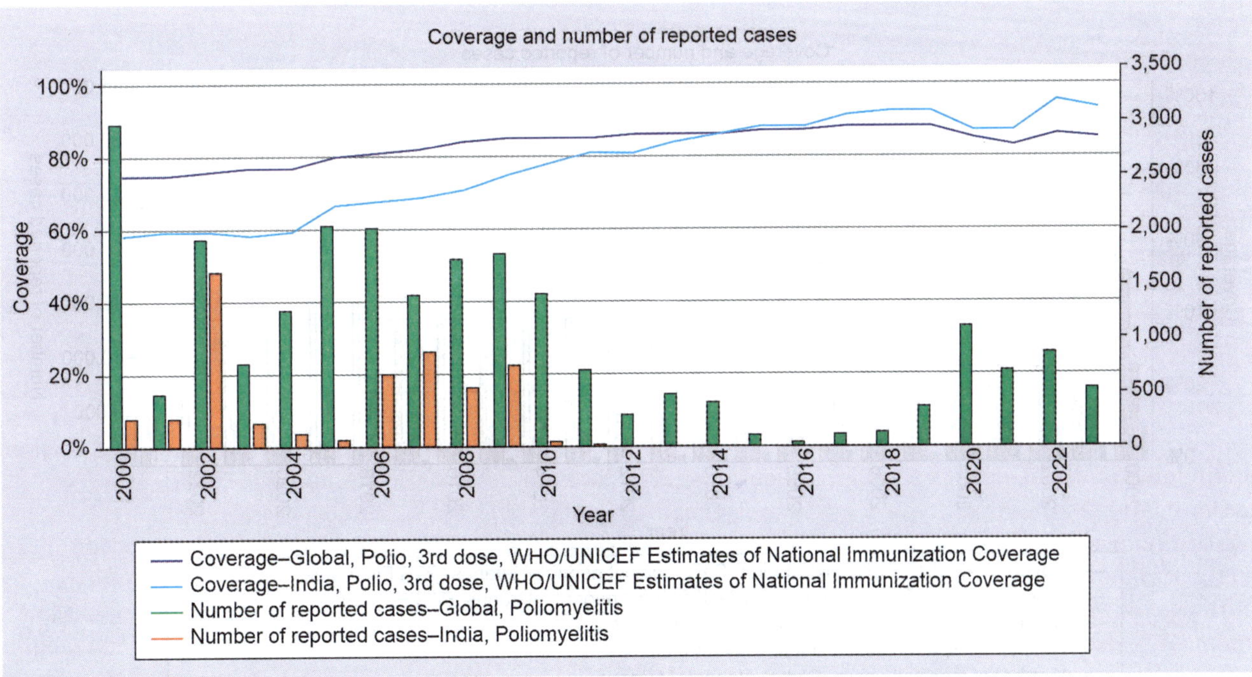

FIG. 7: Number of reported cases of polio globally and in India with coverage of the polio vaccine third dose.[2]

a toxin that can lead to severe disease or death. Neonatal tetanus remains a significant public health problem in around 10 countries, primarily in Africa and Asia.

Figure 9 shows the trend of the number of cases of neonatal tetanus and total tetanus globally and in India and coverage of tetanus vaccination. Globally, cases of tetanus have decreased with few peaks in between. In India, the number of neonatal tetanus and total tetanus both decreased drastically in the recent past.

Pneumococcal

Pneumococcal diseases encompass a range of illnesses, including pneumonia, febrile disease, meningitis, otitis media, and bronchitis. In the year 2023, pneumococcal

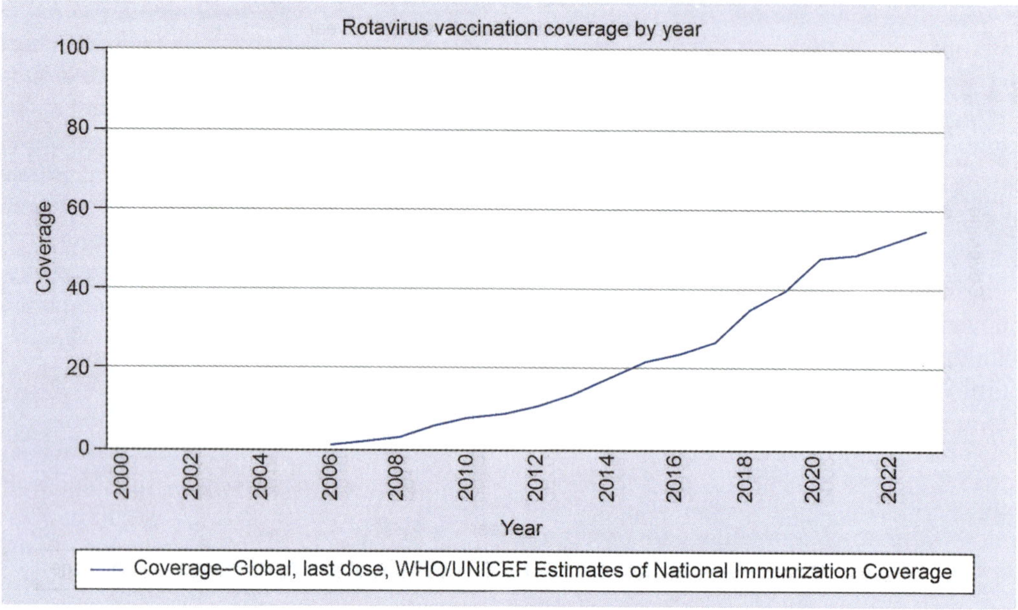

FIG. 8: Global coverage of rotavirus vaccine third dose.[2]

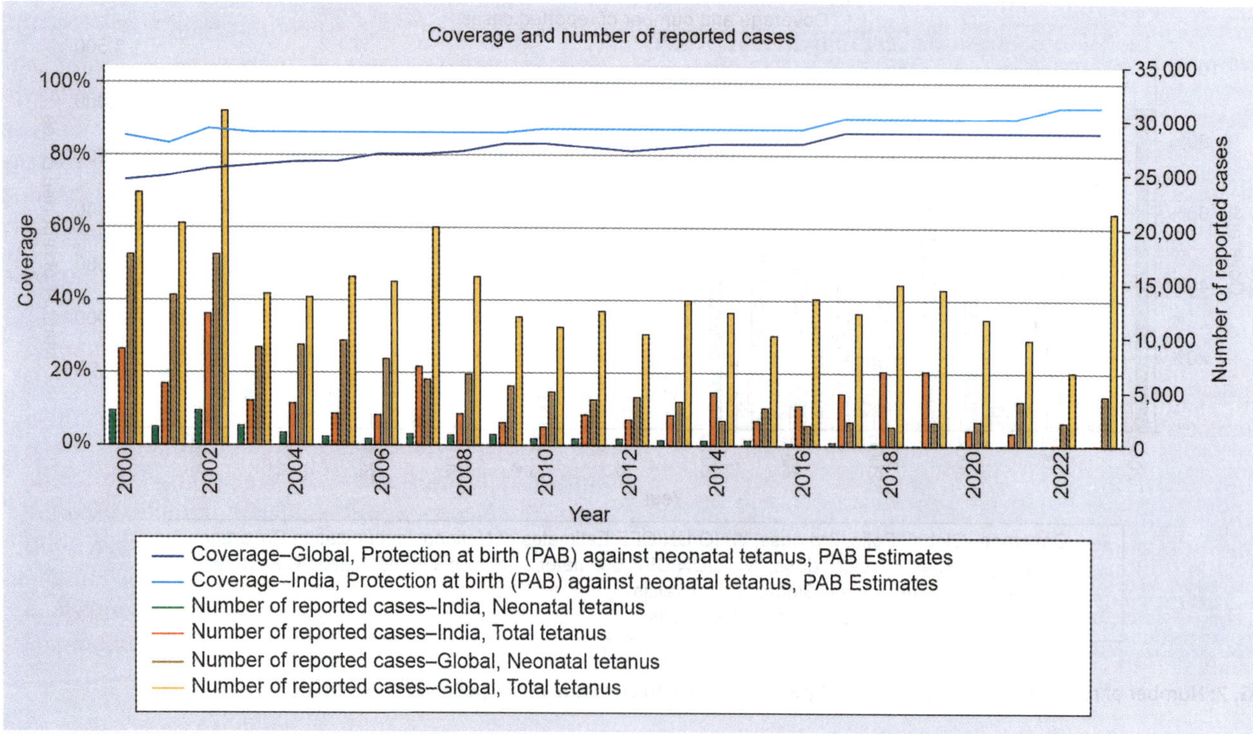

FIG. 9: Number of reported cases of tetanus globally and in India with coverage of the tetanus vaccine.[2]

vaccines are being used in 159 member states, with global coverage for the third dose estimated at 65% **(Fig. 10)**. However, coverage varies widely by region, with the WHO European Region achieving an estimated 86% coverage compared to just 26% in the Western Pacific Region.[6]

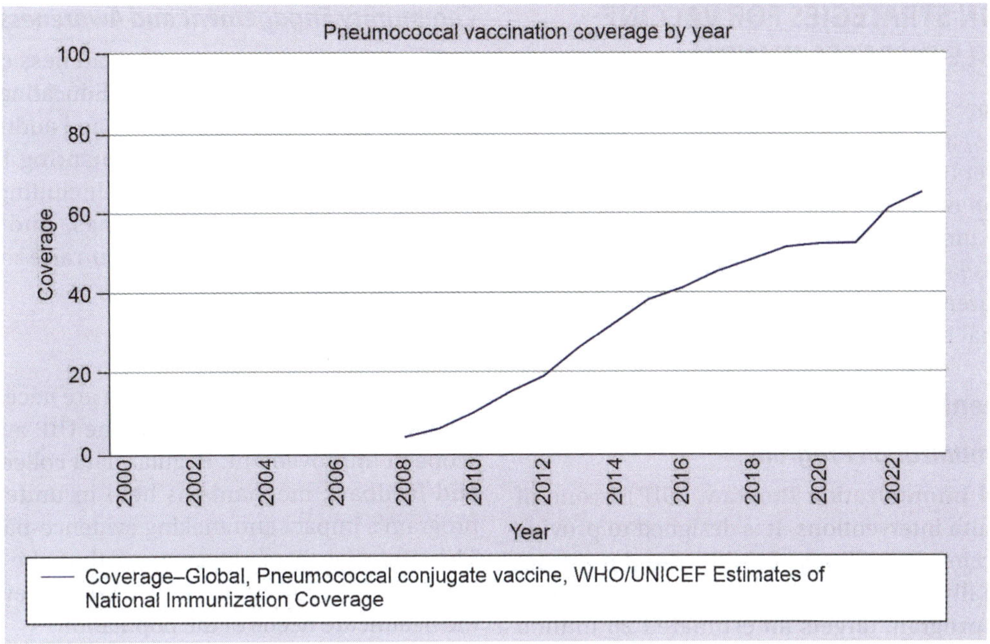

FIG. 10: Global coverage of pneumococcal conjugate vaccine.[2]

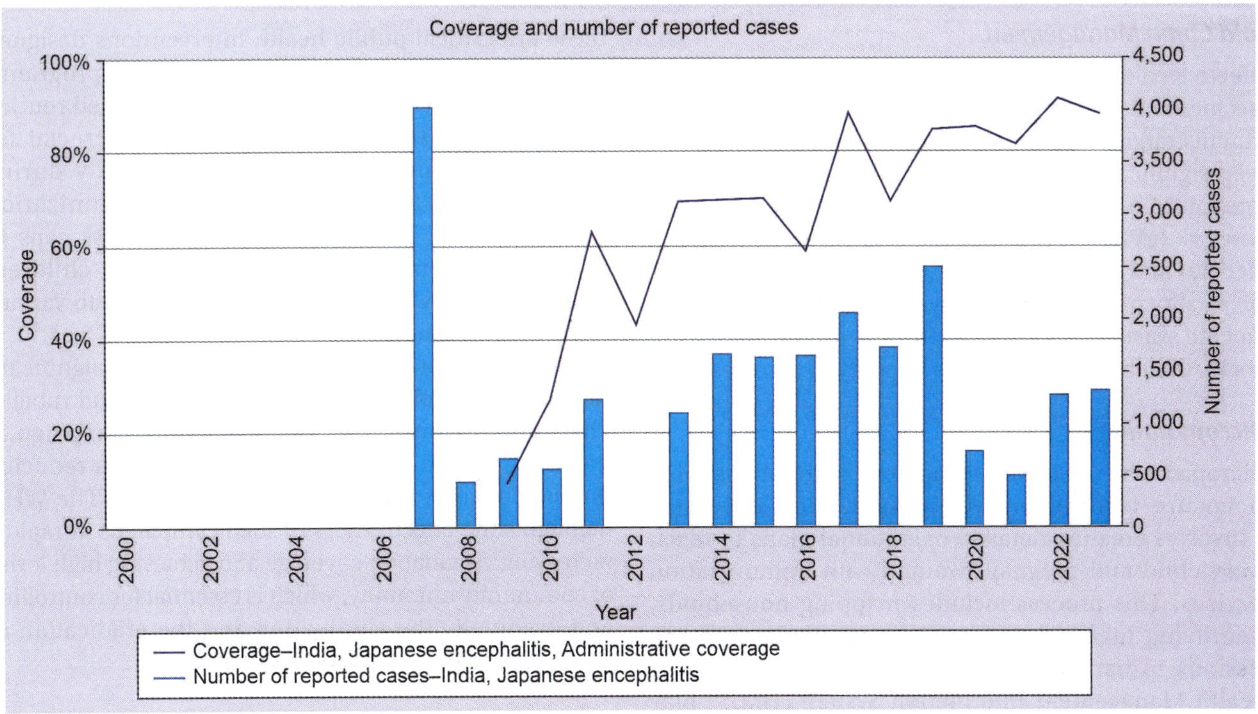

FIG. 11: Number of reported cases of Japanese encephalitis in India with coverage of the Japanese encephalitis vaccine.[2]

Japanese Encephalitis

It is a viral zoonotic disease transmitted by vectors and one of the leading causes of viral encephalitis. It affects nearly all countries across Asia, regardless of climate, and has spread into new regions via the movement of infected vectors. Presently, around 3 billion people in the South-East Asia and Western Pacific Regions are at risk of Japanese encephalitis (JE) **(Fig. 11)**.

ELIMINATION STRATEGIES FOR VACCINE-PREVENTABLE DISEASES IN INDIA

Reduction in prevalence of different vaccine preventable diseases (VPDs) are mainly due to the efforts of the team of health workers in India. Different strategies adopted for the elimination of these VPDs which includes, strengthening routine immunization, intensified immunization campaigns, disease surveillance and monitoring, efforts for public awareness and community engagement, well drafted National Immunization Policy and others.

Strengthening Routine Immunization

Universal Immunization Program

The Universal Immunization Program (UIP) is one of the largest health interventions. It is designed to provide life-saving vaccines to millions of children and pregnant women annually, significantly reducing the burden of VPDs. The program targets an estimated 26 million infants and 30 million pregnant women every year. Under UIP, vaccines are provided free of cost to protect against 12 VPDs.[6]

Cold Chain Management

Effective cold chain management is essential to ensure vaccines remain potent and effective from manufacture to administration. In India, the cold chain infrastructure has been significantly enhanced through various initiatives. One such initiative is Electronic Vaccine Intelligence Network (eVIN). It provides the availability of different vaccines and storage temperatures in real time, ensuring the quality of vaccines. This system helps in preventing vaccine wastage and ensures timely replenishment of stocks, thereby maintaining the integrity of vaccines.[7]

Microplanning

Microplanning is a critical component of the UIP, aiming to ensure comprehensive immunization coverage. It involves creating detailed operational plans to reach every child and pregnant woman with immunization services. This process includes mapping households, identifying high-risk areas, and organizing outreach sessions in hard-to-reach regions. Tools such as the Health Management Information System (HMIS) play a vital role in tracking immunization coverage. These systems help in identifying gaps in coverage and facilitate targeted interventions to improve immunization rates. By leveraging these technologies, health authorities can ensure that immunization services are effectively delivered to the most vulnerable populations.[8]

Community Engagement and Awareness

Community engagement and awareness campaigns are integral to the success of the UIP. Educating communities about the importance of vaccines and addressing vaccine hesitancy are crucial steps in ensuring high immunization rates. Various strategies, including mass media campaigns, community meetings, and involvement of local leaders, are employed to raise awareness and encourage participation.

Monitoring and Evaluation

Proper monitoring and evaluation are necessary to assess the quality and effectiveness of the UIP and identify the scope of improvement. Regular data collection, analysis, and feedback mechanisms help in understanding the program's impact and making evidence-based decisions. This iterative process ensures that the UIP remains responsive to emerging challenges and evolves to meet the healthcare needs of the population.

Intensified Immunization Campaigns

Supplementary Immunization Activities

These are critical public health interventions designed to increase the coverage of immunization programs, particularly targeting children who have missed routine vaccination sessions. These activities are crucial for enhancing community immunity, especially during outbreaks of VPDs. Supplementary immunization activities (SIAs) are implemented to address gaps in routine immunization and ensure that all children, including those who missed vaccinations due to various reasons, receive necessary immunizations.

In India, SIAs have been employed with significant success to control diseases such as measles and rubella. The introduction of the MR vaccination campaign, a notable example of SIAs, has been pivotal in reducing the incidence of these diseases nationwide. The WHO highlights the effectiveness of such campaigns in rapidly increasing vaccination coverage and achieving high levels of community immunity, which is essential for controlling and eventually the elimination and the eradication of these diseases.[9]

National Immunization Days

These are large-scale, mass immunization campaigns that aim to eliminate specific diseases by administering vaccines to a large segment of the population within a defined period. These campaigns are particularly effective for diseases where high vaccination coverage is needed to interrupt transmission. In India, national immunization days (NIDs) have been a cornerstone of the polio eradication efforts. Multiple rounds of NIDs have been conducted as part of the comprehensive strategy to eliminate poliomyelitis, which culminated in India achieving polio-free status in 2014. The success of these campaigns underscores their role in achieving significant public health milestones, such as the eradication of polio.[10]

Disease Surveillance and Monitoring

Surveillance Systems

Robust disease surveillance systems are fundamental for the early detection of disease outbreaks and the effective management of VPDs. The Integrated Disease Surveillance Programme (IDSP) in India represents a decentralized, state-based approach that plays a vital role in monitoring and reporting on epidemic-prone diseases. This program allows for timely identification and response to disease outbreaks, which is essential for controlling the spread of VPDs. The IDSP's structure enables it to provide real-time data and support rapid response efforts, thereby enhancing the overall effectiveness of disease control measures.[11]

Vaccine-preventable Disease Surveillance

Continuous surveillance of diseases is crucial for assessing the impact of immunization programs and identifying areas with insufficient coverage or ongoing outbreaks. Surveillance networks, such as the Measles-Rubella Surveillance Network, are essential for collecting data on VPDs. This data is invaluable for informing targeted interventions and improving vaccination strategies. By monitoring trends and outbreaks, these networks help public health officials to focus efforts where they are most needed, thus enhancing the overall effectiveness of vaccination programs.[12]

Real-time Data Monitoring

The integration of digital tools and platforms, such as eVIN, has significantly advanced the management of immunization programs. eVIN enables real-time monitoring of vaccine stocks, storage temperatures, and immunization coverage, which is important for maintaining the quality and effectiveness of vaccination efforts. By providing timely and accurate data, eVIN supports informed decision-making and efficient resource allocation, thereby enhancing the overall management of immunization programs and ensuring that vaccines are distributed and stored properly.[13]

Public Awareness and Community Engagement

Health Education Campaigns

Public awareness campaigns are essential for educating communities about the importance of vaccination and countering vaccine-related myths and misconceptions. Initiatives such as Mission Indradhanush and its intensified version, Intensified Mission Indradhanush, have been instrumental in raising public awareness and demand for vaccines. These campaigns aim to reach out to underserved populations and ensure that all eligible children receive their vaccinations. The success of these campaigns highlights the necessity of comprehensive health education efforts in increasing immunization coverage and fostering community support for vaccination programs.

Community Mobilization

Engaging community leaders, religious figures, and other influential individuals is a critical strategy for promoting vaccine acceptance and overcoming vaccine hesitancy. Community mobilization efforts in states such as Uttar Pradesh and Bihar have demonstrated significant improvements in immunization coverage. By involving local leaders and influencers, these efforts help to build trust and address concerns about vaccines, leading to higher vaccination rates and better public health outcomes.

Behavioral Change Communication

They are employed to address vaccine hesitancy and misinformation through a variety of communication channels. Behavioral change communication (BCC) involves using mass media, social media, and interpersonal communication to disseminate accurate and compelling information about vaccines. These strategies aim to correct misconceptions, provide clear information about the benefits of vaccination, and encourage positive vaccination behaviors. Effective BCC is crucial for ensuring that the public receives reliable information and feels confident in the safety of vaccines.

Policy and Governance

National Immunization Policy

Formulating and continuously updating national immunization policies, grounded in robust evidence and recommendations from the WHO, are imperative for the successful implementation of vaccination programs. In India, the National Technical Advisory Group on

Immunization (NTAGI) plays an instrumental role in this process. NTAGI provides expert guidance on vaccine schedules, new vaccine introductions, and policy adjustments based on epidemiological data and global health trends.[14] Regular updates ensure that vaccination policies remain aligned with emerging health threats and advancements in vaccine technology.

Multisectoral Collaboration

Effective immunization efforts benefit greatly from multisectoral collaboration. Engaging various sectors such as education, transportation, and local governance can enhance vaccination coverage and program effectiveness. For instance, the School Health Program exemplifies how integrating immunization services with school health initiatives can improve vaccine uptake among school-aged children. By leveraging existing school infrastructure and networks, this approach ensures that children receive all vaccines in a proper manner.[15] Such collaborations also facilitate the development of community-based strategies that address local barriers to vaccination.

Regulatory Framework

A robust regulatory framework is important for ensuring the safety, efficacy, and quality of vaccines. In India, the Central Drugs Standard Control Organization (CDSCO) is responsible for the regulation and approval of vaccines. The CDSCO's mandate includes evaluating vaccine safety and efficacy through rigorous clinical trials, monitoring postmarketing surveillance, and ensuring compliance with quality standards. Strengthening these regulatory processes is essential for maintaining public trust and safeguarding health. Enhanced regulatory mechanisms also support the timely introduction of new vaccines.

Research and Innovation

Vaccine Development

Investment in research is critical for advancing vaccine technology and addressing emerging infectious diseases. The Indian Council of Medical Research (ICMR) are at the forefront of vaccine research in India, contributing to the development of newer vaccines. This research is crucial for responding to evolving public health threats and improving immunization coverage.[16] Collaborative efforts between research institutions and pharmaceutical companies can accelerate the development of innovative vaccines and expand their accessibility.

Operational Research

Operational research plays a key role in optimizing immunization programs by identifying best practices and innovative strategies. Research on vaccine delivery mechanisms, cold chain management, and community engagement provides valuable insights for improving program efficiency and coverage. For example, studies on cold chain logistics can inform strategies to enhance vaccine storage and distribution, thereby reducing vaccine wastage and ensuring that vaccines remain effective throughout the supply chain.[16] Operational research also supports evidence-based decision-making and the implementation of effective vaccination strategies.

Monitoring Vaccine Efficacy

Postmarketing surveillance is crucial for monitoring the long-term efficacy and safety of vaccines. The AEFI surveillance is a key component of this monitoring process, tracking and investigating adverse events to ensure public confidence in vaccination programs. By systematically collecting and analyzing data on vaccine-related adverse events, health authorities can identify potential safety concerns and make informed decisions about vaccine use.[17] Effective surveillance also contributes to the continuous improvement of vaccine safety and efficacy.

Human Resource Development

Capacity Building and Training

Ongoing training and capacity building are vital for maintaining high standards in immunization practices. Regular training programs for healthcare workers focus on vaccine administration techniques, cold chain management, and accurate data entry. These programs ensure that the knowledge and skills of healthcare improve, protocols are maintained, and high-quality services are delivered. Capacity-building initiatives also support the development of leadership skills and the ability to manage immunization programs effectively.

Supportive Supervision

Supportive supervision is an essential component of maintaining high standards in immunization practices. Supervisors provide on-the-job training, monitor performance, and offer constructive feedback to healthcare workers. This approach helps identify and address challenges in real time, promotes adherence to best practices, and supports continuous quality improvement. By fostering a supportive environment, supervisory practices contribute to the overall effectiveness and efficiency of immunization programs.

Capacity Enhancement

Enhancing capacity at all levels, from grassroots health workers to policymakers, strengthens the overall immunization program. Initiatives such as training programs offered by the National Institute of Health and Family Welfare (NIHFW) are instrumental in building the skills and knowledge of health professionals. These programs focus on various aspects of immunization, including program management, data analysis, and community engagement. Strengthening capacity across all levels ensures that immunization programs are well-managed and responsive to emerging challenges.

Financial Sustainability

Government Funding

Adequate government funding is essential for the sustainability of immunization programs. The Government of India allocates substantial resources to the UIP through mechanisms such as the National Health Mission (NHM). This funding supports various aspects of the immunization program, including vaccine procurement, distribution, and program implementation. Ensuring financial sustainability is essential for maintaining program continuity and expanding vaccine coverage.

International Aid

International aid and partnerships play a significant role in supporting immunization efforts. Organizations such as GAVI, the Vaccine Alliance, and WHO provide financial and technical assistance to strengthen immunization programs in India. These partnerships facilitate access to funding, technical expertise, and resources that enhance the effectiveness of vaccination programs. Leveraging international support helps address resource gaps and ensures the successful implementation of immunization initiatives.

Public-private Partnerships

Public-private partnerships (PPPs) can enhance resource mobilization and the delivery of vaccination services. Collaborations with pharmaceutical companies, nongovernmental organizations (NGOs), and private healthcare providers expand the reach and impact of immunization programs. PPPs facilitate the sharing of resources, expertise, and technology, leading to more effective and efficient vaccination services.[18] Encouraging such partnerships supports the achievement of immunization goals and improves program outcomes.

Addressing Equity and Accessibility

Targeting Vulnerable Populations

Ensuring equitable immunization coverage requires special attention to marginalized and hard-to-reach populations. Approaches such as mobile vaccination units and frequent outreach sessions in remote areas address geographical barriers and ensure that underserved populations receive necessary vaccines. Targeting vulnerable groups helps reduce health disparities and improve overall vaccination coverage.[19] Tailored approaches that address specific needs and barriers are essential for achieving equity in immunization.

Mobile Vaccination Units

Mobile vaccination units play an important role in providing immunization services in remote and underserved areas. These units are equipped with cold chain facilities and trained staff to administer vaccines safely and effectively. By overcoming logistical challenges and reaching communities with limited access to healthcare services, mobile vaccination units contribute to improving vaccination coverage and ensuring that no one is left behind.

Inclusive Policies

Formulating inclusive policies that address barriers faced by different socioeconomic groups is essential for achieving equitable immunization coverage. Policies should consider factors such as gender, socioeconomic status, and geographic location to ensure that all individuals have access to vaccination services. Inclusive policies help address systemic inequalities and promote health equity by targeting the needs of diverse populations.

Emergency Preparedness and Response

Outbreak Response Plans

Planning of comprehensive outbreak response is critical for managing VPD outbreaks. These may include strategies for rapid assessment, vaccination campaigns, and community engagement. Effective outbreak response plans ensure timely and coordinated action to control and contain disease outbreaks.[19] Preparedness and response activities are essential for minimizing the impact of outbreaks on public health.

Rapid Response Teams

Establishing rapid response teams is essential for swift action during outbreaks. These teams are trained to conduct rapid assessments, implement vaccination campaigns, and provide technical support to local health authorities. By mobilizing expertise and resources quickly, rapid response teams contribute to effective outbreak management and help mitigate the spread of disease.[19]

Stockpile Vaccines

Maintaining a strategic stockpile of vaccines for emergency use during outbreaks is crucial for timely response. The Government of India, in collaboration with international partners, maintains reserves of vaccines for diseases such as measles and cholera. These stockpiles ensure that vaccines are available when needed and support rapid response efforts during emergencies.[19] Strategic vaccine reserves are a key component of preparedness and response planning.

ADVERSE EVENT FOLLOWING IMMUNIZATION

It is any untoward medical occurrence following immunization. It does not necessarily have a causal relationship with the usage of the vaccine. These events can include any unfavorable or unintended symptom, sign, or abnormal lab result.

Adverse events following immunization (AEFIs) can either be directly related to the vaccine or the vaccination process, or they might be coincidental, happening around the same time as the vaccination but not caused by it.

A vaccine reaction is a person's specific response to the vaccine's properties, which can occur even when the vaccine has been correctly administered, correctly prepared, and properly handled. A list of adverse events known to be associated with vaccines are provided in **Table 1**.

Any adverse medical event after vaccination should be reported as an AEFI, regardless of whether it is directly caused by the vaccine.

Adverse events following immunization may be broadly grouped as under:

- *Adverse events following immunization by the severity of the event:*
  - Minor reactions (common)
  - Serious and severe vaccine reactions (rare)
- *Cause-specific AEFIs:*
  - Vaccine product-related reactions
  - Immunization error-related reactions
  - Vaccine quality defect-related reactions
  - Immunization-triggered stress response (ITSR)

Severe Reactions

The term "severe" reaction is broader and not typically used for regulatory purposes. It encompasses reactions that are more intense than minor reactions but do not necessarily require hospitalization. Severe reactions may cause temporary disability and do not lead to long-term complications.

Severe AEFI:

- Can be disabling
- Most do not lead to long-term complications
- Must also be reported
- *Examples*: Prolonged crying, convulsion, hypotonic hyporesponsive episodes (HHEs), and thrombocytopenia

TABLE 1: List of adverse events known to be associated with vaccines.[7]

Vaccine	Reaction
BCG	• *Local*: Local abscess, keloid, lymphadenitis, and cutaneous lesions • *Systemic*: Osteitis, osteomyelitis, disseminated BCG disease, and immune reconstitution syndrome (HIV patients)
OPV	Vaccine-associated paralytic poliomyelitis (VAPP)
DTwP/pentavalent (DTwP + HiB + HBV)	• Fever > 38°C, irritability, and drowsiness • Prolonged inconsolable crying (>1 hour) • High fever >40.5°C • Acute encephalopathy/encephalitis, HHE, seizure, anaphylaxis/shock
Hepatitis B	Anaphylaxis
Measles/MR	• Fever >39.4°C, rash, and febrile seizure • Thrombocytopenia, anaphylaxis, encephalopathy/encephalitis/encephalomyelitis
Rubella	Arthralgia/arthritis/arthropathy
Mumps	Aseptic meningitis
MMR vaccine	Febrile seizure
Tetanus/Td	Brachial neuritis and anaphylaxis
Rotavirus	Intussusception
Japanese encephalitis	• Serious allergic reactions, seizures, encephalopathy, neuropathy, and encephalitis • Myelitis and aseptic meningitis

(BCG: Bacillus Calmette–Guérin; DTwP: diphtheria, tetanus, and pertussis; HBV: hepatitis B virus; HHE: hypotonic hyporesponsive episode; HiB: *Haemophilus influenzae* type b; MMR: measles-mumps-rubella; MR: measles-rubella; OPV: oral polio vaccine)

Serious Reactions

An AEFI is classified as "serious" if it meets any of the following criteria: It poses a life-threatening risk, requires hospitalization, leads to persistent or significant disability, causes a congenital anomaly, requires intervention to prevent permanent impairment, or may result in death.

Serious AEFI:

- Hospitalization
- Clusters
- Disability
- Congenital anomaly/birth defect
- Death
- Media reports/community or parental concern

Cause-specific Categorization of Adverse Event Following Immunization

- *Vaccine product-related reaction:* An event that is caused due to the inherent properties of the vaccine product.
- *Immunization triggered stress response (previously known as immunization anxiety-related reaction):* An event arising from anxiety regarding injections or vaccination.
- *Vaccine quality defect-related reaction:* A cause by quality defects of the vaccine product, including its administration device.
- *Immunization error-related reaction (previously known as "program error"):* An event that is caused by inappropriate vaccine handling or administration.
- *Coincidental event:* An event that is caused by something other than above all.

Each and every training of health works should encompass this AEFIs also. To minimize these events, focused efforts on training, raising awareness, and ensuring the commitment of health workers are crucial.

CONCLUSION

As one of the world's leading vaccine manufacturers, India continues to expand its National Immunization Schedule by introducing new vaccines and enhancing coverage of existing ones through various strategic approaches. While increasing immunization coverage through the dedicated efforts of health workers, it is equally important to recognize and address Adverse Events Following Immunization (AEFIs). Efforts should focus on minimizing AEFIs through comprehensive training, awareness, and the unwavering commitment of healthcare professionals.

REFERENCES

1. World Health Organization. (2024). BCG vaccine. [online] Available from https://www.who.int/teams/health-product-policy-and-standards/standards-and-specifications/norms-and-standards/vaccines-quality/bcg [Last accessed March, 2025].
2. World Health Organization Dashboard. (2024). [online] Available from https://immunizationdata.who.int/compare [Last accessed March, 2025].
3. World Health Organization. (2024). Diphtheria. [online] Available from https://www.who.int/teams/immunization-vaccines-and-biologicals/diseases/diphtheria [Last accessed March, 2025].
4. World Health Organization. (2024). Immunization Coverage. [online] Available from https://www.who.int/news-room/fact-sheets/detail/immunization-coverage [Last accessed March, 2025].
5. World Health Organization. (2024). Poliomyelitis (polio). [online] Available from https://www.who.int/health-topics/poliomyelitis#tab=tab_1 [Last accessed March, 2025].
6. Ministry of Health and Family Welfare. Universal Immunization Program. [online] Available from https://mohfw.gov.in/sites/default/files/4101639587148966 2752.pdf
7. World Health Organization. Cold Chain Management in Immunization. [online] Available from https://cdn.who.int/media/docs/default-source/searo/india/publications/immunization-handbook-107-198-part2.pdf [Last accessed March, 2025].
8. UNICEF. Microplanning for Immunization. [online] Available from https://www.unicef.org/immunization [Last accessed March, 2025].
9. World Health Organization. (2020). Supplementary immunization activities (SIAs). [online] Available from https://www.who.int/publications/i/item/9789241511254 [Last accessed March, 2025].
10. Polio Eradication Initiative. (2021). National Immunization Days. [online] Available from https://polioeradication.org/who-we-are/polio-endgame-strategy-2019-2023/supplementary-immunization/ [Last accessed March, 2025].
11. Centers for Disease Control and Prevention (CDC). (2022). Integrated Disease Surveillance Programme (IDSP). [online] Available from https://ncdc.mohfw.gov.in/integrated-disease-surveillance-programme/
12. World Health Organization. (2021). Vaccine-Preventable Disease (VPD) Surveillance. [online] Available from https://www.who.int/publications/m/item/global-strategy-for-comprehensive-vaccine-preventable-disease-(vpd)-surveillance [Last accessed March, 2025].
13. Electronic Vaccine Intelligence Network (eVIN). (2020). Real-time Data Monitoring. [online] Available from https://www.undp.org/india/projects/improving-vaccination-systems-evin [Last accessed March, 2025].
14. Ministry of Health and Family Welfare. (2022). National Immunization Policy. Government of India. [online] Available from https://nhm.gov.in/index1.php?lang=1&level=2&sublinkid=824&lid=220.
15. World Health Organization. (2020). School Health Program: Integrating Immunization. [online] Available from https://www.who.int/teams/immunization-vaccines-and-biologicals/essential-

programme-on-immunization/integration/school-vaccination [Last accessed March, 2025].

16. World Health Organization. (2021). Operational Research in Immunization Programs. World Health Organization. [online] Available from https://iris.who.int/bitstream/handle/10665/324962/9789290234173-eng.pdf [Last accessed March, 2025].
17. World Health Organization. (2022). Monitoring Vaccine Efficacy and Safety. World Health Organization. [online] Available from https://www.who.int/news-room/questions-and-answers/item/vaccines-and-immunization-vaccine-safety#:~:text=How%20is%20vaccine%20safety%20monitored,or%20caregivers%2C%20and%20health%20workers. [Last accessed March, 2025].
18. The National Health Systems Resource Centre (NHSRC), New Delhi. (2021). Public-Private Partnerships in Health Care under the National Health Mission in India: A Review. [online] Available from https://nhsrcindia.org/sites/default/files/2022-09/PPP%20BOOK%2027.05.2022_0.pdf [Last accessed March, 2025].
19. Centers for Disease Control and Prevention. (2022). Rapid Response Teams for Outbreak Management. [online] Available from https://www.cdc.gov/globalhealth/healthprotection/errb/global-rrt.htm.

CHAPTER

13

Vaccines for Special Populations

Rajvir Bhalwar, Mandar P Baviskar

MeSH words: Vaccination; vaccination coverage; program; immunization; health disparate minority and vulnerable populations; travel health; occupational health; military medicine; agricultural workers disease; rural health.

INTRODUCTION

Special Populations: Definition and Characteristics

"Special populations" refer to groups of people whose needs are not fully addressed by traditional health services delivery. Greater access to these services, or tailored services, must be provided to reduce inequities in physical and mental healthcare systems.[1] Many different groups have been identified as special populations, based on the fact that the precise definition may vary depending on who is using the terminology. For example, it may refer to individuals who are disabled, or are "vulnerable" to certain socioeconomic hazards, for which the term "vulnerable populations" has also been sometimes used. In our national context, while neonates, infants, children, women and elderly definitely form very important "special populations", their vaccination requirements are being discussed in separate chapters in this book. This chapter will focus on the vaccination requirements of the following "special population groups":

- Populations displaced due to disasters/humanitarian emergencies
- Populations which are part of mass gatherings, fairs, festivals, and pilgrimages
- Healthcare personnel (HCP)
- Agriculturists
- Armed forces personnel
- International travelers
- *Labor workforce*: In industrial, agricultural, construction, and transport sectors, workers who handle wastes, and sex workers
- Persons having chronic diseases or immunocompromised status

Cautionary Remarks

At the very outset, it would be prudent to bear the following aspects in mind:

- Firstly, though vaccination forms a very important component in the overall strategy of preventing and controlling various infectious diseases, it must be combined with various other methods of prevention of communicable diseases, as prevention of overcrowding, use of face mask, water and food hygiene, personal protection and control of insect vectors, etc. Alone and by itself, vaccination may not be able to achieve complete protection from infectious diseases; on the contrary, it may lead to an undesirable sense of complacency toward adoption of a holistic approach for control of infectious diseases.
- Secondly, the material presented in this chapter is based on the latest available guidelines by eminent professional bodies and experts. However, it does not constitute an authority to claim vaccination by any person or group. Actual provisioning of vaccination would be the purview of the Central/State/Local Government or the management of the private organization, as the case may be.
- Thirdly, these recommendations do not supersede the guidelines given by the Government of India or any other governmental authority in their respective Immunization Schedules and in case of any conflict, the guidelines of the governmental body/parental organization will be final authority. In addition, it is strongly recommended that children and pregnant women should be completely immunized as per the provisions of National Immunization Schedule (NIS).

This chapter is divided into two major parts. Part I deals with the recommendations for vaccination of various special population groups. Part II deals with the details of individual vaccines which have been recommended for the various special populations in Part I.

PART I: RECOMMENDATIONS FOR VARIOUS SPECIAL POPULATION GROUPS

Recommended Vaccination for "Displaced Populations" due to Disasters/Humanitarian Emergencies

- A disaster or an acute humanitarian emergency refers to conditions that might arise as a consequence of either man-made or natural events, leading to sudden unplanned displacement of a large proportion of the population away from the place of habitual residence and into any settlement (e.g., refugee camps), resulting in reduced access to healthcare, deterioration of nutritional status or any other breakdown of critical public health or governmental function. Population displaced due to disasters/humanitarian emergencies is very prone to various diseases since they are relocated away from their main habitat, have hardly any finances or wherewithal to meet their needs and are under tremendous psychological pressure, besides having to live under insanitary conditions of overcrowding, inadequate shelters and clothing, lack of protected water supply and hygienic food, and exposure to insect vectors. For this reason, immunization should be accorded high priority for displaced populations.
- The most common vaccine preventable diseases (VPDs) encountered in humanitarian emergencies include measles, polio, meningococcal meningitis, hepatitis A, and cholera. To a lesser extent, pneumococcal pneumonia, rotavirus diarrhea, and chickenpox are also potential problems.
    - The most important step is to ensure, as far as possible, that all children, adolescents, and pregnant women are covered as per the guidelines laid down in the respective NISs. In our NIS, the directives include vaccination against tuberculosis, diphtheria, pertussis, tetanus, polio, hepatitis B, *Haemophilus influenzae* type B, rotavirus disease, pneumococcal disease, measles, rubella, and Japanese encephalitis (JE). In addition, depending on the availability and logistic feasibility, vaccination with injectable typhoid vaccine, oral cholera vaccine, and meningococcal vaccine may be considered. The recommended vaccinations for populations displaced due to disasters/ humanitarian emergencies, based on guidelines of eminent professional organizations,[2-4] are given in **Table 1**.

Recommended Vaccination for Populations which are Part of Mass Gatherings (Pilgrimages, Fairs, and Festivals)

In our country, many pilgrimages, fairs, and festivals involving large human congregations occur all over the country, and at different times of the year. The major

TABLE 1: Recommended vaccination for populations displaced due to disasters/acute humanitarian emergencies.

Disease	Recommendations for vaccination of displaced/disaster affected population
Vaccine preventable diseases (VPDs) covered by the National Immunization Schedule (NIS)	
Diphtheria	It should be ensured that the vaccine coverage of children and women in the disaster affected population as per the guidelines given in NIS is implemented, focusing at maximum coverage of the affected population, with minimum disruption in the supplies of vaccine and logistics. This step itself will go a long way in ensuring that adequate protection is available to the affected population in respect of these VPDs. Coverage of at least 95% for measles and at least 85% for other VPDs should be aimed at, to obviate the occurrence of any outbreak as well as to minimize the vicious circle between infectious diseases and malnutrition to which the displaced populations, particularly children, are very vulnerable
Pertussis	
Tetanus	
Polio	
Hepatitis B	
Haemophilus influenzae type b	
Rotavirus disease	
Measles	
Rubella	
Tuberculosis	
Pneumococcal disease	
Japanese encephalitis	

Continued

Continued

Disease	Recommendations for vaccination of displaced/disaster affected population
Other VPDs which are not covered by the NIS: (Depending on risk assessment, as given below, against individual diseases)	
SARS-CoV-2	Depending on the occurrence of this disease and instructions for vaccinating the population, as issued by Government authorities, displaced populations should be included for vaccination against COVID-19, starting with higher priority for the elderly (aged 60 years and above)
Influenza	Depending on risk assessment when conditions of marked overcrowding, inadequate availability of shelters for displaced population and high transmission potential are expected, immunization with a single dose of trivalent inactivated influenza vaccine (IIV) may be considered for children older than 6 months till 5 years of age (preferably up to 8 years of age) and elderly persons aged 65 years and above (preferably those aged 46 years and above if resources permit)
Meningococcal disease	Polysaccharide vaccine [purified bacterial capsular polysaccharide (PBCP)] 0.5 mL one dose by SC injection may be considered for persons aged 50 years and above, depending on risk assessment when conditions of marked overcrowding, inadequate shelters for displaced population and high transmission potential are expected
Cholera	One oral dose of either inactivated, whole-cell recombinant subunit vaccine or else, live-attenuated vaccine may be considered for persons aged 18 years and above, depending on risk assessment when conditions of marked overcrowding, inadequate supply of safe drinking water and hygienic food, and high transmission potential are expected
Typhoid	Immunization with single dose of Vi polysaccharide vaccine, 0.5 mL IM injection may be considered for persons aged 2 years and above, depending on risk assessment when conditions of marked overcrowding, inadequate supply of safe drinking water and hygienic food, and high transmission potential are expected
Tetanus	In addition to coverage of children and pregnant women under the NIS, adults who have not been earlier adequately immunized against tetanus are recommended to be covered with TT or Td
Pneumococcal disease	Depending on risk assessment when conditions of marked overcrowding, inadequate availability of shelters for displaced population and high transmission potential are expected, immunization is recommended for persons aged 50 years and above with one dose of PCV-13, 0.5 mL IM injection. If stay is prolonged beyond 1 year in the displaced conditions, a dose of PPSV-23, 0.5 mL may be given after 1 year
Other diseases: Rabies and snake bite	Readiness with adequate logistics for postexposure prophylactic treatment (PEP) of rabies and snake bites should be ensured

(PCV: pneumococcal conjugate vaccine; PPSV: pneumococcal polysaccharide vaccine; SARS-CoV-2: severe acute respiratory syndrome coronavirus 2)

TABLE 2: Recommendations for vaccinations during mass gatherings in India.

Disease/Vaccine	Recommendations
Vaccination recommended for all persons, irrespective of duration of stay:	
SARS-CoV-2	Depending on the occurrence of this disease and instructions for vaccinating the population, as issued by Government authorities, persons involved in mass congregations should be included as a high priority group for vaccination against COVID-19, with elderly being given higher priority
Tetanus	Injection TT or Td, as per national policy in vogue. One dose is recommended for all those who have already completed the primary course as a part of NIS.
Influenza	Immunization with a single dose of trivalent vaccine is recommended.
Typhoid	Immunization with single dose of Vi polysaccharide vaccine, IM injection is recommended.
Hepatitis A	Recommended that ideally, two doses of hepatitis A vaccine be given by IM injection, separated by 6–12 months. In case this is not possible due to urgency, at least one dose of hepatitis A vaccine as early as possible before departure for the mass gathering is recommended.

Continued

Continued

Disease/vaccine	Recommendations
Vaccination recommended in case stay is going to be prolonged (>4 weeks) or in special situations:	
Hepatitis B	Ideally, the person should complete the primary schedule of three doses of 1 mL IM injection at 0, 1, and 6 months. In case the person has completed the primary schedule of three doses as part of NIS, one booster dose, if >5 years have passed since completion of the primary schedule or the last booster, is recommended.
Japanese encephalitis	Recommended after proper risk evaluation by local health authorities, taking into consideration the transmission potential in that area and during that particular time
Pneumococcal disease	Recommended for (1) persons aged 50 years and above: one dose of PCV-13, 0.5 mL IM injection, followed by PPSV-23, 0.5 mL after 1 year (2) aged >18 years and having immunocompromised status or chronic diseases as CKD, on hemodialysis, heart disease, lung disease, chronic liver disease, alcoholism, or diabetes mellitus: one dose of PCV-13 followed by one dose of PPSV after 8 weeks.

Note: For recommended vaccination for pilgrims going to other countries, see details given later under recommended vaccination of travelers.

(CKD: chronic kidney disease; NIS: National Immunization Schedule; PCV: pneumococcal conjugate vaccine; PPSV: pneumococcal polysaccharide vaccine; SARS-CoV-2: severe acute respiratory syndrome coronavirus 2)

communicable diseases that are likely during such mass gatherings are orofecal transmitted infections, respiratory infections, vector-borne diseases, and infections following injuries. The following vaccines are recommended **(Table 2)**.[5]

Recommended Vaccination for Healthcare Personnel

Healthcare personnel are frequently exposed to various infectious diseases during the process of direct patient care or during handling of infectious material. The recommendations for vaccination of HCP based on various eminent professional bodies and experts[5-9] are given in **Table 3**.

Recommended Vaccination for Agriculturists (Including Livestock Workers)

Our country is greatly dependent on agriculture and hence agriculturists constitute a very important occupational group. Most of the agriculturists are also associated with livestock, mainly cows, buffaloes, sheep, and goats. In our country, agriculturists are exposed to several infectious diseases specific to agriculture and livestock, as follows:

- Rabies due to bites of wild animals, especially wild canines and felines
- Leptospirosis due to contamination of water-logged soil with urine of infected rodents
- Malaria and lymphatic filariasis due to exposure to biting anopheline and Culicines, along with the fact that agriculturists often remain semi-clad.
- Japanese encephalitis due to exposure to Culicines in water-logged rice fields in endemic areas.
- Anthrax and Brucellosis due to frequent exposure to livestock
- Snake bite is another important hazard necessitating management with antisnake venom (ASV).
- Indian tick typhus due to exposure to ticks which infest cattle
- Scrub typhus due to exposure to wild rodents infested with mites, in agricultural fields
- Tetanus due to frequent injuries along with exposure of wounds to contaminated soil
- Hookworm infestation due to exposure to soil containing infective stage larvae
- Byssinosis and bagassosis due to exposure to cotton and sugarcane dust contaminated with fungi
- Enteric fever, bacillary dysentery, *Escherichia coli* diarrhea, and cholera due to frequent exposure to unprotected drinking water.

The recommended vaccination plan for agriculturists is presented in detail in **Table 4**.

Recommended Vaccination for Military Personnel

Personnel of the Armed Forces need to be considered as a special and vulnerable population from the vaccination point of view. They are at high risk of injuries and exposure to extremes of climatic conditions. Often, they are required to stay in operational areas, in camps where adequate control of water quality, food hygiene, and control of insect vectors is quite difficult. Moreover, they have to often operate within our country, in counter-insurgency operations against terrorists, in densely forested lands, hilly areas, and riverine belts. The overall policy for all aspects of healthcare including vaccination policy is the prerogative of the Military Headquarters and the Director General, Armed Forces Medical services.[10] The suggested vaccination plan for military personnel is given in **Table 5**.

TABLE 3: Vaccination recommendations for healthcare personnel (HCP).[5-9]

Disease	Situations in which recommendation to be given
Part 1: Vaccines recommended to be given to all HCP—	
SARS-CoV-2	Health workers should be included in the highest priority group for vaccination against COVID-19, depending on the occurrence of the disease and instructions for vaccinating, as issued by Government authorities
Hepatitis B	Strongly recommended for all healthcare persons when they start their medical/dental/nursing/paramedical training curriculum, if they have not been earlier successfully immunized against hepatitis B as part of National Immunization Schedule during childhood. For those who are not immunized in childhood and even at the start of their healthcare studies course, it is suggested to immunize them at the start of healthcare job. At least, all those healthcare workers who are at high risk of acquiring infection and who have not been vaccinated previously [healthcare workers including auxiliary workers in surgical disciplines, laboratory workers, those who have risk of exposure to blood and blood products as dialysis personnel, those involved in giving injections or drawing blood samples or blood transfusion, and all healthcare workers (including auxiliary workers) involved in handling biomedical wastes]
Influenza	Health workers are an important group for influenza vaccination. Annual immunization with a single dose of inactivated influenza trivalent vaccine is recommended for: (1) All medical and paramedical personnel working in casualty/emergency department of identified hospitals treating influenza cases; (2) All medical and paramedical personnel working in ICU and isolation wards managing influenza patients; (3) All personnel identified to work in screening centers that would be set up for categorization of patients during seasonal influenza outbreak; (4) All medical and paramedical personnel engaged in treating/managing the high-risk group; (5) Laboratory personnel working in virological laboratories testing suspected influenza samples; (6) Rapid Response Team members identified to investigate outbreaks of influenza; (7) Drivers and staff of vehicles/ambulances involved in transfer of influenza patients[6]
Tetanus	HCPs should be adequately immunized against tetanus using injection TT (or Td, in case it has been introduced locally as part of the national program). For those who have already undergone the primary series, a booster is required once in 10 years. For those who have not undergone the primary course as part of NIS, a primary course of three doses of TT or Td, separated by at least 4 weeks, should be administered
Measles	All health workers should have natural immunity or be vaccinated against measles. Those who have not been adequately immunized against measles earlier and do not have a definite history of having suffered from measles should be offered the measles vaccine
Rubella	If rubella vaccine has been introduced into the national program, as is the case in India, all health workers should have immunity or be vaccinated against rubella, either by earlier natural immunity or through vaccination with MR vaccine
Varicella	It is recommended that countries should consider vaccination of potentially susceptible health workers (i.e., unvaccinated and with no history of varicella) with two doses of varicella vaccine. This should receive special focus for those working in infectious diseases (ID) hospitals or ID wards, those working in pediatric departments and healthcare workers caring for cases during outbreak of chickenpox or health workers working in situations where risk assessment indicates that there is high risk of varicella transmission (as sudden increase in recruits in military training centers, displaced population living in overcrowded conditions)
HPV infection	HPV vaccine may be considered for HCP up to 26 years of age, both males and females. Not to be given to pregnant women
Part 2: Vaccines recommended to be given to HCP under certain specific situations—	
Anthrax	May be considered for healthcare workers working in laboratories which handle anthrax bacilli or spores
Tuberculosis	BCG is recommended for unvaccinated, tuberculin skin test (TST) negative or interferon gamma release assay (IGRA) negative HCP at risk of occupational exposure (health workers working in OPDs and IPDs of TB hospitals/medical colleges/teaching hospitals, microbiology departments, medical and nursing students, and other HCP assessed to be at high risk of occupational exposure)
Diphtheria	Health workers who have not been adequately immunized earlier against diphtheria and who may have occupational exposure to *Corynebacterium diphtheriae* should be vaccinated, especially those working in infectious diseases (ID) hospitals or ID wards, those working in pediatric departments and microbiology laboratory workers
Typhoid	Recommended for HCP involved in direct patient care, laboratory work, handling biomedical waste, house-keeping and sanitary staff, and personnel working in food catering establishments in hospitals

Continued

Continued

Disease	Situations in which recommendation to be given
Pertussis	Those health workers who have not been earlier adequately immunized against pertussis should be prioritized as a group to receive pertussis vaccine, especially those working in infectious diseases (ID) hospitals or ID wards, those working in pediatric departments and laboratory workers
Pneumococcal disease	Recommended for HCP working in infectious diseases (ID) hospitals or ID wards, or HCP who have chronic heart disease, COPD, CKD, diabetes mellitus, or immunocompromised state
Polio	Healthcare workers who are known or suspected to be unvaccinated or incompletely vaccinated (not adequately immunized as per NIS) against polio should receive and complete the polio vaccination series with IPV. Healthcare workers who have completed their polio vaccination but who are at increased risk of exposure to poliovirus may receive one lifetime IPV booster
Meningococcal disease	Health workers assessed to be at continued risk, especially those working in ID hospitals/wards, and during those times when an epidemic is likely to occur in their area of work, should be administered the primary dose followed by one booster dose, 3–5 years after the primary dose
Rabies	HCPs who are likely to come in contact with patients of Rabies as part of direct patient care or handling secretions/ excretions of patients of rabies or handling laboratory material from patients or animals suspected to be having Rabies are recommended to be given pre-exposure prophylaxis as follows:[7] Total three injections, each of either 0.1 mL by ID injection or 1 vial (containing either 1 mL or 0.5 mL depending on manufacturer), by IM injection, on days 0, 7, and either 21 or 28
Japanese encephalitis	Recommended for HCPs working in geographical areas known to be at high risk of transmission and high density of aquatic birds or pigs in the local area
Yellow fever	Recommended for HCP going for working in yellow fever endemic countries
Ebola	Recommended for HCP likely to undertake patient care of confirmed or suspected Ebola patients

(BCG: Bacillus Calmette–Guérin; COPD: chronic obstructive pulmonary disease; CKD: chronic kidney disease; HPV: human papillomavirus; IPV: inactivated polio vaccine; SARS-CoV-2: severe acute respiratory syndrome coronavirus 2)

TABLE 4: Recommendations for vaccination for agriculturists (including livestock workers).

Disease	Recommendations for vaccination
Tetanus	Recommended complete vaccination schedule with adsorbed injection of TT or Td. In case of persons who have completed the primary schedule as a part of NIS, one booster dose once in 10 years is recommended. In case the primary schedule has not been completed, start with primary schedule of three doses of injection TT or Td, 0.5 mL IM injection, separated by 4–8 weeks. In case the immunized person gets an injury which is potentially contaminated, thorough wound toilet and one dose of injection TT or Td should be given
Rabies	Recommended pre-exposure prophylaxis (PrEP) as follows: Total three injections, each of either 0.1 mL by ID injection or one vial (containing either 1 mL or 0.5 mL depending on manufacturer), by IM injection, on days 0, 7, and either 21 or 28. If an animal bite occurs within 3 months of completion of this primary schedule, only thorough wound cleaning is required. If >3 months have passed since completion of primary, thorough wound toilet and two doses (either 0.1 mL by ID injection or 1 vial by IM injection) on days 0 and 3 to be given. Booster may be given as one injection (either ID or IM) after every 2 years for those having continued high risk of exposure
Japanese encephalitis (JE)	Recommended for agriculturists in areas of high endemicity and environmental conditions conducive to high risk of transmission, as high density of Culex vector, paddy cultivation, and increased density of amplification hosts, as pigs and aquatic birds. Primary series consists of two doses each of 0.5 mL by subcutaneous route (for live-attenuated vaccine) or by IM route (for inactivated vaccine), separated by at least 4 weeks. It should not be given to pregnant women and during epidemic season. In addition, children and adults should be vaccinated as per the provisions of NIS in respect of JE
Anthrax	May be considered in a restricted manner for persons closely involved with livestock, in known endemic areas where anthrax transmission has been recorded. Primary vaccination consists of three doses, 0.5 mL each by IM injection at 0, 1, and 6 months followed by a booster after 6 months and thereafter every 12 months
Snake bite	Though it is not for primary (pre-exposure) immunization but rather for post-exposure treatment, it is important that polyvalent antisnake venom derived from both Elapid and Viperid snake families should be made available at the health subcenter level and above, in predominantly agricultural areas

(NIS: National Immunization Schedule)

TABLE 5: Suggested vaccinations for military personnel.

Disease/Vaccine	Recommendations
Tetanus toxoid (TT) or Td*	Recommended for all personnel. Ideally the primary series of vaccination should be undertaken at the time of joining the armed forces. Primary series is recommended to be three doses of 0.5 mL by IM Injection, at 0, 4 weeks, and 1 year. Booster is recommended after every 5 years
Typhoid	Recommended for all personnel. Ideally the primary series of vaccination should be undertaken at the time of joining the armed forces. Primary series consists of only one dose of Vi polysaccharide vaccine, 0.5 mL by IM Injection. Booster is recommended after every 3 years
Hepatitis B	Recommended for all armed forces personnel, including all healthcare personnel (HCP) and auxiliary HCP of armed forces. Recommended schedule is three doses each of 1 mL by IM injection, at 0, 4 weeks, and 6 months. No further boosters are recommended
Chickenpox (varicella)	Recommended for all personnel. Ideally the primary series of vaccination should be undertaken at the time of joining the armed forces. Primary series consists of two doses of 0.5 mL by SC injection, given 4 weeks apart. Booster dose is not required. In addition, healthcare persons who have not still been administered the primary course at the time of joining the armed forces may be considered for administering the primary series, especially those working in direct patient care in infectious diseases wards or working in training centers where recruits of armed forces are initially trained
Hepatitis A	Recommended for personnel deployed in operational and field conditions where standard methods of purification of water supplies are difficult to implement or when personnel are on mobile operations wherein supply of hygienic food and water is difficult to implement
COVID-19	Depending on risk-assessment, as and when directed by the DGAFMS, for all armed forces personnel, with highest priority being given to HCP
Anthrax	In situations where risk assessment indicates possibility of exposure to biological warfare with anthrax spores or when terrorist elements are likely to use anthrax spores in covert manner, as sending the spores by postal letters
Influenza A H1N1 (swine flu)	Recommended for HCP of armed forces who are likely to be exposed to cases of swine flu. Yearly booster is also recommended for such HCP
Japanese encephalitis	Recommended for military personnel engaged in special operations as anti-insurgency missions in geographical areas known to be at high risk of transmission.
Meningococcal meningitis	Depending on risk assessment when conditions of marked overcrowding and influx of young persons occur, as during enhanced recruitment with consequent overcrowding among recruits in military training centers
Polio	One dose of OPV, in case personnel are moving for military duty abroad, to countries where polio transmission is known to be endemic (see Government of India directives for travelers in See **Table 7** later)
Rabies, pre-exposure prophylaxis (PrEP)	For military personnel who work in "Dog Units" of the military and also, depending on risk assessment, for personnel of military veterinary service
Yellow fever	As per international health regulations, for personnel proceeding on military duty to yellow fever endemic countries
Tick-borne encephalitis	Depending on risk assessment, for personnel operating in jungle warfare or military operations in known endemic areas where other preventive measures for insect vector control are difficult to implement

*Tetanus toxoid (TT) or Td as per national policy in vogue.

(DGAFMS: Director General Armed Forces Medical Services; OPV: oral polio vaccine)

Recommended Vaccination for Travelers

Vaccination for travelers can be considered under two categories, viz., travelers coming to India from other countries and travelers going to other countries from India. The recommendations are as follows:[5,11,12]

Recommendations for travelers coming to India from outside countries: The recommendations are given in **Table 6**.

Recommendations for travelers going from India to outside countries: The details are given in **Table 7**.

"Workforce" as a Special Population: Recommendations for Vaccination

India has a substantial proportion of persons in the "workforce" contributing immensely to our national development. Of the workforce, a small proportion is of an

TABLE 6: Recommendations for vaccination for travelers coming to India from outside.*

Disease	Recommended vaccine and details
Mandatory vaccines:	
Yellow fever	Mandatory for persons coming from, or transiting through, yellow fever endemic countries as per list available at the WHO site, including those who have transited through these endemic countries
Polio	Mandatory one dose of oral polio vaccine (OPV) is required for all travelers coming to India from one of the eleven countries. These include six countries which are endemic for poliovirus infection (Afghanistan, Cameroon, Nigeria, Pakistan, Somalia, and Syria) and five countries listed as countries with poliovirus circulation (Malawi, Mozambique, Madagascar, Congo, and DR Congo). This one additional dose of OPV is required regardless of age and vaccination status at least 4 weeks prior to departure to India[12]
SARS-CoV-2	Certificate of successful COVID-19 vaccination is mandatory in case there are regulations specified by Government of India and International Health Regulations are in force at that instant point of time
Desirable, in addition to the mandatory vaccines above:	
Hepatitis A	Recommended that ideally, two doses of hepatitis A vaccine by IM injection, separated by 6–12 months should be taken before travel. In case this is not possible due to urgency, at least one dose of hepatitis A vaccine as soon as possible before departure is recommended. For persons aged >40 years, it is recommended that one dose of hepatitis A vaccine and a dose of immune serum globulin, 0.06 mL/kg body weight may be given as early as possible before departure. In case both hepatitis A vaccine and immunoglobulin are given, they should be injected at different sites
Cholera	One dose of either inactivated, whole-cell recombinant subunit vaccine or else, live attenuated (both given by oral route) is recommended. Booster may be required after 2 years
Hepatitis B	Those who have not undertaken the primary schedule, an accelerated three dose schedule (days 0, 7, and 21) before travel is recommended. This should be followed by a booster after 1 year. No further boosters are required
Japanese encephalitis	For travelers likely to visit areas where risk of transmission is high, primary series of two IM injections of inactivated vaccine at days 0 and 28 is recommended. For those who have undergone the primary series, a booster is required after 1 year of completion of primary series
Meningococcal disease	One dose by IM or SC injection (depending on the specification given by the manufacturer), recommended to be taken 2 weeks before the date of departure. Booster may be required every 3 yearly
Rabies (PrEP)	In case contact with wildlife or domestic/wild dogs is expected, a course of pre-exposure prophylaxis (PrEP) of three injections (at days 0, 7, and 21st or 28th day) with HDCV/PCECV is recommended
Typhoid	Recommended one dose of injectable Vi capsular polysaccharide vaccine. Immunity is likely to last for 2–3 years. Alternatively, four doses of oral live-attenuated typhoid vaccine can be taken, in which case the immunity is likely to last for approximately 5 years

*In addition to the above recommendations, it is also recommended that, in their own interest, travelers coming to India from foreign countries should have already been completely vaccinated with MMR, varicella, pneumococcal, DTaP, and influenza vaccines, as per the immunization schedule prevalent in their respective country.

TABLE 7: Recommendations for vaccination for travelers going from India to other countries.

Disease	Recommended vaccine and details
Mandatory vaccines:	
Yellow fever	Mandatory for persons going to yellow fever endemic countries as per list available at the WHO site
Polio	Indian residents traveling from India to the following eleven polio infected countries are required to receive a dose of OPV at least 4 weeks prior to departure, regardless of age and vaccination status: (1) Six countries which are endemic for poliovirus infection, namely, Afghanistan, Cameroon, Nigeria, Pakistan, Somalia, and Syria, (2) five listed as countries with poliovirus circulation, namely, Malawi, Mozambique, Madagascar, Congo, and DR Congo[12]
SARS-CoV-2	Mandatory in case there are regulations as specified by Government of India and International Health Regulations are in force at that instant point of time
Meningococcal disease	Travelers going to Saudi Arabia for the purpose of Umrah or pilgrimage (Hajj) or for seasonal work are required to submit a certificate of vaccination with the quadrivalent (ACYW135) vaccine against meningitis issued no more than 3 years and no less than 10 days before arrival in Saudi Arabia. Adults and children over the age of 2 years should be vaccinated with 1 dose of the quadrivalent polysaccharide (ACYW135) vaccine

Continued

Continued

Disease	Recommended vaccine and details
Desirable, in addition to the mandatory vaccines above: • Persons traveling from India to other countries should check from the Embassy/consulate of that country regarding specific vaccination requirements of that country, well in advance of the travel and complete the required vaccination process with needful certification • In general, different countries may require one or more of the following vaccinations: DPT/DTaP, hepatitis B, *Haemophilus influenzae* type B, HPV, MMR, meningococcal vaccine, pneumococcal vaccine, polio vaccine, rotavirus vaccine, varicella vaccine, and BCG	

(BCG: Bacillus Calmette–Guérin; DTaP: diphtheria, tetanus, and pertussis; HPV: human papillomavirus; MMR: measles, mumps, and rubella; SARS-CoV-2: severe acute respiratory syndrome coronavirus 2)

TABLE 8: Recommended vaccinations for "workforce".

Vaccine	IW	AW	CW	TW	ESW	FW	SW
COVID-19*	R	R	R	R	R	R	R
Anthrax	NR	SR (N-1)	NR	NR	NR	NR	NR
JE	NR	SR (N-2)	SR (N-2)	NR	NR	NR	NR
Typhoid#,**	R	R	R	R	R	R	R
Td	R	R	R	R	R	R	R
Hepatitis A	NR	NR	NR	NR	R	R	NR
Hepatitis B	R	R	R	R	R	R	R
HPV	NR	NR	NR	NR	NR	NR	R***
Meningitis	SR (N-3)	NR	SR (N-3)	NR	NR	NR	SR (N-3)

*As and when there are instructions issued by the Central/State governments or by the local health authority for COVID-19 vaccination; R: Recommended to be administered; NR: Not required; SR: Under special circumstances only; SR (N-1): For agricultural workforce exposed to livestock in areas where cases of anthrax have been reported; SR (N-2): If staying and working in areas known to be endemic for JE transmission and there is evidence of amplifying host population locally (pigs, water birds).

**Injectable Vi polysaccharide vaccine is preferable due to operational reasons.

#Typhoid Conjugate Vaccine (TCV) can be used if economically viable.

***Females up to 26 years and males up to 21 years; SR (N-3) = In case there is warning of impending epidemic in that area and persons are living in congested/overcrowded conditions.

(HPV: human papillomavirus; JE: Japanese encephalitis)

"organized" nature while a large proportion is of a casual or unorganized nature, including a substantial number of laborers who are "migratory" in nature. While there are a large number of categories of occupations in which our workforce is involved, the major categories include: industrial workers (IW), agricultural workers (AW), construction workers (CW) (who work in various projects ranging from small housing projects to huge projects like dams, townships, highways, etc.), transport workers (TW) (working in railways, road transport including truckers, waterways, etc.), environmental sanitation workers (ESW) (working in sewage works, waterworks, handling solid wastes or nightsoil or both, etc.), food industry workers (FW), and sex workers (SW). Surprisingly, there is hardly any consensus available on the vaccination requirements of this category of special population and with this background, the recommendations are as shown in **Table 8**.

Recommendations for Vaccination in Certain Disease Conditions

Persons suffering from immunocompromised state and chronic diseases form a special population group whose vaccination needs are different from the population at large.[5,8] The recommendations are given in **Table 9**, while the recommendations for vaccination of children with HIV infection[13] are laid out in **Table 10**.

TABLE 9: Vaccination in certain important disease conditions.[5,8]

Disease	Vaccination recommended to be undertaken
PLHIV (adults)	Recommended: COVID-19, Td, hepatitis A, hepatitis B, HPV, influenza (with inactivated or recombinant quadrivalent influenza vaccine but not with live vaccine), meningococcal quadrivalent ACWY135, pneumococcal (PCV-13 or PPSV-23), rabies (if exposure to dogs/cats/wildlife is potential), and shingles (herpes zoster). In addition, injectable typhoid Vi polysaccharide vaccine may be considered if benefits outweigh risk
PLHIV (children)	See **Table 10**
Persons with heart disease, lung disease, diabetes mellitus, CKD, or on hemodialysis	COVID-19, chickenpox (varicella), Td, Hib, hepatitis B, HPV, quadrivalent influenza (inactivated or recombinant), PCV-13 or PPSV-23. Rabies may be given as PEP as part of anti-rabic treatment. In addition, hepatitis A, meningococcal quadrivalent, and herpes zoster (shingles) can be given in case there are additional risk factors such as chronic liver disease, HIV infection, injecting drug use, or MSM

(CKD: chronic kidney disease; HPV: human papillomavirus; PCV: pneumococcal conjugate vaccine; PLHIV: people living with HIV; PPSV: pneumococcal polysaccharide vaccine)

TABLE 10: Recommendations for immunization of HIV-infected children.[13]

Vaccine	Recommendations
BCG	• If asymptomatic, administer birth dose • Do not administer if symptomatic
DTP/TT/Td	Administer as per national immunization schedule (6, 10, 14 weeks, 16–24 months, and 5 years)
Polio vaccine	IPV at 6, 10, 14 weeks, 16–24 months, and 5 years. If IPV is not affordable, give bivalent OPV
MR	• If asymptomatic, administer as per schedule at 9 months and 15–18 months • If symptomatic, administer only if CD4+ count is >15%
Hepatitis B	• If asymptomatic, administer at 0, 1, and 6 months • If symptomatic, give four doses, give double dose and check for seroconversion, give regular boosters
Hib/Pentavalent	Administer as per national immunization schedule at 6, 10, and 14 weeks
Pneumococcal	• If PCV, give at 6, 10, and 14 weeks and 12–15 months • If PPSV-23, give first dose 2 months after PCV, second dose 5 years after 1st dose. Do not give more than 2 doses
Hepatitis A	Can be given. In case of symptomatic, check for seroconversion and administer booster if needed
Influenza	Inactivated influenza vaccine can be given starting at 6 months age, revaccination every year
Typhoid	Injectable Vi polysaccharide vaccine can be given once in 3 years
Varicella	• If asymptomatic, give two doses at interval of 4–12 weeks • If symptomatic, but if CD4+ count is >15%, it can be given as 2 doses, 4–12 weeks apart
Rotavirus	At present, it is not recommended due to lack of data

(BCG: Bacillus Calmette–Guérin; Hib: *Haemophilus influenzae* type B; DTP: diphtheria, tetanus, and pertussis; MR: measles and rubella; PCV: pneumococcal conjugate vaccine; PPSV: pneumococcal polysaccharide vaccine)

PART II: DETAILS OF VACCINES RECOMMENDED FOR SPECIAL POPULATION GROUPS

Ready-reckoner information with respect to vaccines recommended for various special populations in Part I of this chapter is given in subsequent paragraphs.[14-17]

Anthrax

General description: Killed (inactivated) cell-free filtrate vaccine from *Bacillus anthracis*.

Contents: Consists of protective antigen protein, aluminum hydroxide (adjuvant), preservatives, and stabilizers as per formulation.

Commercial name: Not widely marketed in India, but is available through government channels as the anthrax vaccine adsorbed (AVA).

Dose schedule: 3 doses each of 0.5 mL IM (0, 4 weeks, and 6 months), annual booster doses only for those who continue to be at risk of exposure to anthrax.

Side effects and adverse reactions:
- *Minor*: Pain, redness, and swelling, muscle aches, headaches, mild fever
- *Major*: Anaphylaxis, serious injection site reactions, rare neurological events

Contraindications: Severe allergic reaction, pregnant women (unless high risk of exposure)

Cold chain requirements: 2–8°C (36–46°F)

Efficacy of vaccine: The exact efficacy can vary. Likely to provide significant protection, against cutaneous anthrax and inhalation anthrax when used alongside antibiotics.

Cholera

General description: The cholera vaccine available in India is an oral inactivated (killed) vaccine. There are two main types: (1) *Dukoral*, which contains inactivated Vibrio cholerae O1 Inaba classic strain, El Tor strain, and Ogawa classic strain and a recombinant cholera toxin B subunit, and (2) *Shanchol*, which contains inactivated Vibrio cholerae O1 Inaba, Ogawa and O139 strains.

Dose schedule in adults: (1) *Dukoral*: Primary series—two doses, the second dose 1–6 weeks after the first dose. A single booster dose is recommended every 2 years for those at continued risk. (2) *Shanchol*: Primary series—two doses, the second dose 2 weeks after the first dose. A single booster dose is recommended after 2 years for those at continued risk.

Dose schedule in children: (1) *Dukoral*: Children aged 2–6 years: Three doses, the second dose 1–6 weeks after the first dose, and the third dose 1–6 weeks after the second dose. A single booster dose is recommended every 6 months for those at continued risk. (2) *Shanchol*: Children aged 1–6 years—two doses, the second dose 2 weeks after the first dose. A single booster dose is recommended after 6 months for those at continued risk.

Dose and route of administration: (1) *Dukoral*: 3 mL orally; (2) *Shanchol*: 1.5 mL for children and 3 mL for adults, orally

Side effects and adverse reactions:
- *Minor side effects*: Abdominal pain, diarrhea, nausea, vomiting, headache, and fatigue
- *Major adverse reactions*: Rarely severe allergic reactions

Contraindications:
- Severe allergic reaction to a previous dose or to any component of the vaccine
- Acute gastrointestinal illness (vaccination should be postponed)

Cold chain requirements:
- Stored at 2–8°C (36–46°F)
- Should not be frozen.

Precautions during vaccination:
- Individuals with a moderate or severe acute illness should wait until recovery before getting the vaccine.
- It is important to avoid eating or drinking for 1 hour before and 1 hour after taking the vaccine.
- Those with a history of allergic reactions to vaccine components should inform their healthcare provider.

Efficacy of vaccine: Studies suggest that the efficacy of Dukoral ranges from 50 to 85% in the first 6 months after vaccination. Shanchol provides around 65% protection over a 5-year period. The vaccine is particularly effective in reducing the severity of illness and is an important preventive support in cholera-endemic regions.

Tdap/Td

General description: Tdap (tetanus toxoid, diphtheria toxoid, and acellular pertussis) and Td (tetanus and diphtheria toxoids) vaccines are inactivated vaccines.

Contents: Inactivated toxins (toxoids) of tetanus, diphtheria, and acellular pertussis, adjuvants (aluminum salts), preservatives, and stabilizers. Td is included in NIS for pregnant women and for children at 5, 10, and 16 years age. Acellular pertussis vaccine is preferred where there is history of adverse reaction to DPT vaccine which contains killed pertussis bacteria.

Commercial name: Tdap Boostrix (GlaxoSmithKline) and Adacel (Sanofi Pasteur). Td: SII Td-Vac (Serum Institute of India)

Schedule in adults: 0.5 mL IM for Td and Tdap. Single dose for adults who have not previously received Tdap. Two doses recommended for pregnant women during pregnancy. Single dose to be taken if subsequent pregnancy is within 3 years.

Side effects and adverse reactions:
- *Minor*: Pain, redness, and swelling, fever, headache, muscle pain, fatigue
- *Major*: Anaphylaxis, Guillain–Barré syndrome (very rare), Arthus-type hypersensitivity reactions (rare)

Contraindications: Severe allergic reaction to a previous dose or to any component of the vaccine, history of encephalopathy not attributable to another identifiable cause within 7 days of administration of a previous pertussis-containing vaccine (for Tdap).

Cold chain requirements: 2–8°C (36–46°F). They should not be frozen.

Precautions during vaccination: Individuals with acute illness should wait until recovery before getting the vaccine. If Arthus-type hypersensitivity reactions occur, subsequent doses of Td or Tdap should be deferred for at least 10 years.

Efficacy of vaccine: Tdap provides high levels of protection against tetanus, diphtheria, and pertussis. Pertussis protection decreases over time, so it is important to follow the recommended schedule. Td provides high levels of protection; however, booster doses (recommended once in 10 years) are necessary to maintain long-term immunity.

Hepatitis A

General description: The hepatitis A vaccine is an inactivated (killed) virus vaccine.

Contents: Inactivated hepatitis A virus, aluminum hydroxide (adjuvant), preservatives, and stabilizers

Commercial name: Havrix (GlaxoSmithKline), VAQTA (Merck & Co.)

Dose schedule in adults: 0.5 mL IM for those aged 1–18 years, and 1.0 mL for adults. The recommended schedule is 2 injections at 0 and 6–12 months. Booster dose not required.

Side effects and adverse reactions:
- *Minor*: Pain, redness, and swelling, fever, headache, muscle pain, fatigue
- *Major*: Anaphylaxis, neurological events (extremely rare)

Contraindications: Severe allergic reaction to previous dose or to any vaccine component

Cold chain requirements: 2–8°C (36–46°F). It should not be frozen.

Precautions during vaccination: Individuals with acute illness should wait until recovery before getting the vaccine. Pregnant or breastfeeding women should consult with their healthcare provider before vaccination. Those with a history of severe allergic reactions to vaccine components should inform their healthcare provider.

Efficacy of vaccine: Data indicates that the vaccine provides protection in over 95% of individuals who complete the primary series. Long-term immunity is generally achieved, with protection lasting up to 20 years, and possibly lifelong, after completing the recommended doses.

Hepatitis B

General description: The hepatitis B vaccine available in India is a recombinant vaccine.

Contents: Recombinant hepatitis B surface antigen (HBsAg), aluminum hydroxide (adjuvant), preservatives, and stabilizers

Commercial name: Engerix-B (GlaxoSmithKline), Recombivax HB (Merck & Co.), Euvax-B (LG Life Sciences), Shanvac-B (Shantha Biotechnics)

Dose schedule: In adults, 3 injections of 0.5 mL IM at 0, 1, and 6 months. Alternate schedules include accelerated schedule for certain at-risk groups: 0, 1, 2 months, and a booster at 12 months. For chronic renal failure patients, the recommended schedule is 0, 1, 2, and 6 months with higher doses. In children, 4 doses at 0, 6, 10, 14 weeks as part of routine childhood immunization schedules, either as monovalent hepatitis B vaccine or else as pentavalent vaccine.

Side effects and adverse reactions:
- *Minor*: Pain, redness, and swelling, fever, headache, muscle pain, fatigue
- *Major*: Anaphylaxis, neurological events (extremely rare)

Contraindications: Severe allergic reaction to previous dose or any vaccine component

Cold chain requirements: 2–8°C (36–46°F). It should not be frozen.

Precautions during vaccination: Individuals with acute illness should wait until recovery before getting the vaccine. Pregnant or breastfeeding women should consult with their healthcare provider before vaccination. Those with a history of severe allergic reactions to vaccine components should inform their healthcare provider.

Efficacy of vaccine: Data indicate that the vaccine provides protection in over 90% of individuals who complete the primary series. Long-term immunity is generally achieved, with protection lasting at least 20 years, and possibly lifelong, after completing the recommended doses.

Human Papillomavirus Vaccine

General description: The human papillomavirus (HPV) vaccine available in India is a recombinant vaccine. There are two main types of HPV vaccines used in India: bivalent (against HPV types 16 and 18) and quadrivalent (against HPV types 6, 11, 16, and 18).

Contents: Recombinant HPV L1 protein virus-like particles (VLPs), adjuvants (e.g., aluminum hydroxide, AS04), preservatives, and stabilizers

Commercial name: Cervarix (bivalent, GlaxoSmithKline), Gardasil (quadrivalent, Merck)

Dose schedule: 0.5 mL IM for adolescents aged 9–14 years: Two doses at 0 and 6–12 months. For those aged 15 years and older: Three doses at 0, 1, and 6 months.

Side effects and adverse reactions:
- *Minor*: Pain, redness, and swelling, fever, headache, muscle pain, fatigue
- *Major*: Severe allergic reactions (anaphylaxis, very rare), fainting attack (rare)

Contraindications: Severe allergic reaction to a previous dose, pregnancy (vaccination should be postponed)

Cold chain requirements: 2–8°C (36–46°F). It should not be frozen.

Precautions during vaccination: Individuals with a moderate or severe acute illness should wait until recovery before getting the vaccine. Pregnant women should delay vaccination until after pregnancy. Observing the patient for 15 minutes after vaccination is recommended to manage potential syncope.

Efficacy of vaccine: Data indicate that the vaccine provides almost 100% protection against sequelae of HPV types 16- and 18-related cervical pre-cancers and genital warts. Long-term studies suggest sustained protection for at least 10 years, with the expectation of even longer-lasting immunity. Vaccination before the onset of sexual activity is crucial for maximum efficacy.

Influenza Vaccine

General description: The influenza vaccine available in India is an inactivated (killed) vaccine that provides immunity against the influenza virus. There are two main types of influenza vaccines: the trivalent (covers three strains: two influenza A and one influenza B) and the quadrivalent (covers four strains: two influenza A and two influenza B).

Contents: Inactivated influenza virus strains, adjuvants (for some vaccines), preservatives (such as thimerosal in multi-dose vials), and stabilizers

Commercial name: Vaxigrip (Sanofi Pasteur), Fluarix (GlaxoSmithKline), Influvac (Abbott), Fluzone (Sanofi Pasteur), and Agripal (Novartis)

Dose schedule: Single annual dose is recommended based on changing nature of influenza virus strains. Children aged 6 months to 35 months: 0.25 mL IM, children aged 3 years and older, and adults 0.5 mL IM. For children aged 6 months to 8 years receiving the influenza vaccine for the first time, two doses are recommended. The recommended schedule is 0 and 4 weeks apart. For children who have previously received the influenza vaccine, a single annual dose is sufficient.

Side effects and adverse reactions:
- *Minor*: Pain, redness, and swelling, fever, headache, muscle pain, nausea, and fatigue
- *Major*: Anaphylaxis (very rare), Guillain-Barré syndrome (very rare)

Contraindications: Severe allergic reaction, history of severe egg allergy (some influenza vaccines are produced in eggs, though egg-free versions are available)

Cold chain requirements: 2–8°C (36–46°F). It should not be frozen.

Precautions during vaccination: Individuals with acute illness should wait until recovery before getting the vaccine. Pregnant women, elderly individuals, and those with chronic health conditions should consult their healthcare provider before vaccination. Individuals with a history of Guillain-Barré syndrome should inform their healthcare provider.

Efficacy of vaccine: On average, the vaccine reduces the risk of influenza illness by 40–60% when there is a good match with circulating virus strains. Annual vaccination is essential due to the frequent changes in influenza virus strains. The vaccine is effective in preventing severe illness, hospitalization, and death, especially among high-risk groups, as HCP.

Meningococcal Meningitis Vaccines

General description: The meningococcal meningitis vaccine protects against bacterial infections caused by *Neisseria meningitidis*, which can lead to meningitis and septicemia (blood infection).

Contents: Outer membrane proteins (OMPs) or polysaccharides from various meningococcal serogroups (e.g., A, C, W, and Y), adjuvants (for some vaccines), stabilizers, and preservatives.

Commercial name: Menactra (Sanofi Pasteur), Menveo (GlaxoSmithKline), Nimenrix (Pfizer), and NeisVac-C (Janssen)

Dose schedule: 0.5 mL IM single dose followed by booster every 5 years in case of continued risk; however, some countries require a booster within 3 years as a part of their international travel regulations.

Side effects and adverse reactions:

- *Minor*: Pain, redness, and swelling at the injection site, fever, headache, fatigue, and muscle aches
- *Major*: Anaphylaxis (very rare), Guillain-Barré syndrome (rare)

Contraindications: Severe allergic reaction to a previous dose or to any component of the vaccine

Cold chain requirements: 2–8°C (36–46°F). Protection from light or freezing.

Precautions during vaccination: Individuals with a moderate or severe acute illness should wait until recovery before getting the vaccine. Pregnant or breastfeeding women should consult their healthcare provider before vaccination. Travelers to areas with high incidence rates of meningococcal disease should consider vaccination prior to travel.

Efficacy of vaccine: Vaccine efficacy can vary depending on the serogroups covered and the vaccine type (e.g., conjugate vs. polysaccharide). Booster doses may be recommended for individuals at continued risk, such as travelers to regions with high rates of meningococcal disease outbreaks.

Pneumococcal Vaccine

General description: Protects against infections caused by *Streptococcus pneumoniae*, which can lead to pneumonia, meningitis, and bloodstream infections.

Contents: Polysaccharides from various pneumococcal serotypes (for polysaccharide vaccines), polysaccharides conjugated to carrier proteins (for conjugate vaccines), adjuvants (for some vaccines), stabilizers, and preservatives.

Commercial name: Pneumovax 23 (Merck & Co.)—polysaccharide vaccine, Prevnar 13 (Pfizer)—conjugate vaccine

Dose schedule: 0.5 mL IM

Pneumovax 23 (PPSV-23 polysaccharide vaccine): Single dose for adults aged 65 years and more. A second dose may be recommended for certain high-risk individuals after 5 years.

Prevnar 13 (PCV-13 conjugate vaccine): Single dose for adults aged 65 years and older who have not previously received it. Sometimes given to adults aged 19–64 years who are at increased risk of pneumococcal disease. In children, *Prevnar 13* is recommended as part of routine childhood immunization schedules.

Side effects and adverse reactions:

- *Minor*: Pain, redness, and swelling at the injection site, fever, headache, fatigue, and muscle aches
- *Major*: Anaphylaxis (very rare), Guillain-Barré syndrome (rare)

Contraindications: Severe allergic reaction to a previous dose or to any component of the vaccine

Cold chain requirements: 2–8°C (36–46°F). It should not be frozen.

Precautions during vaccination: Individuals with acute illness should wait until recovery before getting the vaccine. Pregnant or breastfeeding women should consult their healthcare provider before vaccination. Those with a history of severe allergic reactions to vaccine components should inform their healthcare provider.

Efficacy of vaccine: The conjugate vaccine (Prevnar 13) provides broader protection, especially in infants and young children, by inducing immune memory and enhancing antibody response. The polysaccharide vaccine (Pneumovax 23) is effective in older adults and high-risk individuals but may not induce long-lasting immunity in young children. Vaccination is recommended based on age, health status, and risk factors for pneumococcal disease.

Injectable Polio Vaccine

General description: The injectable polio vaccine (IPV) is a killed (inactivated) vaccine that provides immunity against poliomyelitis, caused by poliovirus types 1, 2, and 3.

Contents: Inactivated poliovirus strains (types 1, 2, and 3), stabilizers, and preservatives

Commercial name: IPV (generic name for inactivated polio vaccine), Imovax Polio (Sanofi Pasteur), and Poliorix (GlaxoSmithKline)

Dose schedule: 0.5 mL IM at 6 weeks, 10 weeks, and 14 weeks of age, as part of routine childhood immunization schedules. A booster dose of IPV is recommended between 4 and 6 years of age. Fractional dosing (0.1 mL intradermal for each dose) has also found to be effective in resource constraints.

Side effects and adverse reactions:

- *Minor*: Pain, redness, and swelling at the injection site, fever, irritability, fatigue
- *Major*: Anaphylaxis (very rare)

Contraindications: Severe allergic reaction to a previous dose or to any component of the vaccine

Cold chain requirements: 2–8°C (36–46°F). It should not be frozen.

Precautions during vaccination: Individuals with a moderate or severe acute illness should wait until recovery before getting the vaccine. Vaccination can generally be administered to pregnant women and immunocompromised individuals, but individual circumstances should be considered.

Efficacy of vaccine: The IPV is highly effective in preventing polio disease caused by wild poliovirus strains. It induces immunity against all three poliovirus types (1, 2, and 3) and contributes to global efforts to eradicate polio. High vaccine coverage is essential to maintain herd immunity and prevent outbreaks. Booster doses help ensure long-term protection against poliovirus infection.

Oral Polio Vaccine

General description: The oral polio vaccine (OPV) is a live-attenuated vaccine that provides immunity against poliomyelitis.

Contents: Live-attenuated poliovirus strains bivalent (types 1 and 3), trivalent (1, 2, and 3). Trivalent vaccine is not currently in use in India.

Commercial name:
- OPV (generic name for oral polio vaccine)
- *Trivalent OPV*: Contains all three types (1, 2, and 3)
- *Bivalent OPV*: Contains types 1 and 3 (NIS)

Dose schedule: 2 drops orally as part of routine childhood immunization schedules. However, instructions from the manufacturer should be seen regarding the dose, for individual suppliers, 0, 6, 10, 14 weeks, and at 16–24 months age. Additional doses or booster doses may be administered during supplementary immunization campaigns or in response to outbreaks.

Side effects and adverse reactions:
- *Minor*: Mild gastrointestinal symptoms (such as diarrhea), low-grade fever, irritability, or dizziness
- *Major*: Vaccine-associated paralytic poliomyelitis (very rare, primarily associated with the use of the live vaccine containing type-2 virus strain)

Contraindications: Severe immunodeficiency (where live vaccines are contraindicated)

Cold chain requirements: 2–8°C (36–46°F) to maintain its potency. It should not be frozen.

Precautions during vaccination: Careful monitoring is essential to manage any adverse events promptly.

Efficacy of vaccine: Mass vaccination campaigns with OPV have been instrumental in achieving and maintaining polio-free status in many countries. However, in rare cases, the live-attenuated vaccine virus (type-2 strain) can mutate and cause vaccine-derived poliovirus infections, which is a consideration in vaccination strategies and monitoring efforts.

Rabies Vaccine

General description: The rabies vaccine used in India is inactivated rabies virus antigens grown in vero cells or purified chick embryo cells.

Contents: Inactivated rabies virus antigens grown in vero cells or purified chick embryo cells, adjuvants (for some vaccines), stabilizers, and preservatives

Commercial name: Rabipur (Novartis)—vero cell culture, Verorab (Sanofi Pasteur)—vero cell culture, Abhayrab (Zydus Cadila)—chick embryo cell culture, and Indirab (Bharat Biotech)—chick embryo cell culture

Dose schedule: Essen regimen: 0.5 mL IM. Five doses of rabies vaccine are typically administered on days 0, 3, 7, and 14 and 28. Additional booster dose may be given on day 90 for immunocompromised individuals. Modified Thai regimen: 0.1 mL ID on either arm at 0, 3, 7, and 28 days. Pre-exposure prophylaxis (PrEP): Three doses on days 0, 7, and 21, or 28 for individuals at high risk of exposure to rabies (e.g., veterinarians, laboratory workers).

RIG (rabies immunoglobulin) either from equine source (ERIG) (40 IU/kg up to 3,000 IU) or from human source (HRIG) (20 IU/kg) is used for passive immunization in conjunction with rabies vaccine. *Monoclonal antibodies* against rabies virus are used in some cases of rabies exposure, providing specific neutralizing antibodies to the virus. These are used in individuals unable to receive RIG from animal sources due to allergies or other concerns. It is available as "RABISHIELD". The dose is 3.33 IU/Kg body weight and the method of local infiltration/systemic administration is the same as for HRIG.

Side effects and adverse reactions:
- *Minor*: Pain, redness, and swelling at the injection site, fever, headache, fatigue, nausea
- *Major*: Severe allergic reactions (anaphylaxis, very rare)

Contraindications: Severe allergic reaction to a previous dose or to any component of the vaccine

Cold chain requirements: 2–8°C (36–46°F). It should not be frozen.

Precautions during vaccination: Proper administration techniques should be followed to avoid contamination and ensure effective vaccination. Post-exposure prophylaxis should be initiated promptly after potential exposure to rabies.

Efficacy of vaccine: The rabies vaccine is highly effective in preventing rabies infection when administered promptly after exposure. The vaccine is a critical component of rabies control programs and is administered in combination with RIG for individuals with higher risk or severe exposure.

Yellow Fever

General description: The yellow fever vaccine is a live-attenuated vaccine (17D strain).

Contents: Live-attenuated yellow fever virus 17D strain, stabilizers, and preservatives

Commercial name: Stamaril (Sanofi Pasteur), YF-VAX (Sanofi Pasteur)

Dose schedule: 0.5 mL SC single dose. A booster can be given 10 years for individuals at continued risk of exposure although not recommended anymore by International Health Regulations. Fractional dosing can be given in emergencies.

Side effects and adverse reactions:
- *Minor*: Pain, redness, and swelling at the injection site, low-grade fever, headache, muscle aches, and fatigue
- *Major*: Severe allergic reactions (anaphylaxis, very rare), vaccine-associated viscerotropic disease (very rare, more common in individuals aged 60 years and older)

Contraindications: Severe allergic reaction to a previous dose or to any component of the vaccine; immuno-deficiency or immunosuppression (unless benefit outweighs risk)

International health regulations (IHR): International travelers should receive the yellow fever vaccine at least 10 days before travel to, or transiting through, yellow fever-endemic areas.

Cold chain requirements: 2–8°C (36–46°F). It should not be frozen.

Precautions during vaccination: Travelers should consult healthcare providers to determine if yellow fever vaccination is recommended based on travel itinerary and individual health factors.

Efficacy of vaccine: The yellow fever vaccine is considered one of the most effective vaccines available. A single dose provides robust immunity in the majority of recipients. Vaccination not only protects individual travelers but also contributes to global health efforts in preventing yellow fever outbreaks and transmission.

Tick-borne Encephalitis

General description: The tick-borne encephalitis (TBE) vaccine is a viral vaccine that provides protection against TBE virus, which can cause severe neurological disease.

Contents: Inactivated TBE virus antigens, adjuvants (for some vaccines), stabilizers, and preservatives

Commercial name: FSME-IMMUN (Pfizer), Encepur (GlaxoSmithKline), TicoVac (Pfizer)

Dose schedule: 0.5 mL IM. Three doses typically administered at 0, 1–3, and 9–12 months schedule. Booster doses are recommended based on individual risk factors and exposure to TBE virus.

Side effects and adverse reactions:
- *Minor*: Pain, redness, and swelling at the injection site, fever, headache, fatigue, myalgia
- *Major*: Severe allergic reactions (anaphylaxis), neurological complications (both rare)

Contraindications: Severe allergic reaction to a previous dose or to any component of the vaccine

Cold chain requirements: 2–8°C (36–46°F). It should not be frozen.

Precautions during vaccination: Proper administration techniques should be followed to avoid contamination and ensure effective vaccination. Individuals with a history of severe allergic reactions should be closely monitored.

Efficacy of vaccine: The TBE vaccine is highly effective in preventing TBE infection caused by TBE virus. It induces a strong immune response and provides long-term protection against the virus. Booster doses may be recommended based on individual risk factors and exposure to TBE virus. Vaccination is particularly important for individuals residing in or traveling to areas where TBE is endemic or where outbreaks occur.

Typhoid Vaccine

General description: Typhoid vaccines are used to prevent typhoid fever, a bacterial infection caused primarily by *Salmonella typhi* bacteria, transmitted through contaminated food or water.

Types of typhoid vaccines:

- *Typhoid conjugate vaccine (TCV)*: Contains polysaccharide of *S. typhi* conjugated to a protein carrier. *Commercial name*: Typbar-TCV (Bharat Biotech), PedaTyph (Serum Institute of India). *Dose schedule*: 0.5 mL IM single dose for adults and children over 6 months of age.
- *Typhoid Vi polysaccharide vaccine (TYP)*: Contains purified Vi polysaccharide from *S. typhi*. *Commercial name*: Typhim Vi (Sanofi Pasteur). *Dose schedule*: A single dose of 0.5 mL by IM injection for adults and children over 2 years of age. Recommended every 2–3 years for individuals at continued risk.
- *Live oral typhoid vaccine (Ty21a)*: Live-attenuated *S. typhi* strain Ty21a. *Commercial name*: Vivotif (Crucell). *Dose schedule*: Capsules taken on alternate days, completing a total of four capsules. A booster dose every 5 years for continued protection in endemic areas or ongoing risk.

Side effects and adverse reactions:

- *Minor*: Pain, redness, and swelling at the injection site (for injectable vaccines). Mild fever, headache, fatigue, and gastrointestinal symptoms (for oral vaccine).
- *Major*: Severe allergic reactions (anaphylaxis, very rare). Neurological complications (very rare).

Contraindications: Severe allergic reaction to previous dose or any vaccine component.

Cold chain requirements: 2–8°C (36–46°F)

Precautions during vaccination: Proper administration techniques should be followed to ensure vaccine efficacy and minimize adverse events. Travelers to endemic areas should receive the vaccine well in advance of travel to allow for immunity to develop.

Efficacy of vaccine: Typhoid vaccines are effective in preventing typhoid fever caused by *S. typhi*. Vaccine efficacy varies by type but generally is estimated to be about 60%. Booster doses may be recommended based on individual risk factors and ongoing.

Varicella Vaccine

General description: Also known as the Chickenpox vaccine, is a live-attenuated vaccine that provides immunity against the varicella-zoster virus (VZV), which causes chickenpox.

Contents: Live-attenuated VZV, stabilizers, and preservatives

Commercial name: Varivax (Merck & Co.), Varilrix (GlaxoSmithKline)

Dose schedule: 0.5 mL SC. Two doses, first at age of 12–15 months and second at age of 4–6 years. For children aged 7–13 years, the gap between the two doses should be at least 3 months and for adolescents/adults aged >13 years, the minimum gap between the 2 doses should be 4 weeks.

Side effects and adverse reactions:

- *Minor*: Pain, redness, and swelling at the injection site, low-grade fever, rash (mild, transient), fatigue
- *Major*: Anaphylaxis (very rare)

Contraindications: Severe allergic reaction to a previous dose or to any component of the vaccine, pregnant women (should wait until after pregnancy)

Cold chain requirements: 2–8°C (36–46°F). It should not be frozen.

Precautions during vaccination: Individuals with a moderate or severe acute illness should wait until recovery, before getting vaccination. Post-vaccination precautions include observing for any signs of allergic reaction.

Efficacy of vaccine: It provides long-lasting immunity against chickenpox and reduces the severity of the disease even if breakthrough infection occurs. Vaccination also helps prevent complications associated with chickenpox, such as secondary bacterial infections and pneumonia. High vaccine coverage in communities contributes to herd immunity, protecting vulnerable individuals who cannot be vaccinated due to medical reasons.

Rotavirus Vaccine

General description: The rotavirus vaccine is an oral vaccine that provides immunity against rotavirus infection, a common cause of severe diarrhea in infants and young children worldwide.

Contents: Live-attenuated rotavirus strains (e.g., G1, G2, G3, G4, and G9), stabilizers, and preservatives

Commercial name: Rotavac (Bharat Biotech), Rotasiil (Serum Institute of India), Rotarix (GlaxoSmithKline), RotaTeq (Merck & Co.)

Dose schedule: Rotavac 0.5 mL orally, rotasiil either 2 or 2.5 mL orally (see instructions from manufacturer on the carton), Rotarix and RotaTeq 5 drops orally. 3 doses at age of at 6, 10, and 14 weeks.

Side effects and adverse reactions:
- *Minor*: Mild irritability, mild diarrhea, vomiting, and fever
- *Major*: Severe allergic reactions (anaphylaxis, very rare), intussusception

Contraindications: Severe allergic reaction to a previous dose or to any component of the vaccine, history of intussusception

Cold chain requirements: 2–8°C (36–46°F)

Precautions during vaccination: Rotavirus vaccine should not be administered to infants with severe combined immunodeficiency (SCID) or other severe immunodeficiencies.

Efficacy of vaccine: It significantly reduces the burden of rotavirus gastroenteritis in vaccinated children and contributes to the overall reduction in rotavirus-related morbidity and mortality globally.

Covishield

General description: Covishield is a viral vector vaccine against COVID-19, developed by Oxford-AstraZeneca and manufactured by the Serum Institute of India.

Contents: Chimpanzee Adenovirus vector (ChAdOx1) containing the genetic material of the SARS-CoV-2 spike protein, stabilizers, and preservatives

Dose schedule: 0.5 mL IM. Two doses are recommended, typically administered 4–12 weeks apart. A booster dose after 1 year may be recommended based on evolving guidelines and emerging variants.

Side effects and adverse reactions:
- *Minor*: Pain, swelling at the injection site, fever, headache, fatigue, and muscle pain
- *Major*: Severe allergic reactions (anaphylaxis, very rare)

Contraindications: Severe allergic reaction to previous dose or any vaccine component

Cold chain requirements: 2–8°C (36–46°F). It should not be frozen.

Precautions during vaccination: Proper administration techniques should be followed to ensure vaccine efficacy and minimize adverse events. Post-vaccination observation is recommended for any immediate allergic reactions.

Efficacy of vaccine: Covishield has shown efficacy in preventing COVID-19 and reducing severe disease and hospitalizations. Efficacy may vary against different variants of SARS-CoV-2.

Covaxin

General description: Covaxin is an inactivated virus vaccine against COVID-19, developed by Bharat Biotech in collaboration with the Indian Council of Medical Research (ICMR) and the National Institute of Virology (NIV).

Contents: Inactivated SARS-CoV-2 virus particles, adjuvants (for enhancing immune response), stabilizers, and preservatives

Dose schedule: 0.5 mL IM. Two doses are recommended, typically administered 4–6 weeks apart. A booster dose may be recommended after 1 year, based on evolving guidelines and emerging variants.

Side effects and adverse reactions:
- *Minor*: Pain, swelling at the injection site, fever, headache, fatigue, nausea
- *Major*: Severe allergic reactions (anaphylaxis, very rare)

Contraindications: Severe allergic reaction to a previous dose or to any component of the vaccine

Cold chain requirements: 2–8°C (36–46°F). It should not be frozen.

Precautions during vaccination: Post-vaccination observation is recommended for immediate reactions.

Efficacy of vaccine: Covaxin has shown efficacy in preventing COVID-19 and reducing severe disease and hospitalizations. Efficacy may vary against different variants of SARS-CoV-2.

Japanese Encephalitis Vaccine

General description: It is a viral vaccine that provides immunity against JE virus, a mosquito-borne virus that can cause severe inflammation of the brain.

Contents and commercial names: Broadly, two types of vaccines are available—
1. *Inactivated vero cell vaccine*: There are two types of vaccines licensed in India, namely (i) SA-14-14-2 strain manufactured by the name of "JEEV" by Biologicals E and (ii) Kolar-821564XY strain manufactured as "JENVAC" by Bharat Biotech.
2. Live-attenuated (primary hamster kidney cells) vaccine, licensed in India, manufactured by Chengdu Institute, China by name of CDJEVAX, from attenuated SA-14-14-2 strain.

Dose schedule:
- *For live-attenuated vaccine*: 0.5 mL subcutaneous, first dose at 9–12 months age and second dose at 16–24 months age.

- *Inactivated vaccine*: 0.5 mL by IM injection two doses separated by a gap of at least 4 weeks.

Side effects and adverse reactions:
- *Minor*: Pain, redness, and swelling at the injection site, fever, headache, fatigue, nausea
- *Major*: Severe allergic reactions (anaphylaxis, very rare)

Contraindications: Severe allergic reaction to a previous dose or to any component of the vaccine

Cold chain requirements: 2–8°C (36–46°F). It should not be frozen.

Precautions during vaccination: Proper administration techniques should be followed to ensure vaccine efficacy and minimize adverse events. Post-vaccination observation is recommended for any immediate allergic reactions. Live-attenuated vaccine should be avoided during pregnancy and during an actual outbreak of JE.

Efficacy of vaccine: It is recommended for individuals residing in or traveling to areas where JE is endemic or where outbreaks occur, especially during the transmission season. Primary series of two doses should be completed at least 2 weeks before the potential exposure to JE transmission area. Booster doses may be recommended based on ongoing risk factors and individual immunity status.

Measles Vaccine

General description: The measles vaccine is a viral vaccine that provides immunity against measles virus, a highly contagious virus that causes measles, characterized by fever, rash, cough, runny nose, and red eyes.

Contents: Live-attenuated measles virus, stabilizers, and preservatives

Commercial name: MMR (measles, mumps, and rubella), MR (measles and rubella) vaccine (combination vaccine), MMRV (measles, mumps, rubella, and varicella) vaccine (combination vaccine), single antigen measles vaccine (less commonly used now)

Dose schedule: 0.5 mL SC. Adults who have not been vaccinated previously should receive two doses of the measles vaccine if they are at risk of exposure (e.g., healthcare workers, international travelers). A booster dose may be recommended in certain situations, especially for adults at higher risk or during outbreaks. For children two or MR doses should be given at 9–12 months and 16–24 months, according to NIS.

Side effects and adverse reactions:
- *Minor*: Pain, redness, and swelling at the injection site, fever, mild rash, temporary joint pain or stiffness (more common in adults)
- *Major*: Severe allergic reactions (anaphylaxis, very rare)

Contraindications: Pregnancy and severe allergic reaction to a previous dose or to any component of the vaccine.

Cold chain requirements: 2–8°C (36–46°F). It should not be frozen.

Precautions during vaccination: Proper administration techniques should be followed to ensure vaccine efficacy and minimize adverse events. Measles vaccine should not be administered to individuals with severe immunodeficiency or those receiving immunosuppressive therapy.

Efficacy of vaccine: The measles vaccine is highly effective in preventing measles infection and its complications. Two doses of the vaccine provide long-lasting immunity in the majority of recipients. Adult vaccination helps protect against measles and contributes to community immunity, reducing the risk of outbreaks in susceptible populations.

CONCLUSION

Elaborate recommendations are available for immunization of children and pregnant women as well as extensive recommendations for vaccination of adults are available, from various reputed professional bodies such as the Association of Physicians of India (API) and Indian Academy of Pediatrics (IAP), and from esteemed international organizations such as WHO and CDC. However, there is need to have detailed guidelines for various "special populations", i.e., those populations whose health needs are not completely met by the routine healthcare services. In this chapter, the vaccination requirements of these special populations have been submitted, based on the existing recommendations of reputed professional bodies and organizations as well as opinion and experience of experts in Public Health. Vaccination needs of the special populations covered in this chapter include: (1) Populations displaced due to disasters/humanitarian emergencies, (2) Populations which are part of mass gatherings, fairs, festivals, and pilgrimages, (3) HCP, (4) Agriculturists, (5) Armed Forces personnel, (6) International travelers, (7) Labor workforce: Industrial, agricultural, construction, transport labor, waste-handling workers, and sex workers, and (8) Persons having chronic diseases or immunocompromised status.

This chapter is divided into two parts. Part I deals with the recommendations for vaccination of the above-mentioned special populations, while Part 2 gives the ready-reckoner information about the various vaccines recommended for these special populations.

It is reiterated that the material presented in this chapter is recommendatory in nature and does not constitute an authority to claim vaccination by any person or group. Actual provisioning of vaccination would be the purview of the Central/State/Local Government or the Management of the private organization, as the case may be.

REFERENCES

1. Sussman S, Kattari SK, Baezconde-Garbanati L, Glackin SN. The Problems of Grouping All Adversity into a Special Populations Label. Eval Health Prof. 2020;43(1):66-70.
2. World Health Organization. Vaccination in acute humanitarian emergencies: A framework for decision making. WHO: Geneva; 2017.
3. World Health Organisation. (2012). A Framework for Deciding on Vaccinations in Acute Emergencies. [online] Available from https://terrance.who.int/mediacentre/data/sage/SAGE_Docs_Ppt_Apr2012/6_vaccination_humanitarian_emergencies/Apr2012_session6_framework_vaccination_emergencies.pdf [Last accessed March, 2025].
4. Lam E, McCarthy A, Brennan M. Vaccine-preventable diseases in humanitarian emergencies among refugee and internally-displaced populations. Hum Vaccin Immunother. 2015;11(11):2627-36.
5. Mathur G, Vora A. (2024). Indian consensus guideline on adult immunisation. Association of Physicians, India, New Delhi, 2024. [online] Available from https://apiindia.org/reader/Indian%20Consensus%20Guideline%20on%20Adult%20Immunization [Last accessed March, 2025].
6. Government of India, Ministry of Health and Family Welfare. Guidelines for vaccination with influenza vaccine. [online] Available from https://mohfw.gov.in/sites/default/files/Seasonal%20Influenza%20-%20Guidelines%20for%20vaccination%20with%20Influenza%20Vaccine%20%28updated%29.pdf [Last accessed March, 2025].
7. Govternment of India, National Centre for Diseases Control, Ministry of Health and Family Welfare. National Rabies Control Program. (2023). Training Module for Medical Officers. 1st edition. [online] Available from https://ncdc.mohfw.gov.in/wp-content/uploads/2024/02/TRAINING-MODULE-FOR-MEDICAL-OFFICERS.pdf [Last accessed March, 2025].
8. Centres for Disease Control & Prevention (CDC), Atlanta, USA. (2024). Recommended Adult Immunisation Schedule for age 19 and Older. CDC Atlanta. [online] Available from https://www.cdc.gov/vaccines/schedules/downloads/adult/adult-combined-schedule.pdf [Last accessed March, 2025].
9. World Health Organisation. Implementation guide for vaccination of health workers. Geneva: World Health Organization; 2022.
10. Director General, Armed Forces Medical Services, Ministry of Defence, Government of India. Public Health and Preventive Medicine for the Indian Armed Forces (The Red Book). In: Jayaram J, Bhalwar R, Vaidya R, Gupta R, Jindal A, Mukherjee S (Eds). Immunization, 8th edition. New Delhi: Ministry of Defence, Government of India; 2008. Chapter 83. pp. 598-621.
11. Keystone JS, Kozarsky PE. Health recommendations for international travel. In: Jameson JL, Fauci AS, Kasper DL, Hauser SL, Longo DL, Loscalzo J (Eds). Harrison's Principles of Internal Medicine, 20th edition. New York, USA: McGraw Hill; 2018. Chapter 119. pp. 893-900.
12. Government of India, Ministry of Health and Family Welfare. (2024). Requirements of Polio vaccination for international travellers between India and polio infected countries. [online] Available from https://ihpoe.mohfw.gov.in/assets/pdf/Requirement%20of%20Polio%20Vaccination.pdf [Last accessed March, 2025].
13. Choudhury P, Vashishtha VM, Manazir Ali S. Immunization of immunocompromised children. In: Vashishtha VM (Ed). IAP Textbook of Vaccines, 2nd edition. New Delhi: Jaypee Brothers Medical Publisher; 2020. Chapter 64. pp. 700-10.
14. Plotkin SA, Orenstein WA, Offit PA, Edwards KM. Plotkins Vaccines, 7th edition. Philadelphia, USA: Elsevier; 2018.
15. Vashishtha VM. IAP Textbook of Vaccines, 2nd edition. New Delhi: Jaypee Brothers Medical Publishers; 2022.
16. Centres for Disease Control & Prevention (CDC), Atlanta, USA. Recommended Adult Immunisation Schedule for age 19 and Older. CDC Atlanta, 2024. Available at: https://www.cdc.gov/vaccines/schedules/downloads/adult/adult-combined-schedule.pdf (Last accessed : 22 March 2025).
17. Government of India, Ministry of Health and Family welfare. (2023). National Immunisation Schedule, 2023. [online] Available from https://nhm.gov.in/New_Updates_2018/NHM_Components/Immunization/report/National_%20Immunization_Schedule.pdf [Last accessed March, 2025].

CHAPTER 14

Adult Vaccination: Importance and Recommendations

Rajvir Bhalwar

INTRODUCTION

"Adults" have been defined, in our country, both from a legal as well as from a pediatric point of view, as persons aged 18 years and above.[1] Our country, with an estimated current population of 1,443 million, constituting almost 17.78% of the world's total estimated population of 8,119 million, is the most populous country. Of the total population of our country, two-thirds are likely to fall into the legal and healthcare definition of adults, comprising a mammoth 962 million, or say, almost a billion adults in our country. This figure of approximately 1 billion, which would be almost equal to the total population of the USA, Russia, and the European Union countries, put together, also comprises one of the biggest resources which our country needs to be proud of—the Human Resource. Besides the sheer numbers, the socioeconomic, ethnic, occupational, and regional diversities in our country call for concerted efforts for the healthcare of the "adults", vaccination being just one of the various modalities for achieving holistic healthcare.

Another healthcare and demography-related factor which has necessitated the need to focus on vaccination of adult populations is the fact that with improving control of communicable diseases, especially among the children, consequent to large-scale childhood immunization programs, coupled with improvements in water supply and sanitation, there is an increasing "shift" in the incidence of communicable diseases from children to the adult population. A number of diseases which were earlier common in children (and hence adults used to escape due to the long-lasting immunity provided by these infections during childhood) are now occurring in adults, due to adequate protection of children. Moreover, it is also a known fact that a number of communicable diseases which follow a mild course during childhood tend to take a more serious course if they occur during adulthood.

The onset of epidemiological transition, with a consequent increase in noncommunicable diseases (NCDs) vis-à-vis communicable diseases, has also opened up an interesting front in respect of vaccination, in that a number of NCDs [as heart disease, chronic lung disease, chronic liver disease, chronic kidney disease (CKD), etc.] lead to a decline in immune function, as a part of the debilitating disease process, thus increasing the need for appropriate vaccinations among these patients.

Surprisingly, while we have a very well-defined policy and program for vaccination of the pediatric age group, which has been operative for the past nearly half a century, we have not been able to formulate clear-cut policies and recommendations for the adult population of our nation. The focus of this chapter is to suggest recommendations for the vaccination of adults, by reviewing the existing body of knowledge and the recommendations submitted earlier by eminent professional bodies, such as the World Health Organization (WHO), Centers for Disease Control and Prevention (CDC), and Association of Physicians of India (API).[2-5]

It may be noted that within the broad category of "adults," there are "special populations" which refer to groups of people whose needs are not fully addressed by traditional health services delivery. The vaccination requirements of these special populations are covered exclusively in a separate chapter titled "Vaccines for Special Populations" (**Chapter 13**), which covers the following "special population groups":

- Populations displaced due to disasters/humanitarian emergencies
- Populations which are part of mass gatherings, fairs, festivals, and pilgrimages
- Healthcare personnel
- Agriculturists
- Armed forces personnel
- International travelers

- *Labor workforce*: In the industrial, agricultural, construction, and transport sectors, workers who handle wastes and sex workers.

With the above backdrop, the current chapter will be covering the vaccination needs of the "general adult population" (excluding the above-mentioned special populations) in our country.

CAUTIONARY REMARKS

At the very outset, it would be prudent to bear the following aspects in mind:

- Firstly, though vaccination forms a very important component in the overall strategy of preventing and controlling various infectious diseases, it must be combined with various other methods of prevention of communicable diseases, such as prevention of overcrowding, use of face masks, water and food hygiene, personal protection and control of insect vectors, etc. Alone and by itself, vaccination may not be able to achieve complete protection from infectious diseases; on the contrary, it may lead to an undesirable false sense of security, and consequent complacency, toward the adoption of a holistic approach for control of infectious diseases.
- Secondly, the material presented in this chapter is based on the latest available guidelines by eminent professional bodies and experts. However, it does not constitute an authority to claim vaccination by any person or group. Actual provisioning of vaccination would be the purview of the Central/State/local government or the management of the private organization, or the physician in-charge of the individual patient, as the case may be.
- Thirdly, these recommendations do not supersede the guidelines given by the Government of India or any other governmental authority in their respective immunization schedules and in case of any conflict, the guidelines of the governmental body/parental organization will be the final authority. In addition, it is strongly recommended that children and pregnant women should be completely immunized as per the provisions of the National Immunization Schedule (NIS).

This chapter is divided into three parts as follows:

- *Part I*: Vaccination recommended for all adults, irrespective of age, gender, or any other socioeconomic factor
- *Part II*: Vaccination recommended for adults, only in a specific age or gender
- *Part III*: Vaccination recommended for adults, only in certain special situations

VACCINATIONS RECOMMENDED FOR ALL ADULTS, IRRESPECTIVE OF AGE, GENDER (INCLUDING PREGNANCY), OR ANY OTHER SOCIOECONOMIC OR HEALTH-RELATED FACTOR

Vaccinations recommended for all adults, irrespective of their age, gender, pregnancy, or any socioeconomic/health-related factor are: (i) Tetanus, (ii) diphtheria, (iii) pertussis, (iv) influenza, (v) hepatitis B, and (vi) COVID-19. The details are as follows.

VACCINATION AGAINST TETANUS, DIPHTHERIA, AND PERTUSSIS

Description of a Vaccine

Vaccines against tetanus, diphtheria, and pertussis are available in the following formulations:

- *Tetanus toxoid (TT)*: This is a stand-alone TT and is commonly used for tetanus prevention as primary vaccination and also in the event of certain types of injuries.
- *Diphtheria and tetanus toxoids and killed pertussis bacteria (DPT)*: This has been used for long in our national immunization program for infants and children. Each 0.5 mL dose contains: Diphtheria toxoid (Td): 20–30 Lf, TT: 5–25 Lf, pertussis: 4.0 or more IU. It also contains aluminum: >1.25 mg and thiomersal: 0.01%.
- *Tetanus and adult diphtheria toxoid (Td)*: Each 0.5 mL dose contains 5 Lf (limit of flocculation) of TT and 2 Lf of diphtheria toxoid (reduced dose for adults). This has been introduced recently in our national immunization schedule, for booster doses at 10 and 16 years of age for children and for pregnant women, replacing standalone TT which was used earlier in these situations.
- *Tetanus toxoid, diphtheria toxoid, and acellular pertussis (Tdap)*: Each 0.5 mL dose contains 5 Lf TT, 2 Lf diphtheria toxoid, and acellular pertussis antigens (2.5 μg detoxified pertussis toxin). Since it does not contain killed pertussis bacteria, it is free of certain serious side effects of DPT vaccine (such as seizures), which can occur, though rarely, with DPT.

Recommended Beneficiary Population Among Adults

The Indian Consensus as well as the Centers for Disease Control and Prevention (CDC)[3,4] has recommended vaccination against DPT for all adults aged 18 years and above, unless there are specific contraindications as mentioned here.

Dose and Route of Administration

For either of the above-mentioned preparations, the dose is 0.5 mL by intramuscular (IM) injection.

Vaccination Schedule

- Under the National Immunisation Schedule (NIS), all children are required to be immunized with DPT vaccine. The primary vaccination schedule is one dose each at 6, 10, and 14 weeks of age followed by booster doses at 16–24 months of age and at 5 years of age. Thereafter, one booster dose with Td at the ages of 10 and 16 years is to be given as a part of NIS.
- For pregnant ladies, under the NIS, the primary course consists of two doses of Td (or TT, in case Td is not available), the first as early during pregnancy as possible and the second dose after 4 weeks of the first dose (the second dose should preferably be given before completion of 36 weeks of pregnancy but should not be denied if this is not possible and may be given even if the lady is in labor). For pregnant ladies who have been given the aforementioned primary schedule within the past 3 years, one booster dose, preferably before the completion of 36 weeks of pregnancy is to be given. If more than 3 years have elapsed since the completion of the primary course or the last booster, complete the primary schedule of two doses to be given to a pregnant lady.
- For adults who have previously received the above-mentioned primary course series under the NIS: One booster dose of Td (preferably Tdap, if available) every 10 years from the last booster dose.[3,4]
- For adults who have previously *not* received the above-mentioned primary course series under the NIS: One dose of Td (preferably Tdap if available) followed by a second dose of Td (or, Tdap) after 4 weeks, and a third dose of Td (or Tdap, if available) 6–12 months after the second dose, and thereafter, a booster dose of Td (preferably Tdap) after every 10 years.[3,4]
- Tetanus prophylaxis during wound management.[4] This is as per **Table 1**.

Side Effects and Adverse Reactions

- *Minor*: Pain, redness, swelling, fever, headache, muscle pain, and fatigue
- *Major*: Anaphylaxis, Guillain–Barré syndrome (very rare), and Arthus-type hypersensitivity reactions (rare)

Conditions requiring use with precaution (*i.e., vaccination should be generally deferred, but might be indicated if the benefit of protection from the vaccine outweighs the risk for an adverse reaction*).

- Guillain–Barré syndrome within 6 weeks after a previous dose of toxoid-containing vaccine
- History of Arthus-type hypersensitivity reactions after a previous dose of diphtheria toxoid–containing

TABLE 1: Tetanus immuno-prophylaxis in case of injury.

Type of injury/wound	
Clean, minor wound	Potentially contaminated (road accident, war wound, fecal or soil contamination, animal bites, etc.)
Previously fully vaccinated with primary series	
Has received complete primary series with DPT/Td/TT and took the last dose within *previous 10 years*: No further vaccination for tetanus required	Has received complete primary series with DPT/Td/TT and took the last dose *within previous 5 years*: No further vaccination for tetanus required
Has received complete primary series with DPT/Td/TT but took the last dose *more than 10 years back* or unknown status: Give one dose of Td or TT (preferably Tdap)	Has received complete primary series with DPT/Td/TT but took the last dose *more than 5 years back* or unknown status: Give one dose of Td or TT (preferably Tdap)
Previously not fully vaccinated or unknown status	
Give one dose of Td or TT (preferably Tdap) and follow up this dose with full immunization of three doses	Give one dose of Td or Td (preferably Tdap) and also give immunoglobulin (preferably TIG, otherwise EIG), and follow up to complete the immunization schedule with three doses

Note: All wounds must be cleaned thoroughly, remove dirt or any foreign material and remove or debride necrotic material irrespective of tetanus immunization status.

(Td: diphtheria toxoid; Tdap: tetanus toxoid, diphtheria toxoid, and acellular pertussis; DPT: tetanus, diphtheria, and pertussis; TIG: tetanus immune globulin; TT: tetanus toxoid) or tetanus toxoid-containing vaccine; in such cases, defer vaccination until at least 10 years have elapsed since the last tetanus toxoid-containing vaccine

- Current moderate or severe acute illness with or without fever
- *For Tdap only*: Progressive or unstable neurological disorder, uncontrolled seizures, or progressive encephalopathy until a treatment regimen has been established and the condition has been stabilized.

Conditions in Which Vaccination is Contraindicated or not Recommended

- Severe allergic reaction (e.g., anaphylaxis) after a previous dose or to a vaccine component
- *For Tdap only*: Encephalopathy (e.g., coma, decreased level of consciousness, prolonged seizures), not attributable to another identifiable cause, within 7 days of administration of the previous dose of DTP, DTaP, or Tdap.

Storage Recommendations

Store at +2°C to +8°C

VACCINATION AGAINST INFLUENZA

Description of Vaccine

Influenza vaccines are broadly of two types: (i) Inactivated/recombinant influenza vaccine (IIV/RIV) and (ii) live attenuated influenza vaccine (LAIV). The trivalent vaccine (IIV/RIV-3 and LAIV3) covers three strains: Two influenza A (H1N1 and H3N2) and one influenza B (B/Victoria) while the quadrivalent vaccines (IIV4/RIV-4 and the LAIV-4) cover four strains: Two influenza A and two influenza B strains (Yamagata and Victoria). In India, inactivated tetravalent vaccine (IIV4) is available. It contains inactivated influenza virus strains, adjuvants (for some vaccines), preservatives (such as thimerosal in multidose vials), and stabilizers. However, it is recommended that as and when it becomes available, the trivalent vaccine (IIV3) should be preferred over quadrivalent (IIV4) vaccine. This is because the trivalent vaccine contains only the strains linked to B/Victoria lineage, while the tetravalent vaccine contains, in addition, strains linked to B/Yamagata also. Since 2020, B/Yamagata strains have not been identified in India.

Recommended Beneficiary Population

- Influenza vaccine has been recommended for all adults aged 18 years and above by both, the Indian consensus as well as by CDC.[3,4]
- In addition, it is also recommended for certain special populations, as per details given in **Chapter 13**.
- Inactivated or recombinant influenza vaccine (IIV/RIV) can also be given in pregnancy, immunocompromised persons, persons living with HIV (PLHIV), and patients of asplenia, complement deficiencies, CKD, on hemodialysis (HD), heart diseases, lung diseases, alcoholism, chronic liver disease, and diabetes mellitus.
- As per Government of India directives, certain categories of health care personnel (HCP) should be offered the influenza vaccine,[6] the details have been discussed in **Chapter 13**.

Dose and Route of Administration

- IIV is administered as an IM injection in the dose of 0.5 mL.
- LAV is administered as an intranasal spray.

Vaccination Schedule

For adults aged 18 years and above, including pregnant women, one dose of IIV4 (preferably IIV3 if available), *once a year*. Adults aged 50 years and above and pregnant women should *not be given the live attenuated vaccine*. Adults should receive the vaccine, especially during the times when the influenza virus is active in the neighborhood, e.g., before the winter season in North India or before the monsoon season in South India.

Side Effects and Adverse Reactions

- *Minor*: Pain, redness, swelling, fever, headache, muscle pain, nausea, and fatigue
- *Major*: Anaphylaxis (very rare) and Guillain-Barré syndrome (very rare)

Conditions requiring use with precaution (*i.e., vaccination should be generally deferred, but might be indicated if benefit of protection from the vaccine outweighs the risk for an adverse reaction*).

- Guillain-Barré syndrome within 6 weeks after a previous dose of any type of influenza vaccine
- Current moderate or severe acute illness with or without fever

Conditions in Which Vaccination is Contraindicated or not Recommended

- Severe allergic reaction (e.g., anaphylaxis) after the previous dose of any influenza vaccine (i.e., any egg-based IIV, ccIIV, RIV, or LAIV of any valency)
- Severe allergic reaction (e.g., anaphylaxis) to any vaccine component (excluding egg)

- In addition to the above contraindications, LAIV is further contraindicated in the following situations:
  - Anatomic or functional asplenia
  - Immunocompromised due to any cause including, medications and human immunodeficiency virus (HIV) infection
  - Close contacts or caregivers of severely immunosuppressed persons
  - Pregnancy
  - Cochlear implant
  - Active communication between the cerebrospinal fluid (CSF) and the oropharynx, nasopharynx, nose, ear, or any other cranial CSF leak
  - Received influenza antiviral medications oseltamivir or zanamivir within the previous 48 hours, peramivir within the previous 5 days, or baloxavir within the previous 17 days

Storage Recommendations

Store at +2°C to +8°C

VACCINATION AGAINST HEPATITIS B

Description of Vaccine

Hepatitis B vaccines are of two types:

1. Manufactured by using recombinant DNA technology, by inserting HBsAg in yeast cells. These are usually used now.
2. Plasma derived inactivated subunit vaccine. These are only infrequently used now.

Recommended Beneficiary Population

- Vaccination for hepatitis B has been recommended for all adults aged 18 years and above by India Consensus and CDC,[3,4] unless there are specific contraindications as mentioned subsequently.
- It is also recommended for pregnant mothers, immunocompromised persons, PLHIV, injecting drug users (IDU), men who have sex with men (MSM), patients of asplenia, complement deficiencies, CKD, on HD, heart diseases, lung diseases, alcoholism, chronic liver disease, and diabetes mellitus.
- It is also recommended for certain *special population groups* as per details given in **Chapter 13**.

Dose and Route of Administration

- *For newborn and infants under NIS*: 0.5 mL by IM injection in the anterolateral region of the thigh (both for hepatitis B vaccine given at birth and for pentavalent vaccine given at 6, 10, and 14 weeks).
- *For adults*: 1 mL by deep IM injection in the deltoid region; avoid the gluteal region.

Vaccination Schedule

- *For newborns and infants under NIS*: Hepatitis B vaccine given at birth or within 24 hours of birth, followed by pentavalent vaccine given at 6, 10, and 14 weeks.
- For adults, who have not received the complete schedule under NIS during infancy/childhood, 3 doses at 0, 1, and 6 months. The minimum duration between doses 1 and 2 should be 4 weeks and between second and third doses should be 3–6 months.
- Revaccination is advisable, every 5 years, for HCPs and persons with high-risk health conditions such as PLHIV, immunocompromised state, CKD, on HD, injecting drug users (IDU), men who have sex with men (MSM), and chronic liver disease (persons with fatty liver diseases, cirrhosis, hepatitis C, alcoholic liver disease, autoimmune hepatitis, or alanine aminotransferase (ALT) or aspartate transferase (AST) levels higher than twice the upper limit of the normal level.

Side Effects and Adverse Reactions

- *Minor*: Fever, soreness at the injection site, headache, muscle pain, and fatigue
- *Major*: Anaphylaxis and neurological events (rare)

Conditions requiring use with precaution (i.e., vaccination should be generally deferred, but might be indicated if benefit of protection from the vaccine outweighs the risk for an adverse reaction).

- Moderate or severe acute illness with or without fever

Conditions in Which Vaccination is Contraindicated or not Recommended

- Severe allergic reaction (e.g., anaphylaxis) after a previous dose or to Baker's yeast
- *Pregnancy*: Use vaccines other than the following trade names, because there is at present lack of safety data in pregnant persons for these two vaccines: (i) Heplisav-B and (ii) PreHevbrio

Storage Recommendations

Store at +2°C to +8°C

VACCINATION AGAINST COVID-19

Description of Vaccine

Following the onset of COVID-19 pandemic, a large number of vaccines were developed. Details are available on page 26 of the Indian consensus.[3] Basically, these vaccines are dependent on four different types of technologies, as follows:

1. *Inactivated or attenuated virus vaccines*: These use an inactivated or attenuated (weakened) version of the virus that does not cause disease but still generates an immune response. For example, *Covaxin* produced by the Indian company Bharat Biotech in collaboration with ICMR and NIV, Pune.
2. *Protein-based/subunit vaccines*: These contain harmless fragments of proteins or protein shells that mimic the COVID-19 virus to safely generate an immune response. For example, *Novavax*.
3. *Recombinant viral vector vaccines*: These use a safe virus that cannot cause disease but serves as a vehicle to produce coronavirus proteins to generate an immune response. An example is the Sputnik vaccine and Oxford-AstraZeneca vaccine. The latter was manufactured in India under the name of *Covishield*. However, it has not been manufactured since 2021 and there have been reports of thromboembolic phenomena (though rare) following the use of this vaccine. Recently, the Oxford AstraZeneca vaccine has been recalled from the market by the manufacturers.
4. *RNA and DNA vaccines*: These are genetically engineered RNA or DNA which create proteins that safely activate an immune response. For example, the *Pfizer BioNtech* and *Moderna* vaccines are mRNA vaccines, while the *ZyCoV-D* vaccine is a DNA plasmid-based vaccine developed by Cadila, an Indian pharmaceutical company, with support from the Biotechnology Industry Research Assistance Council.

Recommended Beneficiary Population

The vaccine is recommended to be administered only after the specific orders of the National/State government or the local health authority, in the eventuality of an epidemic/pandemic. Usually, the priority will be in the descending order, starting from HCPs and frontline workers, followed by elderly persons aged 60 years and above, and then the other population groups. Vaccination is recommended for pregnant women, persons with adverse health status as PLHIV, immunocompromised state, CKD, on HD, chronic liver disease, asplenia, complement deficiencies, heart diseases, chronic pulmonary disease, alcoholism, diabetes mellitus, special populations as travelers, displaced populations, mass gatherings, and military persons (see **Chapter 13** for details).

Dose and Route of Administration

The dose of COVAXIN (and Covishield which was used during 2021–2022) is 0.5 mL IM injection.

Vaccination Schedule

The schedule of COVAXIN (and Covishield which was used during 2021–2022) is the primary schedule of two doses separated by 4 weeks and a booster after 1 year of the completion of the primary schedule.

Side Effects and Adverse Reactions

- *Minor*: Pain, swelling at the injection site, fever, headache, fatigue, and muscle pain
- *Major*: Severe allergic reactions (anaphylaxis, very rare); reports of thromboembolic phenomena (suspected as a long-term adverse effect)

Conditions requiring use with precaution (*i.e., vaccination should be generally deferred but might be indicated if the benefit of protection from the vaccine outweighs the risk for an adverse reaction*). Depending on the type of COVID-19 vaccine being used, the following conditions should be considered with caution:

- Diagnosed nonsevere allergy (e.g., urticaria beyond the injection site) to a component of a previous dose of COVID-19 vaccine
- Nonsevere, immediate (onset <4 hours) allergic reaction after administration of a previous dose of a COVID-19 vaccine
- Myocarditis or pericarditis within 3 weeks after a previous dose of any COVID-19 vaccine
- Multisystem inflammatory syndrome in children (MIS-C) or multisystem inflammatory syndrome in adults (MIS-A)
- Current moderate or severe acute illness, with or without fever

Conditions in Which Vaccination is Contraindicated or not Recommended

Severe allergic reaction (e.g., anaphylaxis) after a previous dose or to a component of a COVID-19 vaccine.

Storage Recommendations

Store at +2°C to +8°C

VACCINATION RECOMMENDED FOR ONLY CERTAIN SPECIFIC AGE OR GENDER GROUPS OF ADULTS

Certain vaccinations are recommended for adults who are in a specific age or gender group or are a part of special populations. The recommended vaccinations in this category are: (i) Measles/measles and rubella (MR)/measles, mumps, and rubella (MMR), (ii) pneumococcal disease, (iii) typhoid, (iv) herpes zoster (Shingles), (v) meningococcal disease, (vi) polio, (vii) chickenpox, (viii) human papilloma virus (HPV), and (ix) respiratory syncytial virus (RSV) disease. The details are as follows.

VACCINATION WITH MEASLES/MEASLES AND RUBELLA/MEASLES, MUMPS, AND RUBELLA

Description of Vaccine

- The term "measles-containing vaccine" (MCV) is applied to a vaccine which contains live attenuated measles virus for the purpose of immunization. MMR vaccine contains live, attenuated viruses of measles (Edmonston strain), mumps (Jeryll Lynn strain), and rubella (RA 27/3 strain). Vaccines which contain only measles virus (M) or a combination of measles and rubella are also available. The lyophilized live MMR vaccine should be reconstituted and administered as recommended by the manufacturers.
- In the NIS in India, earlier only the measles (M) vaccine was being used, but recently it has been changed to MR, with a view to give lifelong immunity to children against rubella (German measles), primarily to protect the in utero child from developing congenital rubella syndrome (CRS), during their pregnancy. Giving rubella components to male children carries the advantage that it cuts down transmission of rubella from male children or adults to females of childbearing age, thus further helping in the prevention of CRS.
- For vaccination of adults in our country at present, measles is the basic vaccine that should be offered, wherever recommended as under; MR or MMR can be given in place of the measles vaccine if financial, logistics, and operational considerations permit.

Recommended Beneficiary Population

- Infants and children as per the directives laid down in NIS
- For adults, recommended up to 50 years of age. Presently, not recommended for adults above 50 years of age, unless there is a specific additional consideration, such as certain special populations such as HCP. Also, *not* recommended in case there are any contraindications to its administration, as per the details given here.
- One dose for adult women of childbearing age provided she is not pregnant and should avoid pregnancy for at least 3 months after receiving the dose.
- Can be given to an adult (if there is no contraindication), within 3 days of exposure to a case of measles, in which case it can prevent the development of clinical measles, since the development of protective immunity takes 7 days after vaccination, while the clinical diseases take 10 days of incubation period following exposure to a case of measles.
- Recommended for adults having asplenia, and complement deficiencies.
- Can be given, after weighing the benefits of vaccinating versus risk, as decided by the individual physician on a case-to-case basis, in cases of CKD, patients on HD, heart diseases, lung disease, alcoholism, liver disease, and diabetes mellitus.
- Recommended for certain special populations (see **Chapter 13**)

Dose and Route of Administration

- 0.5 mL by subcutaneous injection
- Use a sterile syringe free of preservatives, antiseptics, and detergents for each injection and/or reconstitution of the vaccine because these substances may inactivate the vaccine viruses. To reconstitute the vaccine, withdraw the entire volume of the supplied sterile diluent from the vial and slowly inject it into the lyophilized vaccine vial. Gently agitate to dissolve completely.
- Discard if the lyophilized vaccine cannot be dissolved. Visually inspect the vaccine before and after reconstitution prior to administration. Before reconstitution, the lyophilized vaccine is a light yellow compact crystalline plug and after reconstitution is a clear yellow liquid. Do not use the reconstituted vaccine if particulates are present or if it appears discolored. Withdraw and administer the entire volume of the reconstituted vaccine, or 0.5 mL if it is a multidose vial. Administer the vaccine immediately after reconstitution, within 4 hours, and discard any leftover, since "Open vial policy" is not allowed for M/MR/MMR vaccine.

Vaccination Schedule

- For children under NIS, 2 doses, first at 9–12 months of age and second at 16–24 months of age, each dose 0.5 mL subcutaneous injection

- For adults, two doses, at least 4 weeks apart, each dose 0.5 mL subcutaneous injection

Side Effects and Adverse Reactions

- Local pain, fever, and mild rash
- Temporary pain and stiffness in the joints, mostly in teenage or adult women who did not already have immunity to the rubella component of the vaccine

Conditions requiring use with precaution (i.e., vaccination should be generally deferred, but might be indicated if the benefit of protection from the vaccine outweighs the risk for an adverse reaction).

- Moderate or severe acute illness with or without fever
- History of receiving antibody-containing blood product within the past 11 months; in such cases, wait for 3 months
- History of thrombocytopenia or thrombocytopenic purpura
- *Suspicion of suffering with TB*: First investigate for TB[4]
- If two or more of the following live virus vaccines (namely, MMR, LAIV, varicella, shingles, and yellow fever) are to be given, then they can be given on the same day but by different syringes and at different sites. If they are not given on the same day, then keep a duration of 28 days between them (30 days for yellow fever vaccine).

Conditions in Which Vaccination is Contraindicated or not Recommended

- *Pregnancy*: However, if a pregnant woman receives MMR by oversight, then there is no need to terminate the pregnancy only for this reason since there is no proof that MMR vaccine carries a teratogenic risk. Also, pregnant women may receive the MMR vaccine during measles or rubella outbreaks since the possible advantages of vaccination outweigh the danger.[3]
- Severe allergic reaction after a previous dose or to a vaccine component
- Severe immunodeficiency (e.g., hematologic and solid tumors, receipt of chemotherapy, congenital immunodeficiency, long-term immunosuppressive therapy, or patients with HIV infection who are severely immunocompromised)
- Family history of altered immunocompetence, unless verified clinically or by laboratory testing as immunocompetent

Storage Recommendations

Store at +2°C to + 8°C

VACCINATION AGAINST PNEUMOCOCCAL DISEASE

Description of Vaccine

Presently available pneumococcal vaccines are broadly of two types: (i) Pneumococcal conjugate vaccines (PCV) and (ii) Pneumococcal polysaccharide vaccine (PPSV)

- *Pneumococcal conjugate vaccines*:
  - *PCV-13*: Pneumococcal conjugate, 13-valent vaccine (PCV-13) consists of polysaccharides from the capsule of *Streptococcus pneumoniae* that are conjugated to a carrier protein. Unlike the PPSV, the pneumococcal conjugate vaccine also protects children <2 years of age. It protects against severe forms of pneumococcal diseases, such as pneumonia, meningitis, and bacteremia. A 0.5 mL dose contains polysaccharides from each of 13 serotypes, 30 µg of CRM197 carrier protein (a genetically detoxified mutant of diphtheria toxin), 1.55 mg L-histidine, 1 mg of polysorbate 20, 4.50 mg sodium chloride, and 125 µg of aluminum phosphate adjuvant. The vaccine does not contain any preservatives.
  - *PCV15 and PCV 20*: These are 15 and 20-valent vaccines, respectively, but presently are not available in India.
- *Pneumococcal polysaccharide vaccine (PPSV23)*: It includes purified preparations of pneumococcal capsular polysaccharide. PPSV23 contains polysaccharide antigens from 23 types of pneumococcal bacteria. It contains 25 µg of each antigen per dose and contains 0.25% phenol as a preservative. Studies have revealed that a good immunological response occurs if PPSV23 is administered after an initial dose of PCV13 has been administered. However, the reverse is not true, and thus PCV13 given after PPSV23 in fact results in a reduced response. For this reason, PPSV can be given after an initial dose of PCV13 has been given, but PCV13 should not be given after an initial dose of PPSV23 has been given.

Recommended Beneficiary Population

- Recommended for all adults aged 50 years and above
- For age <50 years, it can be offered to patients who have certain additional risk factors such as immunocompromised states, PLHIV, asplenia, complement deficiencies, diabetes mellitus, CKD, HD, heart diseases, lung disease, alcoholism, or liver disease, on individual case-to-case basis, after weighing benefits against risks.

- It can also be considered for certain special populations or under certain circumstances as HCPs, travelers, mass gatherings, displaced pollutions, and military personnel (*For details, see* ***Chapter 13*** *on "Vaccination of Special Populations"*).
- PCV is also included in NIS, as per the schedule mentioned here.

Dose and Route of Administration

- *PCV13*: 0.5 mL, IM injection
- *PPSV*: 0.5 mL IM or subcutaneous injection

Vaccination Schedule

- *For adults with no other diseases*: First dose with PCV13 followed by one dose of PPSV after 1 year
- *For adults having other diseases as specified above*: First dose with PCV13 followed by one dose of PPSV after 8 weeks
- Adults can receive PCV13 or PPSV23, on the same day along with the shingles vaccine and/or influenza vaccine
- Under NIS, PCV has been introduced in selected states/districts, in the dose of 0.5 mL IM injection, at the age of 6 weeks and 14 weeks, and a booster at 9–12 months of age.

Side Effects and Adverse Reactions

- Side effects are uncommon and include swelling or pain at the injection site, mild to moderate fever, tiredness, and loss of appetite.

Conditions requiring use with precaution (i.e., vaccination should be generally deferred but might be indicated if the benefit of protection from the vaccine outweighs the risk for an adverse reaction).

- Moderate or severe acute illness with or without fever

Conditions in Which Vaccination is Contraindicated or not Recommended

- *For PCV and PPSV*: Severe allergic reaction (e.g., anaphylaxis) after a previous dose or to a vaccine component
- *Additionally, for PCV*: Severe allergic reaction (e.g., anaphylaxis) to any diphtheria-toxoid-containing vaccine

Storage Recommendations

Store at +2°C to +8°C

VACCINATION AGAINST TYPHOID (ENTERIC) FEVER

Description of Vaccine

- Typhoid fever is still an important cause of morbidity in our country. Worldwide, 10–12 million cases and approximately 1.25 lakh deaths are reported. Approximately 2 million cases are reported annually in our country as per the National Health Profile; the actual occurrence may be much higher due to underdiagnosis and underreporting. A parenteral heat-phenol-inactivated whole-cell vaccine was first licensed in 1952; it was associated with high rates of fever and systemic reactions and has been discontinued now. At present, the following three types of typhoid vaccines are available, the overall efficacy being 60–70% for either of them and possibly up to 80% for typhoid conjugate vaccine (TCV).
  - Typhoid conjugate vaccine contains polysaccharides of *Salmonella* typhi conjugated to TT. While Vi capsular polysaccharide of *Salmonella* typhi (see below) alone elicits B-cell responses, however, the conjugation of bacterial polysaccharide to a protein carrier provides foreign peptide antigens that are presented to the immune system eliciting antigen-specific CD4+ Th cells, referred to as T-dependent antibody responses. A hallmark of T-dependent responses, which are also elicited by toxoids, is to induce both higher-affinity antibodies and long-term immune memory. TCV vaccine has been recommended by WHO for use in children above 6 months of age and among adults. The efficacy of TCV may be higher (approximately 80%) compared to Vi polysaccharide and oral Ty21a vaccine whose efficacy is between 60% and 70%. This vaccine is available under the trade name of "TYPBAR-TCV", manufactured in India by Bharat Biotech.
  - Injectable Vi capsular polysaccharide vaccine, which can be given to children above 2 years of age. It is available under the trade name of "Typhim-Vi"
  - Oral live-attenuated vaccine from the Ty21a strain of *Salmonella* serotype Typhi which can be given to children above 6 years of age and adults. It is available under the trade name "Typhoral". Ty21a vaccine can be administered simultaneously or at any interval before or after other live vaccines (injectable or intranasal) or immune globulin if indicated. However, being a live vaccine, it is contraindicated or should be used with caution in certain groups (Contraindications are given later in the next page)

Recommended Beneficiary Population

Vaccination is recommended for the following groups of adult populations:

- Unvaccinated adults aged 18–45 years living in endemic areas, as per decision of the Central/State/Local governmental health authority or the physician in-charge of healthcare of the concerned person/population
- Special populations such as military persons, travelers to endemic areas, healthcare persons or household contacts exposed to patients of typhoid and other infectious diseases, certain categories of laboratory workers, displaced populations due to humanitarian emergencies, food handlers, etc., (see **Chapter 13** for vaccination of special populations).
- Based on the recommendations of SAGE, in 2017, WHO recommended the introduction of TCV for infants and children over 6 months of age in typhoid-endemic countries. This recommendation needs to be considered in our country for implementation in the NIS.
- Typhoid vaccine is also recommended in following adult populations, on a case-to-case basis, after appropriately weighing the benefits against the risks: Pregnancy (do not use live vaccine), PLHIV, persons having immunocompromised states, asplenia, complement deficiencies, CKD, on HD, heart disease chronic liver diseases, diabetes mellitus, alcoholism, and chronic lung diseases.

Dose and Route of Administration

- *Oral Ty21a vaccine*: One capsule orally as per the schedule below
- *Injectable Vi polysaccharide vaccine*: 0.5 mL (containing 25 μg) IM injection
- *Injectable typhoid conjugate vaccine*: 0.5 mL (containing 25 μg) IM injection

Vaccination Schedule

- *Oral Ty 21a vaccine*: one capsule orally is taken every alternate day for a total of four capsules. Booster, if required, to be given after every 5 years, repeating the same primary schedule of four capsules.
- *Injectable Vi polysaccharide vaccine*: Single dose. The booster also as a single dose after every 3 years if risk persists
- *Injectable TCV*: Single dose. The booster also as a single dose after every 3 years if risk persists

Side Effects and Adverse Reactions

These are rare and mild. They include pain and swelling at the injection site, fever, local erythema, muscle aches, headache, urticaria, nausea, and abdominal pain.

Conditions requiring use with precaution (i.e., vaccination should be generally deferred but might be indicated if the benefit of protection from the vaccine outweighs the risk for an adverse reaction).

- In pregnancy, Vi polysaccharide or TCV should be given only if the benefits outweigh the risk. Oral Ty21a should *not* be given in pregnancy.
- Ty21a should not be given until at least 3 days after the last dose of antimicrobial agent and, if possible, antimicrobial agents should not be started within 3 days of the last dose of Ty21a vaccine. A longer interval should be considered for long-acting antimicrobials (e.g., azithromycin).

Conditions in Which Vaccination is Contraindicated or not Recommended

- Oral Ty21a should not be administered to persons during an acute febrile illness or acute gastroenteritis
- Oral Ty21a should not be administered during pregnancy
- All three vaccines (TCV, Vi polysaccharide, and Ty21a) are contraindicated in patients with a history of hypersensitivity to any component of the vaccine.
- Live-attenuated oral Ty21a vaccine should not be used by immunocompromised persons. The TCV and injectable Vi polysaccharide vaccines are theoretically safer for this group.

Storage Recommendations

Store at +2°C to +8°C

VACCINATION AGAINST POLIOMYELITIS

Description of Vaccine

- There are two types of vaccines against poliomyelitis: The live oral polio vaccine (OPV) and the inactivated polio vaccine (IPV). There are three types of polioviruses, types 1, 2, and 3. Type 2 wild poliovirus was declared eradicated in September 2015. The last detection of type 2 was in India, in 1999. Type 3 wild poliovirus was declared eradicated in October 2019. It was last detected in November 2012. Only type 1 wild poliovirus remains in natural circulation.

- OPV also known as Sabin's vaccine is a live attenuated vaccine, administered orally. Earlier, trivalent vaccines containing all three types (trivalent or tOPV, containing poliovirus types type I, II, and III) were in use. However, since 2016, only bivalent vaccines (bOPV) containing types I and III have been available since the type II virus has been eradicated and, moreover, the type II virus in OPV was associated with vaccine-associated paralytic poliomyelitis. bOPV is being used in the NIS in India and many other countries. Monovalent OPV, containing only type I is also available.
- IPV is also known as Salk's vaccine and is an inactivated formulation that contains all the three types of poliovirus individually grown in Vero cells on microcarriers using eagle MEM modified medium, supplemented with newborn calf serum, with 2-phenoxy-ethanol as the preservative. It has been added in NIS in India to supplement bOPV among children. In a number of developed countries such as the USA, IPV is the only vaccine available for immunization against polio.

Recommended Beneficiary Population

- Vaccination of children against poliomyelitis has been in force in India for almost 50 years. Under the NIS in India, as per the schedule described later.
- Once completely immunized as per the above schedule, immunity against poliomyelitis is considered to be lifelong, and no further immunization against polio during adulthood is required, unless there are situations as mentioned here.
- Adults aged 18 years and above, who are known or suspected to be unvaccinated or incompletely vaccinated against polio should complete a primary vaccination series with IPV. Such adults requiring a primary polio vaccination series should receive a total of three doses of IPV as per the schedule given later.
- Since the polio vaccination program of children as part of the expanded program on immunization (EPI) and later universal immunization program (UPI) has been in place for almost 50 years by now in our country, there should be clear reasons to believe that the concerned adult has not been immunized against poliomyelitis during childhood before adult vaccination with IPV is considered.
- Adults who have earlier received a primary series of tOPV or IPV in any combination (e.g., as per the schedule in our NIS) but who are at increased risk for exposure to poliovirus may receive one additional dose of IPV as a single lifetime booster dose. Available data do not indicate the need for more than a single lifetime booster dose with IPV for adults. Such adults who might be at increased risk for exposure to poliovirus include travelers to countries where polio is epidemic or endemic, laboratory and healthcare workers who handle specimens that might contain polioviruses, healthcare workers or other caregivers who have close contact with patients in a community with polio outbreak, and other adults who are identified by public health authorities as being part of a group or population at increased risk for exposure to poliovirus because of an outbreak. (Also see **Chapter 13** for details of vaccination of "special populations").
- In case an adult woman who is pregnant needs to be given a polio vaccine, then vaccination with IPV should preferably be delayed till the completion of the pregnancy period. OPV should *not* be given to pregnant women.
- Mandatory one dose of OPV is required for all travelers coming to India from, or Indian residents traveling from India to, the following eleven polio-infected countries or countries with poliovirus circulation. These include: Afghanistan, Cameroon, Nigeria, Pakistan, Somalia, Syria, Malawi, Mozambique, Madagascar, Congo, and DR Congo. This one additional dose of OPV is required regardless of age and vaccination status at least 4 weeks prior to departure from/to India.[7]
- At present, polio vaccination is *not recommended* for the following categories of adults: Immunocompromised persons, PLHIV, patients of asplenia, complement deficiencies, CKD, heart diseases, chronic lung diseases, chronic liver disease, on HD, diabetes mellitus, or alcoholism.

Dose and Route of Administration

- OPV is administered orally in dose of two drops.
- IPV is administered by IM injection in a dose of 0.5 mL.
- "Fractional IPV" (fIPV) is a concept in which one-fifth of the usual dose of IPV, i.e., 0.1 mL is administered by intradermal injection. It is likely to induce as good immunity as the regular dose of 0.5 mL given by IM route, and can be used instead of regular IPV injections, provided the person administering the dose is adequately trained in administering intradermal injections

Vaccination Schedule

- *For children, under the NIS*: OPV at birth, a 3-dose primary schedule at 6-, 10- and 14-week of age, followed by a booster at the age of 16–24 months. This is supplemented with two doses of "fractional IPV" at the ages of 6 and 14 weeks. The National Technical Advisory Group on Immunisation (NTGI) in India has also recommended that children receive a third dose of fIPV at 9–12 months of age, in addition to the two doses at 6 and 14 weeks.

- *For adults who have been adequately immunized earlier but are at particular risk*: One dose of IPV by IM injection as a single lifetime booster dose (or fIPV if facilities for giving intradermal injection are adequately available).
- *Adults who are known or suspected to be unvaccinated or incompletely vaccinated against polio*: Three doses of IPV are as follows: First dose whenever they come in contact with the healthcare system, followed by the second dose administered after 4–8 weeks, and, a third dose should be administered 6–12 months after the second dose. There is no need to restart the series if the interval between doses exceeds the recommended interval. If three doses of IPV cannot be administered within the recommended interval before protection is needed (e.g., before travel to a country with endemic polio), an accelerated schedule can be undertaken, based on the amount of time available.

Side Effects and Adverse Reactions

Side effects are rare and usually resolve in 24–48 hours. They include pain, swelling, and redness at the injection site, fever, decreased appetite, and vomiting.

Conditions requiring use with precaution (i.e., vaccination should be generally deferred but might be indicated if the benefit of protection from the vaccine outweighs the risk for an adverse reaction).

- Moderate or severe illness with or without fever, or with diarrhea/vomiting
- *Pregnancy*: OPV should *not* be used. IPV should be better delayed till pregnancy is over; however, if necessary use it with caution.

Conditions in Which Vaccination is Contraindicated or not Recommended

- *Inactivated polio vaccine*: History of a severe allergic reaction (e.g., anaphylaxis) following any previous administration of IPV or to any component of IPV. Avoid or at least use with caution during pregnancy
- *OPV*: It should not be used in pregnancy and immunocompromised states.

Storage Recommendations

Store +2°C to +8°C at the point of use in the healthcare system. If long-term storage (>3 months) is required, keep it at minus 20°C. OPV vial, once opened should be used within 4 hours and any leftover should be discarded.

VACCINATION AGAINST CHICKENPOX

Description of Vaccine

Chickenpox vaccine is a live attenuated vaccine containing the OKA strain of varicella-zoster virus (VZV). It is available as a monovalent varicella vaccine and as a polyvalent vaccine in the form of measles, mumps, rubella, and varicella (MMRV) vaccine.

Recommended Beneficiary Population

- Recommended for adults aged 18–49 years of age who do not have any evidence of immunity, either through previous varicella vaccination or through chickenpox disease
- Recommended for adults who have evidence of only partial immunity (had only one dose and not two complete doses of the vaccine)
- Recommended for special populations, such as HCPs, laboratory workers, military recruits, and persons living in overcrowded, congested conditions (see **Chapter 13** for details).
- Can be administered to adults having certain health-risk factors such as asplenia, complement deficiencies, HD, CKD, heart disease, chronic lung disease, chronic liver disease, alcoholism, and diabetes mellitus
- CDC Atlanta as well as the Indian consensus[3,5] recommend that after being exposed to varicella or herpes zoster, people with no evidence of immunity and who are eligible for vaccination should get the varicella vaccine. Ideally, the vaccine should be given within 3–5 days after the person is exposed. This may either prevent the development of varicella disease or result in milder disease. CDC also recommends that even if it has been >5 days, the vaccine can still be offered. This will provide protection against varicella if a person is exposed again in the future and the previous exposure did not result in infection.
- *Not* to be given during pregnancy, in immunocompromised persons, persons on immunosuppressives, PLHIV, and children <12 months of age.

Dose and Route of Administration

0.5 mL by IM injection.

Vaccination Schedule

- Primary schedule consists of two doses separated by at least 4–8 weeks.
- For those who have already been given one dose earlier, one more dose at least 4 weeks after the first dose.

- Children should get their first dose at 12–15 months and the second dose at 4–6 years.
- No booster is required after the successful completion of the primary schedule of two doses.

Side Effects and Adverse Reactions

- Usually rare and mild, as pain at the injection site, fever, mild arthralgia. Sometimes, rarely, serious side effects such as severe rash, febrile seizures, and hepatitis can occur.

Conditions requiring use with precaution (i.e., vaccination should be generally deferred but might be indicated if the benefit of protection from the vaccine outweighs the risk for an adverse reaction).

- Recent (≤11 months) receipt of antibody-containing blood product (specific interval depends on the product)
- Receipt of specific antiviral drugs (acyclovir, famciclovir, or valacyclovir) 24 hours before vaccination (avoid use of these antiviral drugs for 14 days after vaccination)
- Use of aspirin or aspirin-containing products
- Moderate or severe acute illness with or without fever

Conditions in Which Vaccination is Contraindicated or not Recommended

- Pregnancy
- Severe allergic reaction (e.g., anaphylaxis) after a previous dose or to a vaccine component
- Severe immunodeficiency (e.g., hematologic and solid tumors, receipt of chemotherapy, and congenital immunodeficiency).
- Long-term immunosuppressive therapy or patients with HIV infection who are severely immunocompromised
- Family history of altered immunocompetence, unless verified clinically or by laboratory testing as immunocompetent

Storage Recommendations

Store +2°C to +8°C at the point of use in the healthcare system. Do not expose to hot conditions or direct sunlight.

VACCINATION AGAINST HERPES ZOSTER (SHINGLES)

Description of Vaccine

Varicella-zoster virus (species *Human herpesvirus 3*) is a member of the genus *varicella virus* of the family *Herpesviridae*. Other alpha-herpes viruses that infect humans include herpes simplex viruses 1 and 2 (HSV-1 and HSV-2), against whom vaccines are not available at present. Vaccines against shingles are of following types:

- Recombinant zoster vaccine (RZV) (Shingrix) for prevention of herpes zoster (shingles) is a recombinant, adjuvanted vaccine. After reconstitution, one dose (0.5 mL) contains: 50 μg of varicella zoster virus 1 glycoprotein E produced in Chinese hamster ovary (CHO) cells by recombinant DNA technology and adjuvanted with AS01B.[8]
- The other vaccine is the live attenuated zoster vaccine which is available as two products: (i) Zostavax for the prevention of shingles in immunocompetent people over the age of 50 years, and (ii) varivax for the prevention of chickenpox in persons aged 12 months and older. While the two vaccines contain the same immunological components (lyophilized preparation of live, attenuated Oka/Merck strain of varicella-zoster virus) and provide protection against the same virus, Zostavax contains a higher dose and is therefore used in older adults to prevent the development of shingles and postherpetic neuralgia. At present, the RZV vaccine is preferred over the live attenuated vaccine.

RZV should not be used for children and should not be used in place of varicella vaccine. Also, the varicella vaccine should not be used in place of Shingrix.

Recommended Beneficiary Population

- Recombinant zoster vaccine is recommended for all immunocompetent adults aged 50 years and older:
    - Whether or not they report a prior episode of herpes zoster.
    - Whether or not they report a prior dose of live attenuated vaccine (Zostavax).
    - It is not necessary to screen, either verbally or by serology, for evidence of prior chickenpox infection.
- *For immunocompromised adults, including PLHIV, 18 years and older*: RZV is recommended for the prevention of shingles and related complications in adults aged 18 years and above, who are or will be immunodeficient or immunosuppressed because of disease or therapy.
- For persons suffering from asplenia, complement deficiencies, CKD, on HD, heart diseases, chronic liver disease, chronic lung disease, alcoholism, and diabetes mellitus, administration of RZV should be considered on case-to-case basis by the physician, depending on additional risk factors.

Dose and Route of Administration

- Each dose is 0.5 mL. RZV, to be injected intramuscularly in the deltoid region.
- Subcutaneous injection is a vaccine administration error and should be avoided. However, if RZV has been inadvertently administered subcutaneously, that dose is still considered valid and does not need to be repeated. If a subcutaneous vaccine administration error occurs on the first dose of Shingrix, a second dose is still required after 2–6 months.[9]
- At the time of vaccination, RZV is prepared by reconstituting the antigen component with the adjuvant suspension component. Thereafter, it should be administered immediately or stored in the refrigerator and used within 6 hours of reconstitution. Otherwise, it should be discarded.

Vaccination Schedule

- Two doses of RZV should be given. The second dose of RZV should typically be given 2–6 months after the first.
- However, for persons who are or will be immunodeficient or immunosuppressed and who would benefit from completing the series in a shorter period, the second dose can be administered 1–2 months after the first.

Side Effects and Adverse Reactions

- Common side effects include redness, pain, and swelling at the site of injection, muscle pain, fatigue, headache, shivering, fever, and gastrointestinal symptoms. These side effects are mild and temporary and usually resolve on their own in a couple of days.

Conditions requiring use with precaution (i.e., vaccination should be generally deferred but might be indicated if the benefit of protection from the vaccine outweighs the risk for an adverse reaction).

- Any moderate or severe acute illness with or without fever

Conditions in Which Vaccination is Contraindicated or not Recommended

- Severe allergic reaction (e.g., anaphylaxis) after a previous dose or to a vaccine component
- Persons who are suffering from an episode of herpes zoster. In such cases, postpone RZV till the time the person is free of all signs/symptoms of herpes zoster.
- *Pregnancy*: Though clear guidelines are not available, the consensus is not to give RZV during pregnancy and postpone it till the pregnancy is over. There is *no* contraindication for giving RZV to a breastfeeding lady.

Storage Recommendations

Store +2°C to +8°C at the point of use in the healthcare system. Do not expose to hot conditions or direct sunlight.

VACCINATION AGAINST HUMAN PAPILLOMA VIRUS

Description of Vaccine

- Epidemiological and clinical studies have identified HPV infection, both internationally and in India, as a major risk factor for the development of cervical cancer, which is one of the leading causes of morbidity and mortality among women. The majority of HPV-associated cancers are caused by HPV 16 or 18 and can be controlled using vaccination. The vaccine also protects against genital warts and some other cancers such as anal, vulval vaginal, penile, and oropharyngeal cancers as well some cancers of the head and neck.
- HPV vaccines are based on the recombinant DNA technology and purified L-1 protein that is assembled to form HPV empty shells. The existing vaccines are delivered via the IM route, resulting in rapid access to draining lymph nodes and are adjuvanted to induce a proinflammatory milieu conducive to initiating a strong humoral response with robust memory.
- At present, there are three types of HPV vaccines that are available in our country: Cervarix (bivalent, types 16 and 18), Gardasil (quadrivalent, types 6, 11, 16, and 18) and, very recently, Serum Institute of India (SII) has launched India's indigenous vaccine, Cervavac, which is a quadrivalent HPV vaccine (HPV types 6, 11, 16, and 18). HPV vaccines are highly immunogenic, with seroconversion at 5 years after giving a complete course of at least two vaccines, estimated to be >95%.

Recommended Beneficiary Population

- Human papilloma virus vaccination has been recently introduced in the NIS of our country. The beneficiary population is girls between the ages of 9 and 14 years, to be covered with two doses given 6 months apart.
- For adults, HPV vaccination has been recommended for all adult women up to the age of 26 years and all adult males up to the age of 21 years,[3,4] in a three-

dose schedule (0, 1, and 6 months) unless there are contraindications (see later).
- For certain adults who have additional risk factors, such as immunocompromised persons, PLHIV, patients of asplenia, complement deficiencies, CKD, on HD, heart disease, chronic lung disease, chronic liver disease, and diabetes mellitus, HPV vaccine is recommended up to the age of 45 years, in a three-dose schedule (0, 1, and 6 months).

Dose and Route of Administration

- Each dose is 0.5 mL by IM injection. The vaccine should be used as supplied; no dilution or reconstitution is necessary.

Vaccination Schedule

- Under the NIS, for girls aged 9–14 years, two doses are placed 6 months apart.
- For adults, three doses at 0, 1, and 6 months.

Side Effects and Adverse Reactions

- Local side effects include pain, which may be severe in rare cases, redness, and swelling at the injection site. Bivalent vaccines may result in more adverse events at the injection site than quadrivalent vaccines.
- Mild systemic adverse events include headache, dizziness, myalgia, arthralgia, and gastrointestinal symptoms (nausea, vomiting, and abdominal pain). Systemic reactions are generally mild and self-limiting.

Conditions requiring use with precaution (i.e., vaccination should be generally deferred but might be indicated if the benefit of protection from the vaccine outweighs the risk for an adverse reaction).
- Moderate or severe acute illness with or without fever

Conditions in Which Vaccination is Contraindicated or not Recommended

- *Pregnancy*: HPV vaccination is not recommended
- Severe allergic reaction (e.g., anaphylaxis) after a previous dose or to a vaccine component

Storage Recommendations

Human papilloma virus vaccines should be maintained at 2–8°C, not frozen and protected from light. They should be administered as soon as possible after being removed from the refrigerator.

VACCINATION AGAINST RESPIRATORY SYNCYTIAL VIRUS

Description of Vaccine

- Two types of vaccines are available. Both are lyophilized, protein-subunit vaccines, one with adjuvant and the other without adjuvant:
  i. Lyophilized antigen (protein subunit, as a sterile white powder) *without adjuvant*, (ABRYSVO), supplied with vials containing sterile water diluent. Reconstitute the lyophilized antigen component with the sterile water diluent component. *Only this type of vaccine is to be used for pregnant women.* It can also be used for persons aged >60 years.
  ii. Lyophilized antigen (protein subunit) *with adjuvant* (AREXVY). It is available as an injectable suspension. AREXVY is supplied as a single-dose vial of lyophilized antigen component to be reconstituted with the accompanying vial of the adjuvant suspension component. A single dose after reconstitution is 0.5 mL. This vaccine can be used for persons >60 years of age but *not for pregnant women.*
- Both of the above vaccines are US FDA approved. However, at present none is available in India, but AREXVY can be imported on the production of the following documents: (i) A valid prescription from a qualified doctor, (ii) the patient's diagnostic reports, and (iii) the patient's identity proof (issued by the government of India).

Recommended Beneficiary Population

- Recommended for prevention of lower respiratory tract disease (LRTD) among persons aged 60 years and above.
- For pregnant women, the objective is to prevent RSV infection among the infant, through maternal antibodies developed by vaccination. Individual benefits of protecting against RSV infection are to be weighed against risks, and the decision is to be taken on case-to-case basis. Only *nonadjuvant* vaccines should be used in pregnant women. Alternatively, infant immunization with nirsevimab (RSV monoclonal antibody) may be considered.

Dose and Route of Administration

Reconstitute immediately before use. Dose 0.5 mL by IM injection.

Vaccination Schedule

- Only one dose is recommended. There is no need of taking annual doses (compared to recommendations for the influenza vaccine).
- If considered during pregnancy, one dose between the 32nd and 36th week of gestation.

Side Effects and Adverse Reactions

- Common side effects include pain at the injection site, fatigue, and headache. They are usually mild and last for a day or two.
- Rarely, Guillain-Barré syndrome has been reported.

Conditions requiring use with precaution (i.e., vaccination should be generally deferred but might be indicated if the benefit of protection from the vaccine outweighs the risk for an adverse reaction).

- Moderate or severe acute illness with or without fever

Conditions in Which Vaccination is Contraindicated or not Recommended

History of severe allergic reaction (e.g., anaphylaxis) to a vaccine component.

Storage Recommendations

Store +2°C to +8°C at the point of use in the healthcare system.

VACCINATION AGAINST TUBERCULOSIS

Description of Vaccine

The Bacillus Calmette-Guérin (BCG) vaccine is a live vaccine, supplied as a lyophilized (freeze-dried) preparation in the vacuum-sealed, multidose, amber-colored vial. It must be reconstituted with "BCG-only" diluents supplied by the manufacturer as the diluents are specifically designed for the needs of that vaccine, with respect to volume, pH, and chemical properties. Reconstituted BCG vaccine must be used within 4 hours of reconstitution. The reconstituted BCG vaccine is highly heat sensitive and must be protected from light and heat.

Recommended Beneficiary Population

- In the NIS, BCG vaccination is stipulated for all infants, preferably within 24 hours of birth, otherwise anytime till completion of 1 year of age. In the NIS, it is not recommended if the child has completed 1 year of age.
- As per the WHO status paper of 2024, BCG is recommended for unvaccinated, tuberculin skin test (TST) negative or interferon-gamma release assay (IGRA) negative older children, adolescents, and adults with settings of high incidence of TB and/or high leprosy burden, those moving from low to high TB incidence/leprosy burden settings, and persons with risk of occupational exposure in low and high TB incidence areas (as HCPs working in OPDs and IPDs of TB hospitals/medical colleges/teaching hospitals, microbiology departments, medical and nursing students, and other persons like prison workers assessed to be at high risk of occupational exposure).[2]
- After a careful review of the literature and available evidence, the Ministry of Health and Family Welfare, Government of India, along with ICMR, is planning to conduct a program implementation research study of BCG vaccination in adults. The study will focus on adults aged 18 years and above, who fulfill any of the six defined inclusion criteria and are willing to take the vaccine.[10]

Dose and Route of Administration

- *For neonates up to 4 weeks of age*: 0.05 mL by intradermal injection
- *For infants more than 4 weeks till 1 year of age*: 0.10 mL by intradermal injection
- *For children >1 year of age and adults*: 0.10 mL by intradermal injection

Vaccination Schedule

One dose only, irrespective of age group.

Side Effects and Adverse Reactions

- Painful axillary lymphadenitis, pain, and redness at the site of injection, fever, dysuria, nausea, vomiting, ulceration, or abscess at the injection site.

Conditions requiring use with precaution (i.e., vaccination should be generally deferred but might be indicated if the benefit of protection from the vaccine outweighs the risk for an adverse reaction).

- Avoid in persons currently sick due to any reason (postpone vaccination till cured)

Conditions in Which Vaccination is Contraindicated or not Recommended

- Individuals with a known history of immunodeficiency or on immune suppressive drugs
- Recipients of any procedure interfering with immune status or transplant or malignancy
- History of known severe reaction to BCG or any other vaccines
- Pregnant or lactating women

Storage Recommendations

- *At the point of healthcare delivery*: Store in ice lined refrigerator (ILR) at +2°C to +8°C.
- In the ILR, the BCG vaccine lot should be kept just above the lot of MR and just below the rotavirus vaccine and at the same level as the JE vaccine.
- The diluent for BCG can be stored at room temperature but should be kept in the topmost layer of ILR for at least 24 hours before use.
- After reconstitution, use as early as possible and within 4 hours of reconstitution. It should be protected from heat and direct sunlight while giving the vaccination.

VACCINATION RECOMMENDED FOR ADULTS, ONLY IN CERTAIN SPECIAL SITUATIONS

Certain vaccinations are recommended for adults who are a part of special populations. These include populations displaced due to disasters/humanitarian emergencies; populations which are part of mass gatherings, fairs, festivals, and pilgrimages; healthcare personnel; agriculturists and livestock workers; armed forces personnel; international travelers; and, labor work-force. The vaccination requirements of these special populations are as follows:

- Anthrax (agriculturists, livestock workers, abattoir workers, and military personnel exposed to bioterrorism).
- Meningococcal disease (persons living in overcrowded conditions, military recruits, healthcare persons (HCPs) working in infectious diseases wards, and laboratory workers)
- Cholera (HCPs, laboratory workers, displaced populations, travelers, and armed forces personnel on disaster management duties)
- HAV (international travelers, persons working in specific laboratories, persons exposed to insanitary conditions).
- Japanese encephalitis (travelers and agriculturists in known endemic areas with high density of reservoir and amplification hosts)
- Rabies (PEP) (veterinarians and dog handlers)
- Yellow fever (travelers to endemic countries)

The details of adult vaccination requirements of the above-mentioned special populations have already been covered in detail in ***Chapter 13*** *(Vaccines for special populations).*

CONCLUSION

The topic of immunization of adults has remained, relatively, a back-bencher, apparently and very rightly so, because of the importance accorded to childhood immunization. However, now there is a felt need to visit this area and draw guidelines, due to various epidemiological and sociodemographic reasons, as follows:

- Firstly, in our country, almost a billion population, comprising two-thirds of the total population of India, are likely to fall into the legal and healthcare definition of adults. This huge population is our gold-mine of human resources and their health must be looked after to ensure their full potential as well as for ensuring their highest possible quality of life.
- Secondly, with improving control of communicable diseases, especially among the children, consequent to large scale childhood immunization programs, coupled with improvements in water supply and sanitation, there is an increasing "shift" in the incidence of communicable diseases from children to the adult population. A number of diseases which were earlier common in children (and hence adults used to escape due to the long-lasting immunity provided by these infections during childhood) are now occurring in adults, due to adequate protection of children. Moreover, a number of communicable diseases which follow a mild course during childhood tend to take a more serious course if they occur during adulthood, and hence the need to focus on prevention of communicable diseases among adults.
- Thirdly, the onset of epidemiological transition and consequent increase in noncommunicable diseases (NCDs) vis-à-vis communicable diseases has also opened up an interesting front in respect of vaccination, in that a number of NCDs (as heart disease, chronic lung disease, chronic liver disease, CKD, T2D, etc) lead to a decline in immune function, as a part of the debilitating disease process, thus increasing the need for appropriate vaccinations among these patients.

It was against the backdrop of above-mentioned epidemiological features, that the present chapter has been composed, with a view to forward recommendations for vaccination of adults, by reviewing the existing body of knowledge and the available guidelines of eminent professional bodies, as the WHO, CDC, and API.

ACKNOWLEDGMENTS

The authors acknowledge the contribution of Brig. VK Bhatti (Prof and Head), Maj. Sumeet Singh (Assistant Professor), Maj. Chandan Panigrahi (PG JR), and Maj. Needhi Rana (PG JR), Department of Community Medicine, Armed Forces Medical College, Pune, for their valuable inputs and prepublication review of this chapter.

REFERENCES

1. John T. IAP Policy for age of children for Paediatric care. Indian Paediatr. 1999;36:461-3.
2. World Health Organization. (2024). Summary of WHO Position Papers - Recommendations for Routine Immunization. [online] Available from https://www.who.int/publications/m/item/table1-summary-of-who-position-papers-recommendations-for-routine-immunization (Last accessed March, 2025).
3. Mathur G, Vora A (Eds). Indian consensus guideline on adult immunisation. Association of Physicians, India, New Delhi; 2024.
4. Centres for Disease Control and Prevention. (2024). Recommended Adult Immunisation Schedule for Ages 19 and Older. [online] Available from https://www.cdc.gov/vaccines/schedules/downloads/adult/adult-combined-schedule.pdf (Last accessed March, 2025).
5. Centers for Diseases Control. (2024). CDC – ACIP Recommendations for Vaccinations. [online] Available from https://www.cdc.gov/vaccines/hcp/acip-recs/index.html [Last accessed March, 2025].
6. Government of India, Ministry of Health and Family Welfare. Guidelines for vaccination with influenza vaccine. [online] Available from https://mohfw.gov.in/sites/default/files/Seasonal%20Influenza%20-%20Guidelines%20for%20vaccination%20with%20Influenza%20Vaccine%20%28updated%29.pdf (Last accessed on March 24, 2025).
7. Government of India, Ministry of Health and Family Welfare. (2024). Requirements of Polio vaccination for international travellers between India and polio infected countries. [online] Available from https://mohfw.gov.in/?q=diseasealerts-5 (Last accessed on 16 July 2024)
8. Shingrix Vaccine for Herpes Zoster. GSK Pharma. [online] Available from https://india-pharma.gsk.com/media/7399/shingrix.pdf (Last accessed March, 2025).
9. CDC, Atlanta, USA. Shingles vaccine recommendations. Available at: https://www.cdc.gov/shingles/hcp/vaccine-considerations/index.html (Last accessed on March, 24, 2025).
10. Government of India, Ministry of Health and Family Welfare. (2024). Standard Operating Procedures for Adult BCG vaccination under pragmatic implementation study in India. [online] Available from https://figshare.com/articles/online_resource/Standard_Operating_Procedures_for_Adult_BCG_Vaccination_under_programmatic_implementation_study_in_India/25272181?file=44647885 (Last accessed March, 2024).

SUGGESTED READINGS

1. Plotkin SA, Orenstein WA, Offit PA, Edwards KM (Eds). Plotkins Vaccines, 7th edition. Philadelphia: Elsevier; 2018.
2. Vashishtha VM (Ed). IAP Textbook of Vaccines, 2nd edition. New Delhi: Jaypee Brothers Medical Publishers Pvt Ltd; 2022.
3. Government of India, Ministry of Health and Family Welfare. (2023). National Immunisation Schedule. [online] Available from https://nhm.gov.in/New_Updates_2018/NHM_Components/Immunization/report/National_%20Immunization_Schedule.pdf (Last Accessed March, 2025).
4. American Public Health Association. Control of Communicable Diseases Manual, 21st edition. Washington DC: A.P.H.A. Press; 2022.

CHAPTER 15

Focus on Specific Vaccines

Anit Kujur

INTRODUCTION

Vaccines play a crucial role in preventing infectious diseases and protecting public health. By stimulating the body's immune system to recognize and fight harmful pathogens, vaccines have significantly reduced or eradicated life-threatening diseases. While immunization programs cover a wide range of vaccines, focusing on specific vaccines allows for a detailed exploration of their unique benefits, mechanisms, and challenges.

Each vaccine is developed with a targeted approach to combat specific infectious diseases, utilizing different scientific methodologies such as live-attenuated, inactivated, messenger ribonucleic acid (mRNA), vector-based, or protein subunit technologies. Some vaccines, like those for measles and polio, have been instrumental in near-elimination efforts, while others, require ongoing adaptation due to evolving pathogens. Additionally, vaccines against diseases like human papillomavirus (HPV) and hepatitis B play a crucial role in preventing certain types of cancer, highlighting their broader impact beyond infectious disease control.

Focusing on specific vaccines also helps address concerns regarding their safety, effectiveness, and accessibility. Misinformation and vaccine hesitancy remain significant challenges, making it essential to provide clear, evidence-based information on how these vaccines work and their role in protecting individuals and communities.

This chapter will delve into key vaccines, examining their development, mechanism of action, real-world impact, and future advancements. By understanding the significance of specific vaccines, we can appreciate their contributions to public health and reinforce the importance of immunization in global disease prevention efforts.

DEVELOPMENT OF THE HUMAN PAPILLOMAVIRUS VACCINE

BACKGROUND ON HUMAN PAPILLOMAVIRUS

Human papillomavirus (HPV) is a group of >200 related viruses, of which about 40 types are transmitted through direct sexual contact. HPV is the most common sexually transmitted infection globally and is associated with several types of cancer, particularly cervical cancer, as well as other conditions like genital warts. The discovery that persistent infection with certain high-risk HPV types (especially HPV-16 and -18) could lead to cervical cancer was a pivotal moment in understanding the role of the virus in carcinogenesis.

EARLY RESEARCH AND VACCINE DEVELOPMENT

The development of the HPV vaccine began with research in the 1980s and 1990s that identified HPV as the cause of nearly all cervical cancers. Scientists sought to create a vaccine that could prevent the virus from infecting individuals. The main challenge was that HPV is a virus that does not enter the bloodstream directly, making it harder for the immune system to recognize and combat.

Researchers developed a vaccine using virus-like particles (VLPs), which mimic the outer shell of the actual virus without containing its DNA, making them noninfectious. These VLPs trigger an immune response in the body, leading to the production of antibodies that can neutralize the virus if a person is exposed to it in the future.

CLINICAL TRIALS AND APPROVAL

Clinical trials for the first HPV vaccine began in the late 1990s. The trials involved tens of thousands of participants and were conducted in multiple phases to assess safety, immunogenicity (the ability to provoke an immune response), and efficacy (the ability to prevent infection and disease). The trials showed that the vaccine was highly effective in preventing infections with the high-risk HPV types 16 and 18, which are responsible for about 70% of cervical cancers.

In 2006, the first HPV vaccine, Gardasil (also known as Silgard in some countries), was approved by the US Food and Drug Administration (FDA). Gardasil was a quadrivalent vaccine, meaning it protected against four HPV types: 16, 18, and two low-risk types, 6 and 11, which are responsible for most cases of genital warts. Cervarix, a bivalent vaccine protecting against HPV types 16 and 18, was approved shortly afterward.[1]

EFFICACY OF THE HUMAN PAPILLOMAVIRUS VACCINE

Protection Against Human Papillomavirus and Cancer

The HPV vaccine is highly effective in preventing infections with the HPV types it targets, especially when administered before individuals are exposed to the virus, typically before they become sexually active. Studies have shown that the vaccine is almost 100% effective in preventing precancerous cervical lesions caused by HPV types 16 and 18.

Long-term studies have also demonstrated that the vaccine's protection is long-lasting, with studies showing no significant decrease in efficacy for at least 10 years after vaccination. The vaccine's success has led to a substantial reduction in the prevalence of the targeted HPV types and a corresponding decrease in the incidence of cervical and other HPV-related cancers in vaccinated populations.

Broader Impact

In addition to protecting against cervical cancer, the HPV vaccine also provides protection against other types of cancer caused by HPV, including cancers of the anus, oropharynx (throat), penis, vulva, and vagina. The vaccine's impact on genital warts has also been significant, with a marked reduction in cases in vaccinated populations.

Herd Immunity

The widespread use of the HPV vaccine has led to the development of herd immunity in some populations, where even unvaccinated individuals benefit from the reduced circulation of the virus. This is particularly important in the context of HPV, as it is a sexually transmitted infection, and reducing its prevalence in the population can significantly lower the overall risk of HPV-related diseases.

USE OF THE HUMAN PAPILLOMAVIRUS VACCINE

Vaccination Recommendations

The HPV vaccine is recommended for both females and males, typically starting at the ages 11 or 12 years, although it can be given as early as age of 9 years. The vaccine is most effective when administered before individuals become sexually active, as it prevents infection with HPV types to which they have not yet been exposed. The vaccine is also recommended for catch-up vaccination in older adolescents and young adults up to age of 26 years who were not vaccinated earlier.

The vaccination schedule originally consisted of three doses, but subsequent research has shown that two doses are sufficient for those who start the vaccination series before age of 15 years. For individuals who begin the series at the age of 15 years or older, the three-dose schedule is still recommended.[2]

GLOBAL IMPLEMENTATION

The HPV vaccine has been introduced in national immunization programs in many countries around the world. However, access to the vaccine varies widely, with higher coverage rates in high-income countries compared to low- and middle-income countries. Efforts are ongoing to improve global access to the HPV vaccine, particularly in regions with high rates of cervical cancer.

CHALLENGES AND CONTROVERSIES

Despite its proven efficacy and safety, the HPV vaccine has faced challenges and controversies. Some of these include:

- *Vaccine hesitancy:* Concerns about vaccine safety, misinformation, and cultural or religious beliefs have led to vaccine hesitancy in some populations. This hesitancy has affected vaccination rates in certain regions, potentially limiting the public health impact of the vaccine.
- *Cost and access:* The cost of the vaccine has been a barrier to widespread implementation in some low-income countries, although efforts by organizations like Gavi, the Vaccine Alliance, have helped increase access in some of these regions.
- *Misconceptions about sexual behavior:* There have been concerns that vaccinating young people against

HPV might lead to riskier sexual behaviors. However, studies have shown that the vaccine does not increase sexual activity or change sexual behavior patterns.

CONCLUSION

The development of the HPV vaccine represents a significant achievement in public health, offering protection against a virus that causes a substantial burden of cancer worldwide. Its efficacy in preventing HPV-related cancers and genital warts has been well established, and its use in immunization programs has led to a significant reduction in the prevalence of high-risk HPV types. Continued efforts to increase vaccine coverage, particularly in low-income countries, and to address vaccine hesitancy are essential to fully realizing the potential of the HPV vaccine in reducing the global burden of HPV-related diseases.

OVERVIEW OF HUMAN PAPILLOMAVIRUS VACCINES

As of now, there are three primary vaccines available for the prevention of HPV infections: (1) Gardasil, (2) Gardasil 9, and (3) Cervarix. Each of these vaccines targets different strains of HPV, offering varying degrees of protection against the virus and related conditions, such as cervical cancer and genital warts.[3]

Gardasil (Quadrivalent HPV Vaccine)

Composition and Targeted Human Papillomavirus Types

Gardasil, the first HPV vaccine approved by the FDA in 2006, is known as a quadrivalent vaccine. It targets four types of HPV:

- *HPV-16 and HPV-18*: These are high-risk types responsible for approximately 70% of cervical cancers and a significant proportion of other HPV-related cancers, such as those affecting the vulva, vagina, anus, and oropharynx.
- *HPV-6 and HPV-11*: These are low-risk types responsible for about 90% of genital warts and other benign conditions, such as respiratory papillomatosis.

Mechanism of Action

Gardasil is made using VLPs that resemble the outer shell of the HPV virus but do not contain viral DNA, rendering them noninfectious. These VLPs stimulate the immune system to produce antibodies that can neutralize the actual virus if the person is exposed to it later.

Efficacy

Gardasil has shown high efficacy in preventing infections with the four targeted HPV types, particularly when administered before individuals are exposed to the virus. Clinical trials demonstrated nearly 100% efficacy in preventing precancerous cervical lesions caused by HPV-16 and HPV-18. Additionally, Gardasil has been highly effective in reducing the incidence of genital warts caused by HPV-6 and HPV-11.

Use and Approval

Gardasil is approved for use in both females and males, typically starting at the ages 11 or 12 years, but it can be administered as early as age of 9 years. It was initially given as a three-dose series, but research later showed that a two-dose schedule is sufficient for those who begin the vaccination before age of 15 years.

Gardasil has been widely used in national immunization programs in many countries, contributing to a significant reduction in the prevalence of the targeted HPV types and associated diseases.[4]

Gardasil 9 (Nonavalent HPV Vaccine)

Composition and Targeted HPV Types

Gardasil 9 is an advanced version of the original Gardasil vaccine, approved by the FDA in 2014. It is known as a nonavalent vaccine because it targets nine HPV types:

- *HPV-16 and HPV-18*: High-risk types that cause most HPV-related cancers.
- *HPV-6 and HPV-11*: Low-risk types that cause genital warts.
- *HPV-31, HPV-33, HPV-45, HPV-52, and HPV-58*: These additional high-risk types account for approximately 15–20% of cervical cancers not covered by the original Gardasil.

Mechanism of Action

Like Gardasil, Gardasil 9 is based on VLPs that stimulate the immune system to produce antibodies. By including additional high-risk HPV types, Gardasil 9 offers broader protection against cervical and other HPV-related cancers.

Efficacy

Gardasil 9 has demonstrated very high efficacy, similar to the original Gardasil vaccine, in preventing infections and diseases caused by the nine targeted HPV types. Clinical studies have shown that Gardasil 9 is nearly 100% effective in preventing precancerous lesions caused by these types. The vaccine also offers protection against a broader range of HPV-related cancers compared to the original Gardasil.

Use and Approval

Gardasil 9 is approved for use in both females and males from ages 9 to 45 years. It is administered in either a two-dose or three-dose schedule, depending on the age at which vaccination begins. It has largely replaced the original Gardasil vaccine in many national immunization programs due to its broader protection.[5]

Cervarix (Bivalent HPV Vaccine)

Composition and Targeted HPV Types

Cervarix, approved by the FDA in 2009, is known as a bivalent vaccine. It targets two high-risk HPV types:

- *HPV-16 and HPV-18*: These types are responsible for the majority of cervical cancers and a significant proportion of other HPV-related cancers.

Mechanism of Action

Cervarix, like the other HPV vaccines, is based on VLPs. However, it uses a different adjuvant system (AS04) that enhances the immune response. This adjuvant system has been shown to produce a stronger and more sustained immune response than some other vaccines.

Efficacy

Cervarix is highly effective in preventing infections and diseases caused by HPV-16 and HPV-18. Clinical trials demonstrated nearly 100% efficacy in preventing cervical precancers caused by these types. Additionally, Cervarix has shown cross-protection against certain other high-risk HPV types not specifically targeted by the vaccine, such as HPV-31 and HPV-45.

Use and Approval

Cervarix is approved for use in females, typically from ages 9 to 25 years, to prevent cervical cancer and precancerous lesions. The vaccine is administered in a two-dose or three-dose schedule, depending on the age at the start of vaccination.

Cervarix has been widely used in some regions, particularly in low- and middle-income countries, due to its effectiveness and the cross-protection it offers against additional high-risk HPV types.[6]

Comparative Summary

- *Gardasil*:
  - *Types covered:* 6, 11, 16, and 18
  - *Focus:* Cervical cancer, genital warts, and other HPV-related cancers
  - *Use:* Both males and females, ages 9–26 years
- *Gardasil 9*:
  - *Types covered:* 6, 11, 16, 18, 31, 33, 45, 52, and 58
  - *Focus:* Cervical cancer, genital warts, and other HPV-related cancers
  - *Use:* Both males and females, ages 9–45 years
- *Cervarix*:
  - *Types covered:* 16 and 18
  - *Focus:* Cervical cancer and some cross-protection against other high-risk types
  - *Use:* Primarily females, ages 9–25 years

GLOBAL IMPACT AND CONSIDERATIONS

- *Herd immunity:* The widespread use of these vaccines, especially Gardasil and Gardasil 9, has led to significant reductions in the prevalence of targeted HPV types and associated diseases, contributing to herd immunity.
- *Access and cost:* The cost of these vaccines, especially Gardasil 9, can be a barrier to widespread use in low-income countries. However, initiatives like Gavi, the Vaccine Alliance, have helped to improve access in some of the world's poorest regions.
- *Vaccine hesitancy:* Despite the vaccines' proven safety and efficacy, vaccine hesitancy due to misinformation, cultural beliefs, and concerns about side effects remains a challenge in some regions. Efforts to increase education and awareness are crucial to improving vaccination rates.
- *Future developments:* Research continues into developing even more comprehensive HPV vaccines, potentially covering additional HPV types or requiring fewer doses to achieve the same level of protection.[7]

KEY POINTS

- The development and widespread adoption of the HPV vaccine, including Gardasil and Cervarix, have significantly reduced the prevalence of high-risk HPV types and related cancers, particularly cervical cancer.
- Gardasil 9, approved in 2014, expanded coverage to nine HPV types, providing broader protection against various cancers compared to its predecessors.
- Studies have consistently demonstrated the near 100% efficacy of HPV vaccines in preventing infections caused by the targeted HPV types, highlighting their role in cancer prevention.
- Despite the success of these vaccines, challenges such as vaccine hesitancy, cost, and access, particularly in low-income countries, remain barriers to achieving universal coverage.

DEVELOPMENT, EFFICACY, AND USE OF THE HEPATITIS A VACCINE

INTRODUCTION TO HEPATITIS A

Hepatitis A is a liver disease caused by the hepatitis A virus (HAV), which is primarily transmitted through the ingestion of contaminated food or water or through direct contact with an infectious person. HAV infection is typically self-limiting and does not result in chronic infection, but it can cause significant morbidity and, in some cases, lead to fulminant hepatitis, which can be fatal. The development of vaccines against hepatitis A has played a crucial role in reducing the incidence of the disease, particularly in regions where the virus is endemic.[8]

DEVELOPMENT OF THE HEPATITIS A VACCINE

The development of the hepatitis A vaccine began in the late 20th century, driven by a need to control outbreaks and prevent the spread of the virus in populations at high risk of infection.

Inactivated Hepatitis A Vaccines

The first hepatitis A vaccines were inactivated vaccines, created by growing the virus in cell cultures, inactivating it with formalin, and then purifying it. The inactivated virus cannot cause disease, but it can stimulate an immune response that provides protection against future infection. The two most widely used inactivated hepatitis A vaccines are as follows:

1. *Havrix (GlaxoSmithKline)*: The first hepatitis A vaccine, Havrix, was developed in the early 1990s and was licensed in several countries by the mid-1990s.
2. *Vaqta (Merck)*: Another inactivated hepatitis A vaccine, Vaqta, was also developed around the same time and licensed for use.

Both vaccines are highly purified and contain aluminum hydroxide as an adjuvant to enhance the immune response. The vaccines are administered in two doses, typically 6–12 months apart.[9]

Live Attenuated Hepatitis A Vaccines

In addition to inactivated vaccines, live attenuated hepatitis A vaccines have been developed, particularly in China. These vaccines contain a weakened form of the virus that can still replicate but does not cause disease in healthy individuals. Examples include:

- *H2 vaccine (China)*: A live attenuated vaccine used primarily in China. It has been shown to be effective in preventing hepatitis A infection, with a single dose providing long-term immunity.

EFFICACY OF THE HEPATITIS A VACCINE

The efficacy of hepatitis A vaccines has been demonstrated through numerous clinical trials and real-world studies. Both inactivated and live attenuated vaccines have been shown to be highly effective in preventing hepatitis A infection.

Inactivated Hepatitis A Vaccines

- Clinical trials of Havrix and Vaqta have demonstrated over 95% efficacy in preventing hepatitis A infection following the complete two-dose series.
- Immunity is typically achieved within 2–4 weeks after the first dose, and long-term protection is provided after the second dose.
- Studies have shown that the vaccine-induced immunity can last for at least 20 years, and potentially lifelong, although ongoing research is assessing the need for booster doses.[10]

Live Attenuated Hepatitis A Vaccines

- The live attenuated H2 vaccine has shown similar efficacy to inactivated vaccines in preventing hepatitis A infection.
- A single dose of the live attenuated vaccine has been found to provide long-term protection, although it is primarily used in specific regions.

Herd Immunity

The widespread use of hepatitis A vaccines has contributed to the development of herd immunity, which helps protect unvaccinated individuals by reducing the circulation of the virus in the population.

USE OF THE HEPATITIS A VACCINE

The hepatitis A vaccine is recommended for various groups, including:

Routine Childhood Immunization

In many countries, including the United States and some European nations, the hepatitis A vaccine is included in the routine childhood immunization schedule. The first dose is usually administered at 12–23 months of age, with the second dose given 6–18 months later.[11]

High-risk Populations

The vaccine is recommended for individuals at high risk of infection, including travelers to regions with high hepatitis A endemicity, men who have sex with men (MSM), people with chronic liver disease, users of injection drugs, and individuals who work with HAV-infected primates or with HAV in research settings.

Outbreak Control

During hepatitis A outbreaks, vaccination is used to control the spread of the virus. Postexposure prophylaxis (PEP) with the hepatitis A vaccine is also recommended for individuals who have been exposed to the virus and are not already immune.

Global Use

The introduction and widespread use of the hepatitis A vaccine in national immunization programs have significantly reduced the incidence of hepatitis A in many countries. In regions where the vaccine has been widely implemented, there has been a dramatic decline in the number of reported cases.[12]

Challenges and Considerations

- Despite its efficacy, the hepatitis A vaccine faces challenges related to access in low-resource settings, where the cost of vaccination programs may be prohibitive. Efforts are ongoing to improve access to the vaccine in these regions.
- Vaccine hesitancy, while less pronounced than with some other vaccines, still exists and can affect coverage rates in certain populations.

CONCLUSION

The development of the hepatitis A vaccine has been a major public health success, significantly reducing the burden of the disease worldwide. The vaccine is highly effective and safe, providing long-term protection against hepatitis A infection. Its use in routine immunization programs and for high-risk populations has led to substantial declines in the incidence of hepatitis A, contributing to improved global health outcomes. Continued efforts to expand access to the vaccine, particularly in low-income countries, are essential to further reducing the global burden of hepatitis A.[13]

DETAILED OVERVIEW OF HEPATITIS A VACCINES AND THEIR SIDE EFFECTS

Hepatitis A vaccines are highly effective in preventing infection caused by the HAV. There are two main types of hepatitis A vaccines: (1) inactivated (killed) vaccines and (2) live attenuated vaccines. Each type has different characteristics, uses, and side effects.

Inactivated Hepatitis A Vaccines

Inactivated vaccines contain killed virus particles that cannot cause disease but can stimulate an immune response to protect against future infection. The two most widely used inactivated hepatitis A vaccines are:

Havrix (GlaxoSmithKline)

Composition and Administration

- Havrix is an inactivated vaccine containing formalin-inactivated HAV, adsorbed onto aluminum hydroxide as an adjuvant to enhance the immune response.
- The vaccine is administered intramuscularly (IM) in two doses, with the second dose given 6–12 months after the first.
- The vaccine is available in two formulations: (1) pediatric [720 enzyme-linked immunosorbent assay (ELISA) units] and (2) adult (1440 ELISA units), with different dosing schedules for each age group.

Efficacy

- Clinical trials have demonstrated that Havrix is over 95% effective in preventing hepatitis A infection after the complete two-dose series.
- The first dose provides substantial protection within 2 weeks, with long-term immunity established after the second dose.[14]

Side Effects

- *Common side effects*: Most side effects are mild and short-lived. These include:
  - Pain, redness, or swelling at the injection site
  - Fatigue
  - Headache
  - Low-grade fever
  - Nausea
- *Less common side effects*:
  - Muscle pain
  - Diarrhea
  - Upper respiratory tract infections
- *Rare side effects*: Serious side effects are very rare but can include:
  - Allergic reactions (e.g., anaphylaxis)
  - Guillain–Barré syndrome (GBS) (a very rare autoimmune disorder)
  - Thrombocytopenia (low platelet count)[15]

Vaqta (Merck)

Composition and Administration

- Vaqta is another inactivated vaccine that contains formalin-inactivated HAV, adsorbed onto aluminum hydroxyphosphate sulfate as an adjuvant.

- Like Havrix, Vaqta is administered IM in two doses, with the second dose given 6–18 months after the first.
- Vaqta is available in pediatric (25 units) and adult (50 units) formulations.

Efficacy

- Vaqta has been shown to be over 95% effective in preventing hepatitis A infection after the complete two-dose series.
- The vaccine induces a strong immune response, providing long-term protection that is likely to last for at least 20 years, and potentially lifelong.[16]

Side Effects

- *Common side effects*:
    - Injection site reactions (pain, redness, and swelling)
    - Fatigue
    - Headache
    - Mild fever
    - Loss of appetite
- *Less common side effects*:
    - Nausea
    - Vomiting
    - Abdominal pain
    - Upper respiratory tract infections
- *Rare side effects*:
    - Hypersensitivity reactions, including anaphylaxis
    - Vasculitis (inflammation of blood vessels)
    - Very rare reports of neurological conditions like GBS

Live Attenuated Hepatitis A Vaccines

Live attenuated vaccines contain a weakened form of the virus that is capable of replicating but does not cause disease in healthy individuals. These vaccines are primarily used in certain regions, such as China.[17]

H2 Vaccine (China)

Composition and Administration

- The H2 vaccine is a live attenuated hepatitis A vaccine derived from a weakened strain of HAV. It is grown in human diploid cells and then attenuated to reduce virulence.
- This vaccine is administered as a single dose, typically subcutaneously.

Efficacy

- The H2 vaccine has been shown to be highly effective in preventing hepatitis A infection, with a single dose providing long-term immunity.
- It is particularly effective in populations where hepatitis A is endemic and where rapid immunization is needed to control outbreaks.

Side Effects

- *Common side effects*:
    - Local reactions at the injection site, such as pain, redness, or swelling
    - Mild fever
    - Fatigue
- *Less common side effects*:
    - Gastrointestinal symptoms, such as nausea and vomiting
    - Mild rash
- *Rare side effects*:
    - Allergic reactions
    - As it is a live vaccine, there is a theoretical risk of viral shedding and transmission, though this has not been widely reported.[18]

Comparative Summary of Hepatitis A Vaccines and Side Effects

- *Havrix and Vaqta (inactivated vaccines)*:
    - Generally well-tolerated with mild, transient side effects
    - Serious side effects are extremely rare.
    - Suitable for a wide range of populations, including children, adults, and those with compromised immune systems.
    - Requires two doses for long-term immunity.
- *H2 vaccine (live attenuated vaccine)*:
    - Also well-tolerated with mild side effects, though live vaccines are generally not recommended for individuals with weakened immune systems.
    - A single dose is sufficient for long-term immunity.
    - Mainly used in specific regions like China.[19]

CONCLUSION

The hepatitis A vaccines, whether inactivated or live attenuated, are highly effective and generally safe. They play a crucial role in preventing hepatitis A infection, particularly in regions with high endemicity or in populations at increased risk. The side effects of these vaccines are typically mild and transient, with serious adverse events being extremely rare. The use of these vaccines has led to a significant reduction in the global burden of hepatitis A, contributing to improved public health outcomes.[20]

HEPATITIS B VACCINES: HISTORY, DEVELOPMENT, EFFICACY, SIDE EFFECTS, USES, AND INDICATIONS

Hepatitis B is a viral infection that affects the liver and can lead to both acute and chronic disease. It is caused by the hepatitis B virus (HBV), which is transmitted through contact with infectious body fluids, such as blood, semen, and vaginal secretions. Chronic HBV infection is a major global health problem, leading to liver cirrhosis and hepatocellular carcinoma. The development and widespread use of hepatitis B vaccines have been pivotal in reducing the incidence of HBV infection and its associated complications.[21]

HISTORY AND DEVELOPMENT OF HEPATITIS B VACCINES

The development of hepatitis B vaccines has evolved over several decades, from the first plasma-derived vaccines to the more advanced recombinant DNA vaccines used today.

Plasma-derived Hepatitis B Vaccines

History

The first hepatitis B vaccine, developed in the early 1980s, was a plasma-derived vaccine. It was produced by isolating the hepatitis B surface antigen (HBsAg) from the blood of chronic HBV carriers. This antigen was then purified and inactivated to create the vaccine.

Development

Heptavax-B (Merck & Co): The first commercially available hepatitis B vaccine was Heptavax-B, licensed in 1981. It was a plasma-derived vaccine that was effective in preventing HBV infection, but its use was limited due to concerns about safety and the potential risk of transmitting other blood-borne pathogens, despite rigorous purification processes.

Transition to Recombinant DNA Vaccines

Due to these concerns, there was a shift toward the development of recombinant DNA vaccines, which are produced in a controlled environment using genetic engineering techniques. These vaccines do not carry the same risks as plasma-derived vaccines.[22]

Recombinant DNA Hepatitis B Vaccines

History

Recombinant DNA technology allowed for the production of safer and more effective hepatitis B vaccines. These vaccines contain the HBsAg produced by yeast or mammalian cells into which the gene for HBsAg has been inserted.

Development

- *Engerix-B (GlaxoSmithKline):* Licensed in 1986, Engerix-B was one of the first recombinant hepatitis B vaccines. It is produced using yeast cells (*Saccharomyces cerevisiae*) that have been genetically modified to produce HBsAg.
- *Recombivax HB (Merck & Co):* Also licensed in 1986, Recombivax HB is another recombinant vaccine produced using similar technology.

Recent Advances

Heplisav-B (Dynavax Technologies): Approved by the FDA in 2017, Heplisav-B is a more recent recombinant hepatitis B vaccine that includes a novel adjuvant (CpG 1018) designed to enhance the immune response. It is administered as a two-dose series, completed within 1 month, offering a more rapid schedule compared to traditional vaccines.

EFFICACY OF HEPATITIS B VACCINES

Hepatitis B vaccines are highly effective in preventing HBV infection. The efficacy varies slightly depending on the vaccine type and the population being immunized, but in general, these vaccines provide excellent protection.[23]

Efficacy in General Population

- Both Engerix-B and Recombivax HB have been shown to be over 90% effective in preventing HBV infection when the full vaccine series is completed.
- Heplisav-B has demonstrated similar efficacy, with studies showing that it provides seroprotection in over 95% of adults after the two-dose series.

Long-term Protection

Immunity conferred by hepatitis B vaccination is long-lasting. Studies indicate that protection can last for at least 20 years, and likely for a lifetime, especially in those who respond well to the initial vaccine series.

Booster Doses

In most cases, booster doses are not necessary for those who have completed the full vaccination series, although they may be recommended for certain high-risk individuals, such as healthcare workers or those with weakened immune systems.

SIDE EFFECTS OF HEPATITIS B VACCINES

Hepatitis B vaccines are generally safe, with most side effects being mild and transient. Serious side effects are very rare.

Common Side Effects[24]

- *Injection site reactions:* Pain, redness, or swelling at the injection site are the most common side effects.
- *Systemic reactions:* Mild fever, fatigue, headache, and muscle aches can occur following vaccination.

Less Common Side Effects

- *Gastrointestinal symptoms:* Some individuals may experience nausea, vomiting, or diarrhea.
- *Upper respiratory symptoms:* Mild symptoms such as a sore throat, cough, or runny nose may occur.

Rare Side Effects

- *Severe allergic reactions:* Anaphylaxis is a very rare but serious allergic reaction that can occur following any vaccine. The incidence is estimated to be about 1 in 1.1 million doses.
- *Neurological reactions:* Rarely, there have been reports of neurological conditions such as GBS following hepatitis B vaccination, though a causal relationship has not been definitively established.

Safety in Special Populations

- *Pregnancy:* Hepatitis B vaccines are generally considered safe for use during pregnancy, particularly in women at high risk for HBV infection.
- *Immunocompromised individuals:* While these individuals may have a reduced response to the vaccine, hepatitis B vaccination is still recommended as it can provide some level of protection.

USES AND INDICATIONS OF HEPATITIS B VACCINES

Hepatitis B vaccines are used for both routine immunization and for specific high-risk groups.

Routine Immunization

- *Infants:* Hepatitis B vaccination is recommended for all infants as part of the routine immunization schedule. The first dose is typically given at birth, with subsequent doses at 1–2 months and 6–18 months.
- *Children and adolescents:* For those not vaccinated as infants, catch-up vaccination is recommended.[25]

High-risk Adults

- *Healthcare workers:* Individuals working in healthcare settings are at increased risk of exposure to HBV and should be vaccinated.
- *People with chronic liver disease:* Those with chronic liver conditions are at higher risk of severe outcomes if infected with HBV and should receive the vaccine.
- *People with multiple sexual partners:* Individuals with multiple sexual partners or those with a history of sexually transmitted infections should be vaccinated due to the higher risk of HBV transmission through sexual contact.
- *Men who have sex with men:* MSM are at higher risk for HBV and are recommended to receive the vaccine.
- *Injection drug users:* Those who use injection drugs are at increased risk of HBV infection through shared needles and should be vaccinated.
- *Household contacts of HBV-infected individuals:* Those living with someone who is chronically infected with HBV are at higher risk and should be vaccinated.
- *Travelers to endemic areas:* People traveling to regions with high rates of HBV infection should receive the vaccine if they are not already immune.[26]

Postexposure Prophylaxis

Hepatitis B vaccine is used in combination with hepatitis B immune globulin (HBIG) for PEP in individuals who have been exposed to HBV through needlestick injuries, sexual contact, or perinatal exposure.[27]

CONCLUSION

The development of hepatitis B vaccines has been a significant milestone in public health, drastically reducing the incidence of HBV infection and its associated complications worldwide. The vaccines are highly effective, safe, and are a critical component of routine immunization programs globally. Continued efforts to expand vaccination coverage, particularly in high-risk populations and regions with high endemicity, are essential to further reduce the global burden of hepatitis B.

HEPATITIS E VACCINES: BURDEN, HISTORY, DEVELOPMENT, INDICATIONS, EFFICACY, AND USES

Hepatitis E is a viral infection caused by the hepatitis E virus (HEV), primarily transmitted through the fecal-oral route, often via contaminated water. The disease is particularly common in regions with poor sanitation, and it can lead to acute liver failure, especially in pregnant women and immunocompromised individuals. Although hepatitis E is typically self-limiting, it can cause significant morbidity and mortality, particularly in endemic areas. The development of vaccines against hepatitis E represents a critical step in preventing outbreaks and reducing the global burden of the disease.

BURDEN OF HEPATITIS E

Hepatitis E is a significant public health concern, particularly in Asia, Africa, and parts of the Middle East, where outbreaks are common. The World Health Organization (WHO) estimates that hepatitis E causes approximately 20 million infections each year, leading to about 3.3 million symptomatic cases and 44,000 deaths globally. The virus is a leading cause of acute viral hepatitis in adults in these regions. Pregnant women are particularly vulnerable, with a mortality rate as high as 25% in the third trimester.[28]

HISTORY AND DEVELOPMENT OF HEPATITIS E VACCINES

The development of a vaccine against hepatitis E was challenging due to the complexity of the virus and its various genotypes. However, significant progress has been made in recent years, resulting in the development of the first licensed hepatitis E vaccine.

Recombinant Hepatitis E Vaccines

The primary approach to developing hepatitis E vaccines has been through recombinant technology, where a portion of the virus (usually the capsid protein) is produced using genetic engineering techniques.

Development

Hecolin (Xiamen Innovax Biotech): Hecolin, the first and currently the only licensed hepatitis E vaccine, was developed by Xiamen Innovax Biotech in China. The vaccine is based on recombinant technology and contains the HEV 239 protein (a truncated form of the HEV ORF2 protein), which is expressed in *Escherichia coli*. The vaccine was approved for use in China in 2011 and has been primarily used to control outbreaks in the country.

INDICATIONS AND USES OF HEPATITIS E VACCINES

The hepatitis E vaccine is primarily indicated for use in populations at high risk of infection, particularly in endemic regions. Its use is also recommended for specific groups who are at an increased risk of severe disease if infected with HEV.

Indications

- *Endemic regions:* In areas where hepatitis E is endemic, the vaccine is recommended to prevent outbreaks, especially in settings with poor sanitation where waterborne transmission is common.
- *Pregnant women:* Given the high risk of severe disease and mortality in pregnant women, especially in the third trimester, vaccination is recommended in endemic regions.
- *Immunocompromised individuals:* People with weakened immune systems, such as organ transplant recipients or those with chronic liver disease, are at higher risk for severe outcomes from hepatitis E infection and are candidates for vaccination.
- *Travelers to endemic areas:* Individuals traveling to regions where hepatitis E is common may benefit from vaccination, particularly if they plan to stay for extended periods or are at risk of consuming contaminated water or food.[29]

EFFICACY OF HEPATITIS E VACCINES

The efficacy of the Hecolin vaccine has been well documented through clinical trials and postmarketing surveillance.

Clinical Efficacy

A large phase III clinical trial conducted in China demonstrated that the Hecolin vaccine has an efficacy of approximately 95% in preventing symptomatic hepatitis E infection after the completion of the three-dose series. The study included over 100,000 participants and provided robust evidence of the vaccine's protective effect.[30]

Duration of Protection

Follow-up studies have shown that the Hecolin vaccine provides long-lasting protection. Immunity persists for at least 4.5 years after vaccination, with ongoing research suggesting that protection may last even longer.

Booster Doses

Currently, there is no recommendation for booster doses, as the primary series appears to provide sufficient long-term protection.

SIDE EFFECTS OF HEPATITIS E VACCINES

The Hecolin vaccine has been shown to be safe, with most side effects being mild and transient.[31]

Common Side Effects

- *Injection site reactions:* Similar to other vaccines, the most common side effects include pain, redness, or swelling at the injection site.
- *Systemic reactions:* Mild fever, headache, and fatigue have been reported following vaccination.

Rare Side Effects

Serious side effects are very rare. There have been no significant safety concerns reported in the large-scale trials or postmarketing surveillance.

USES OF HEPATITIS E VACCINES

The use of the hepatitis E vaccine is primarily focused on preventing outbreaks in endemic regions and protecting high-risk populations. However, its broader use is limited by the fact that it is currently only licensed in China.

Routine Vaccination

In China, the Hecolin vaccine is used for routine vaccination in high-risk populations, particularly in regions with frequent outbreaks.[32]

Outbreak Control

The vaccine has been used to control outbreaks in settings such as refugee camps or during natural disasters, where the risk of hepatitis E transmission is elevated due to poor sanitation.

Global Considerations

While the Hecolin vaccine is currently only licensed in China, there is ongoing research and interest in expanding its use to other countries, particularly those in South Asia, Africa, and the Middle East, where hepatitis E is a significant public health issue.

CONCLUSION

The development of the hepatitis E vaccine marks a significant advancement in the fight against hepatitis E, particularly in endemic regions where the disease is a major public health concern. The Hecolin vaccine, the first and only licensed hepatitis E vaccine, has demonstrated high efficacy and safety in preventing HEV infection. While its use is currently limited to specific regions, the vaccine holds great potential for broader global application, especially in preventing outbreaks and protecting high-risk populations.

DETAILED OVERVIEW OF HEPATITIS E VACCINES

Hepatitis E is a significant public health issue in many parts of the world, particularly in regions with poor sanitation. HEV causes this liver disease, which can lead to severe complications, especially in pregnant women and immunocompromised individuals. Vaccination against HEV is a critical strategy to control the spread of the virus and prevent outbreaks.

Currently, there is one licensed vaccine against hepatitis E: Hecolin. Below is a detailed overview of this vaccine, including its history, development, efficacy, safety, indications, and uses.[33]

Hecolin (Hepatitis E Vaccine)

- *Manufacturer:* Xiamen Innovax Biotech Co., Ltd.
- *Type:* Recombinant protein vaccine (based on HEV 239 antigen)
- *Licensed:* China, 2011.

History and Development

Background

Hecolin is the first and only vaccine licensed to prevent hepatitis E. The vaccine was developed in response to the need for an effective preventive measure against HEV, particularly in regions where the virus is endemic and where outbreaks frequently occur due to contaminated water supplies.[34]

Development Process

- The vaccine development began with identifying the HEV capsid protein, which is critical for inducing an immune response. Researchers focused on the *ORF2* gene of the HEV, which codes for the viral capsid protein. A truncated version of this protein, called HEV 239, was selected for use in the vaccine because

it retains the antigenic properties necessary to trigger immunity without requiring the full virus.
- The HEV 239 antigen was produced using recombinant DNA technology, where the gene coding for this protein was inserted into an *E. coli* bacterial system, which then produced the protein in large quantities.
- Preclinical studies demonstrated the safety and immunogenicity of the vaccine, leading to human trials.

Clinical Trials

- Hecolin underwent extensive clinical testing, including a phase III trial conducted in China involving over 100,000 participants. The trial results were published in The Lancet in 2010, showing an efficacy of 94–100% in preventing symptomatic hepatitis E after the full vaccine series was administered.
- The Chinese regulatory authorities approved the vaccine in 2011, making it the first vaccine against hepatitis E to be licensed for use.[35]

Efficacy

General Efficacy

The Hecolin vaccine has demonstrated high efficacy in preventing symptomatic HEV infections. The large phase III trial indicated that the vaccine was about 95% effective at preventing symptomatic disease after the completion of the three-dose series.

Long-term Efficacy

Follow-up studies have shown that the vaccine provides long-lasting protection, with immunity persisting for at least 4.5 years postvaccination. Ongoing studies suggest that the protection may last even longer.

Booster Doses

Currently, booster doses are not routinely recommended as the initial vaccination series provides long-term protection. However, research is ongoing to determine whether boosters might be necessary after many years.

Safety and Side Effects

General Safety Profile

The Hecolin vaccine has been shown to be safe and well tolerated in clinical trials. Most adverse events reported were mild and temporary.[30]

Common Side Effects

- *Injection site reactions:* Pain, redness, and swelling at the injection site are the most commonly reported side effects.
- *Systemic reactions:* Some individuals experience mild fever, headache, fatigue, and muscle aches after vaccination.

Rare Side Effects

Serious side effects are rare. There have been no significant safety concerns identified in the postmarketing surveillance or clinical trial.

Use in Pregnancy

The vaccine has not been widely studied in pregnant women, although it may be recommended in high-risk areas due to the significant risk hepatitis E virus poses during pregnancy. However, the decision to vaccinate should be made on a case-by-case basis, considering the potential risks and benefits.

Indications and Uses

Primary Indications

The Hecolin vaccine is indicated for use in individuals who are at high risk of hepatitis E infection, particularly in regions where the virus is endemic, such as South Asia, parts of Africa, and the Middle East.[36]

High-risk Groups

- *Residents in endemic areas:* People living in regions with high rates of hepatitis E transmission.
- *Travelers:* Individuals traveling to endemic regions may be advised to receive the vaccine before departure.
- *Immunocompromised individuals:* Those with weakened immune systems, such as organ transplant recipients or individuals with chronic liver disease, may benefit from vaccination.
- *Pregnant women in endemic areas:* Given the high mortality risk from HEV infection during pregnancy, vaccination may be considered, although the safety data is limited.

Outbreak Control

The vaccine is also used in outbreak settings to quickly immunize high-risk populations and prevent the spread of the virus.

Potential Global Expansion

While Hecolin is currently only licensed in China, there is interest in expanding its use globally, particularly in other endemic regions. The WHO and other public health agencies are considering strategies for broader vaccine deployment.[37]

Other Hepatitis E Vaccines (Under Development)

Global Efforts

Several research groups and pharmaceutical companies have been working on developing additional hepatitis E vaccines. However, none have progressed to the point of being licensed or widely available outside China.

Challenges

The major challenges in developing and licensing new hepatitis E vaccines include the need for extensive clinical trials, the genetic variability of HEV genotypes, and the regulatory hurdles associated with bringing a new vaccine to market.

Current Research

Ongoing research focuses on developing vaccines that are effective across different HEV genotypes and can be produced at a lower cost to facilitate broader access, particularly in low- and middle-income countries.[37]

CONCLUSION

The development of the Hecolin vaccine represents a significant milestone in the fight against hepatitis E, providing an effective tool to prevent the disease in high-risk populations. The vaccine's success in China offers hope for broader global applications, particularly in regions where hepatitis E is a significant public health concern. Ongoing research and potential new vaccines may further expand the options available for controlling and preventing hepatitis E worldwide.

INTRODUCTION TO RABIES AND RABIES VACCINES

Rabies is a fatal viral disease caused by the Rabies *Lyssavirus*, which affects the central nervous system, leading to neurological symptoms and eventually death. The development of effective rabies vaccines has been crucial in preventing the spread of this deadly disease in both humans and animals. Over the years, different types of rabies vaccines have been developed, each with unique characteristics, development histories, and uses.[38]

NERVE TISSUE VACCINES

Development

Nerve tissue vaccines (NTVs) were among the earliest rabies vaccines, developed in the early 20th century. They were made from the brain tissue of infected animals, such as sheep or goats. The virus was inactivated using phenol or other chemicals, and the vaccine was administered to patients who had been exposed to rabies.

Efficacy

Nerve tissue vaccines were initially effective in preventing rabies, but they had significant drawbacks. The presence of neural tissue in the vaccine often led to severe neurological side effects, such as GBS. Moreover, the immune response triggered by NTVs was relatively weak compared to modern vaccines. Due to these issues, NTVs have largely been phased out and replaced by safer alternatives.

Uses

Nerve tissue vaccines were widely used in many developing countries until the late 20th century. However, due to the development of safer and more effective vaccines, their use has been discontinued in most parts of the world.[39]

DUCK EMBRYO VACCINES

Development

Duck embryo vaccines (DEVs) were developed as an alternative to NTVs in the mid-20th century. These vaccines were produced by growing the rabies virus in the embryos of ducks and then inactivating the virus. The use of duck embryos reduced the risk of neurological complications associated with NTVs.

Efficacy

Duck embryo vaccines were safer than NTVs, with fewer side effects. However, the immunogenicity of DEVs was still not optimal, requiring multiple doses to achieve adequate protection. Despite this, DEVs were a significant improvement over NTVs and were used in many countries for several decades.[40]

Uses

Duck embryo vaccines were used primarily in regions where NTVs were phased out, particularly in countries with limited access to more advanced vaccines. However, with the advent of cell culture vaccines, the use of DEVs has also declined significantly.

HUMAN DIPLOID CELL VACCINE

Development

The human diploid cell vaccine (HDCV) was developed in the 1960s and became commercially available in the 1970s. HDCV was the first rabies vaccine developed using the human diploid cell line WI-38, which was originally derived from fetal lung tissue. The rabies virus is cultured in these cells and then inactivated using β-propiolactone.[41]

Efficacy

Human diploid cell vaccine is highly immunogenic and provides strong, long-lasting immunity against rabies.

It is considered the gold standard for rabies vaccination, with a seroconversion rate of nearly 100% after the full vaccination course. HDCV has a favorable safety profile, with only minor side effects such as local pain and mild fever.

Uses

Human diploid cell vaccine is used both as a preexposure prophylaxis (PrEP) for individuals at high risk of rabies exposure (e.g., veterinarians and laboratory workers) and as PEP for individuals who have been exposed to the rabies virus. It is widely used in developed countries and is the preferred vaccine in many settings.

Schedule and Eligibility

- *Preexposure prophylaxis:* For individuals at high risk of rabies exposure, such as veterinarians, laboratory workers, and travelers to endemic areas. The schedule consists of three doses administered on days 0, 7, and 21 or 28.[42]
- *Postexposure prophylaxis:* For individuals exposed to the rabies virus, the schedule is four doses administered on days 0, 3, 7, and 14. For immunocompromised individuals, a fifth dose on day 28 is recommended. If the patient has previously been vaccinated with HDCV, only two doses on days 0 and 3 are required.

Brand names: Imovax Rabies (Sanofi Pasteur)

Regimens

- *Preexposure prophylaxis*:
  - *Standard regimen*:
    - *Dosage:* 1.0 mL IM
    - *Schedule:* Three doses on days 0, 7, and 21 or 28
  - *Booster doses:* For those at continuous risk of rabies exposure, a booster dose is recommended every 2–3 years. Regular serological testing can determine the need for boosters.[43]
- *Postexposure prophylaxis*:
  - Previously unvaccinated individuals:
    - *Dosage:* 1.0 mL IM
    - *Schedule:* Four doses on days 0, 3, 7, and 14
    - *Rabies immune globulin (RIG):* Administered on day 0, along with the first vaccine dose, at a dosage of 20 IU/kg, infiltrated into and around the wound if possible, with the remainder given IM.
  - Previously vaccinated individuals:
    - *Dosage:* 1.0 mL IM
    - *Schedule:* Two doses on days 0 and 3
    - *RIG:* Not required for previously vaccinated individuals

Considerations

Human diploid cell vaccine (HDCV) is suitable for all age groups and is recommended for both primary immunization and booster doses. It is generally well-tolerated, with minor side effects such as pain at the injection site, fever, and headache.[44]

PURIFIED CHICK EMBRYO CELL VACCINE

Development

The purified chick embryo cell vaccine (PCECV) was developed as an alternative to HDCV and became available in the 1980s. PCECV is produced by growing the rabies virus in chick embryo cells, followed by purification and inactivation with β-propiolactone.

Efficacy

Purified chick embryo cell vaccine has efficacy comparable to that of HDCV, providing strong and long-lasting immunity. It is well-tolerated, with a similar safety profile to HDCV. PCECV has become a widely used rabies vaccine, especially in regions where poultry-based production is more feasible than human cell-based production.

Uses

Purified chick embryo cell vaccine is used for both PrEP and PEP, similar to HDCV. It is commonly used in Europe, Asia, and Latin America. The vaccine is particularly useful in areas with poultry industries, as the infrastructure for producing chick embryo-based vaccines is often already in place.

Schedule and Eligibility

- *Preexposure prophylaxis:* Similar to HDCV, three doses on days 0, 7, and 21 or 28.
- *Postexposure prophylaxis:* Four doses on days 0, 3, 7, and 14. In cases of severe exposure or in immunocompromised patients, a fifth dose on day 28 may be considered. For previously vaccinated individuals, only two doses on days 0 and 3 are required.[45]

Brand Names

- Rabipur (Bavarian Nordic)
- RabAvert (GlaxoSmithKline)

Regimens

- *Preexposure prophylaxis*:
  - Standard regimen:

    - *Dosage:* 1.0 mL IM
    - *Schedule:* Three doses on days 0, 7, and 21 or 28.
  - *Booster doses:* For those at continuous risk, booster doses are recommended every 2–3 years, with serological testing to guide the timing.
- *Postexposure prophylaxis*:
  - Previously unvaccinated individuals:
    - *Dosage*: 1.0 mL IM
    - *Schedule*: Four doses on days 0, 3, 7, and 14.
    - *RIG:* Administered on day 0 at 20 IU/kg, with as much as possible infiltrated into the wound.
  - Previously vaccinated individuals:
    - *Dosage:* 1.0 mL IM
    - *Schedule:* Two doses on days 0 and 3.
    - *RIG:* Not required for previously vaccinated individuals.

Considerations

Purified chick embryo cell vaccine is recommended for use in both adults and children. It is often preferred in areas where the infrastructure for poultry-based production exists. Side effects are generally mild and include local reactions at the injection site, such as redness, swelling, and pain.[46]

VERO CELL RABIES VACCINE

Development

The Vero cell rabies vaccine (VCRV) was developed in the 1980s using the Vero cell line, derived from African green monkey kidney cells. VCRV production involves the cultivation of the rabies virus in Vero cells, followed by inactivation with β-propiolactone.

Efficacy

Vero cell rabies vaccine is highly immunogenic and provides excellent protection against rabies, with a safety and efficacy profile similar to HDCV and PCECV. The vaccine is well tolerated and has become an important tool in rabies prevention, particularly in developing countries.

Uses

Vero cell rabies vaccine is used for both PrEP and PEP and is widely distributed in many parts of the world, including Africa, Asia, and South America. It is particularly favored in regions where Vero cell production facilities are established.

Schedule and Eligibility

- *Preexposure prophylaxis:* Three doses administered on days 0, 7, and 21 or 28.
- *Postexposure prophylaxis:* Typically involves a four-dose regimen on days 0, 3, 7, and 14. A fifth dose may be recommended for immunocompromised patients or in cases of severe exposure. For those previously vaccinated with VCRV, two doses on days 0 and 3 suffice.

Brand Names

- Verorab (Sanofi Pasteur)
- Indirab (Bharat Biotech)

Regimens

- *Preexposure prophylaxis*:
  - *Standard regimen*:
    - *Dosage*: 0.5 or 1.0 mL IM (depending on the product)
    - *Schedule*: Three doses on days 0, 7, and 21 or 28.
  - *Booster doses*: Recommended every 2–3 years for those at continuous risk, guided by serological testing.
- *Postexposure prophylaxis*:
  - Previously unvaccinated individuals:
    - *Dosage*: 0.5 or 1.0 mL IM
    - *Schedule*: Four doses on days 0, 3, 7, and 14.
    - *RIG:* Administered on day 0, with the full dose infiltrated around the wound site.
  - Previously vaccinated individuals:
    - *Dosage*: 0.5 or 1.0 mL IM
    - *Schedule*: Two doses on days 0 and 3.
    - *RIG*: Not required for previously vaccinated individuals.

Considerations

Vero cell rabies vaccine is suitable for all age groups, including children, and is widely used in regions where cell culture production is accessible. Side effects are generally mild, including local pain, erythema, and occasional fever.[47]

DNA-BASED RABIES VACCINES

Development

DNA-based rabies vaccines represent a novel approach to vaccination, with research and development ongoing since the late 1990s. These vaccines involve the insertion of rabies virus genes into a plasmid, which is then introduced into host cells to induce an immune response.

Efficacy

Early studies of DNA-based rabies vaccines have shown promising results, with the potential for strong and long-lasting immunity. These vaccines may offer advantages such as ease of production, stability, and the ability to induce both humoral and cell-mediated immune responses.

Uses

DNA-based rabies vaccines are still in the experimental stage, with ongoing clinical trials. If proven effective, they could become a valuable addition to the rabies vaccine arsenal, particularly in regions where traditional vaccine production is challenging.

Schedule and Eligibility

As these vaccines are still under development, the exact vaccination schedule and eligibility criteria are yet to be established. They are expected to follow a similar regimen to existing vaccines once they reach the market.

ADSORBED RABIES VACCINE

Brand names: Rabivax-S (Serum Institute of India)

Regimens

- *Preexposure prophylaxis*:
    - *Standard regimen*:
        - *Dosage*: 1.0 mL IM
        - *Schedule*: Three doses on days 0, 7, and 21 or 28.
    - *Booster doses*: Booster doses are recommended every 2–3 years, with periodic serological testing.
- *Postexposure prophylaxis*:
    - Previously unvaccinated individuals:
        - *Dosage:* 1.0 mL IM
        - *Schedule:* Four doses on days 0, 3, 7, and 14.
        - *RIG:* Administered on day 0, infiltrated into the wound.
    - Previously vaccinated individuals:
        - *Dosage:* 1.0 mL IM
        - *Schedule:* Two doses on days 0 and 3.
        - *RIG:* Not required for previously vaccinated individuals.

Considerations

DNA-based rabies vaccines have the potential to revolutionize rabies prevention, especially in regions where traditional vaccine production is challenging. They may offer advantages such as stability, ease of production, and a strong immune response.

Considerations for Specific Populations

- *Children:* Rabies vaccines are generally safe for use in children, with the same dosages and schedules as adults. The only difference may be in the administration technique, especially in younger children, where the anterolateral thigh is preferred over the deltoid for IM injections.
- *Immunocompromised individuals:* These patients may require an additional dose of rabies vaccine (fifth dose) during PEP and should have their antibody titers monitored to ensure adequate immune response. They should receive the full course of vaccine and RIG even if they were previously vaccinated.
- *Pregnancy:* Rabies vaccines, including HDCV, PCECV, and VCRV, are considered safe during pregnancy, especially in cases where the risk of rabies exposure is high. The benefits of vaccination far outweigh the potential risks.[48]

CONCLUSION

The development of rabies vaccines has evolved significantly from the early NTVs to modern cell culture and DNA-based vaccines. Each vaccine type has contributed to the overall goal of reducing rabies incidence and preventing rabies-related deaths. The continued advancement in vaccine technology holds the promise of even more effective and accessible rabies prevention strategies in the future.

CONCLUSION

The role of vaccines in safeguarding public health cannot be overstated. By targeting specific diseases, vaccines have helped control outbreaks, reduce mortality rates, and improve overall quality of life. Their development and deployment represent a triumph of medical science, turning once-deadly infections into preventable conditions.However, the success of vaccination programs relies not only on scientific advancements but also on public trust, equitable access, and continuous research. As new health challenges emerge, the refinement and adaptation of vaccines remain critical in combating evolving threats.

Ultimately, focusing on specific vaccines highlights their individual and collective impact on global health. By supporting immunization efforts and staying informed, society can ensure that vaccines continue to protect present and future generations from preventable diseases.

REFERENCES

1. Soliman M, Oredein O, Dass CR. Update on Safety and Efficacy of HPV Vaccines: Focus on Gardasil. Int J Mol Cell Med. 2021;10(2):101-13.
2. World Health Organization (WHO). (2024). Human papillomavirus (HPV) and cervical cancer. [online] Available from https://www.who.int/news-room/fact-sheets/detail/cervical-cancer [Last accessed March, 2025].
3. Centers for Disease Control and Prevention. HPV vaccine recommendations [Internet]. CDC. 2021. Available from: https://www.cdc.gov/vaccines/vpd/hpv/hcp/recommendations.html [last assessed March 2025].
4. National Cancer Institute (NCI). HPV and Cancer. [online] Available from https://www.cancer.gov/about-cancer/causes-prevention/risk/infectious-agents/hpv-and-cancer. [Last accessed March, 2025].
5. Serrano B, Brotons M, Bosch FX, Bruni L. Epidemiology and burden of HPV-related disease. Best Pract Res Clin Obstet Gynaecol. 2018;47:14-26.
6. Joura EA, Giuliano AR, Iversen OE, Bouchard C, Mao C, Mehlsen J, et al. A 9-valent HPV vaccine against infection and intraepithelial neoplasia in women. N Engl J Med. 2015;372(8):711-23.
7. Garland SM, Hernandez-Avila M, Wheeler CM, Perez G, Harper DM, Leodolter S, et al. Quadrivalent vaccine against human papillomavirus to prevent anogenital diseases. N Engl J Med. 2007;356(19):1928-43.
8. Fiore AE, Wasley A, Bell BP. Prevention of Hepatitis A through active or passive immunization: Recommendations of the Advisory Committee on Immunization Practices (ACIP). MMWR Recomm Rep. 2006;55(RR-7):1-23.
9. André FE, Zuckerman AJ. Review: Protective efficacy of Hepatitis A vaccines. J Med Virol. 1994;44(4):452-8.
10. Zhang L, Xu A, Wang X, Wang J, Zhang L. Efficacy and safety of live attenuated and inactivated hepatitis A vaccines in children: A meta-analysis. Vaccine. 2017;35(35 Pt B):4508-14.
11. Cuthbert JA. Hepatitis A: Old and new. Clin Microbiol Rev. 2001;14(1):38-58.
12. Murphy TV, Feinstone SM, Bell BP. Hepatitis A vaccine: a decade of experience. Clin Infect Dis. 2003;37(9):1266-73.
13. Jacobsen KH, Wiersma ST. Hepatitis A virus seroprevalence by age and world region, 1990 and 2005. Vaccine. 2010;28(41):6653-57.
14. Advisory Committee on Immunization Practices (ACIP). Update: Prevention of Hepatitis A after Exposure to Hepatitis A Virus and in International Travelers. Recommendations of the Advisory Committee on Immunization Practices (ACIP). MMWR Morb Mortal Wkly Rep. 2007;56(41):1080-4.
15. André FE. Overview of a 7-year experience with Havrix: the world's first inactivated hepatitis A vaccine. J Hepatol. 1995;22 (1 Suppl):12-8.
16. Shouval D, Roggendorf M, Roggendorf H. Enhanced immunity against hepatitis A by a two-dose regimen of a formalin-inactivated hepatitis A vaccine: a comparison with human immunoglobulin. Vaccine. 1993;11(8):877-81.
17. Lemon SM, Shapiro CN. The value of immunization against hepatitis A. Infect Agents Dis. 1994;3(1):38-49.
18. Wasley A, Fiore A, Bell BP. Hepatitis A in the era of vaccination. Epidemiol Rev. 2006;28:101-11.
19. Cui F, Hadler SC, Zheng H, Wang F, Zhenhua W, Yuansheng H, et al. Hepatitis A surveillance and vaccine use in China from 1990 through 2007. J Epidemiol. 2009;19(4):189-95.
20. Nelson NP, Link-Gelles R, Hofmeister MG, Romero JR, Moore KL, Ward JW, et al. Update: Recommendations of the Advisory Committee on Immunization Practices for Use of Hepatitis A Vaccine for Postexposure Prophylaxis and for Preexposure Prophylaxis for International Travel. MMWR Morb Mortal Wkly Rep. 2018;67(43):1216-20.
21. Zuckerman JN, Zuckerman AJ. Hepatitis B: Overview. Vaccine. 2006;24(49-50):4907-10.
22. McMahon BJ. The influence of hepatitis B vaccine doses and timing on immunogenicity and duration of protection: A meta-analysis. Vaccine. 2017;35(31):3978-85.
23. Shouval D. Hepatitis B vaccines. J Hepatol. 2003;39 Suppl 1: S102-5.
24. Heplisav-B [package insert]. Berkeley, CA: Dynavax Technologies Corporation; 2017.
25. Centers for Disease Control and Prevention (CDC). A comprehensive immunization strategy to eliminate transmission of hepatitis B virus infection in the United States: recommendations of the Advisory Committee on Immunization Practices (ACIP). Part II: immunization of adults. MMWR Recomm Rep. 2006;55(RR-16):1-33.
26. West DJ. The risk of hepatitis B infection among health professionals in the United States: a review. Am J Med Sci. 1984;287(2):26-33.
27. FitzSimons D, François G, De Carli G, Shouval D, Prüss-Ustün A, Puro V, et al. Hepatitis B virus, hepatitis C virus and other blood-borne infections in healthcare workers: guidelines for prevention and management in industrialised countries. Occup Environ Med. 2008;65(7):446-51.
28. Zhang J, Zhang XF, Huang SJ, Wu T, Hu YM, Wang ZZ, et al. Long-term efficacy of a hepatitis E vaccine. N Engl J Med. 2015;372(10):914-22. [Erratum in: N Engl J Med. 2015;372(15):1478.]
29. Zhu FC, Zhang J, Zhang XF, Zhou C, Wang ZZ, Huang SJ, et al. Efficacy and safety of a recombinant hepatitis E vaccine in healthy adults: a large-scale, randomised, double-blind placebo-controlled, phase 3 trial. Lancet. 2010;376(9744):895-902.
30. Hepatitis E vaccine: WHO position paper, May 2015. Wkly Epidemiol Rec. 2015;90(18):185-200.
31. Shrestha MP, Scott RM, Joshi DM, Mammen MP Jr, Thapa GB, Thapa N, et al. Safety and efficacy of a recombinant hepatitis E vaccine. N Engl J Med. 2007;356(9):895-903.
32. Zhang J, Shih JW, Wu T, Li SW, Xia NS. Development of the hepatitis E vaccine: from bench to field. Semin Liver Dis. 2013;33(1):79-88.
33. Cao D, Meng XJ. Molecular biology and replication of hepatitis E virus. Emerg Microbes Infect. 2012;1(8):e17.
34. Rein DB, Stevens GA, Theaker J, Wittenborn JS, Wiersma ST. The global burden of hepatitis E virus genotypes 1 and 2 in 2005. Hepatology. 2012;55(4):988-97.
35. Aggarwal R, Goel A. Hepatitis E: epidemiology, clinical course, prevention, and treatment. Gastroenterol Clin North Am. 2014;43(3):623-34.
36. Cao Y, Bing Z, Guan S, Zhang Z, Wang X. Development of new hepatitis E vaccines. Hum Vaccin Immunother. 2018;14(9): 2254-62.
37. World Health Organization (WHO). (2023). Hepatitis E. [online] Available from https://www.who.int/news-room/fact-sheets/detail/hepatitis-e [Last accessed March, 2025].
38. Manning SE, Rupprecht CE, Fishbein D, Hanlon CA, Lumlertdacha B, Guerra M, et al. Human rabies prevention--United States, 2008:

recommendations of the Advisory Committee on Immunization Practices. MMWR Recomm Rep. 2008;57(RR-3):1-28.
39. Wilde H, Hemachudha T, Jackson AC. Rabies: still a silent killer targeting the poor. Vaccine. 2015;33(49):6545-8.
40. Hemachudha T, Laothamatas J, Rupprecht CE. Human rabies: a disease of complex neuropathogenetic mechanisms and diagnostic challenges. Lancet Neurol. 2002;1(2):101-9.
41. Warrell MJ, Warrell DA. Rabies and other lyssavirus diseases. Lancet. 2004;363(9413):959-69.
42. World Health Organization. Rabies vaccines: WHO position paper—April 2018. Wkly Epidemiol Rec. 2018;93(16):201-20.
43. Jackson AC. Rabies: Scientific Basis of Disease and Its Management, 3rd edition. Oxford, UK: Academic Press; 2013.
44. Fooks AR, Cliquet F, Finke S, Freuling C, Hemachudha T, Mani RS, et al. Rabies. Nat Rev Dis Primers. 2017;3:17091.
45. World Health Organization. (2018). WHO Expert Consultation on Rabies: third report (WHO Technical Report Series). [online] Available from https://iris.who.int/bitstream/handle/10665/272364/9789241210218-eng.pdf [Last accessed March, 2025].
46. Rupprecht CE, Hanlon CA, Hemachudha T. Rabies re-examined. Lancet Infect Dis. 2002;2(6):327-43.
47. Plotkin SA, Orenstein WA, Offit PA, Edwards KM. Plotkin's Vaccines, 7th edition. Philadelphia, PA: Elsevier; 2018.
48. Huang G, Liu H, Cao Q, Liu B, Pan H, Fu C. Safety of post-exposure rabies prophylaxis during pregnancy: A follow-up study from Guangzhou, China. Human Vaccines & Immunotherapeutics. 2013;9(1):177-83.

CHAPTER 16

Vaccine Development

Pankaj B Shah

INTRODUCTION

Vaccines are commonly used in public health. Vaccine development used to be lengthy process like any drug development during the pre-COVID era, and the complete process got expedited during the COVID era all over the world **(Table 1)**.

The mentioned aspects very well indicate that inactivated vaccines are tested model in India compared to different development and implementation process for newer technology like mRNA and DNA vaccines.

VARIOUS PHASES OF VACCINE DEVELOPMENT

Discovery and Preclinical Development

- *Target identification*: The first step is identifying a pathogen or antigen that could elicit an immune

TABLE 1: Technical differences in the development of various types of vaccines in India.

Aspect	Inactivated virus vaccines	mRNA vaccines	Viral vector vaccines	Protein subunit vaccines
Technology	Uses killed or inactivated virus	Uses mRNA to instruct cells to produce proteins	Uses a virus vector to deliver pathogen genes	Uses purified proteins from the pathogen
Production process	Virus cultivation, inactivation, and formulation	mRNA synthesis, encapsulation in lipid nanoparticles	Vector virus engineering, production, and formulation	Protein expression, purification, and formulation
Preclinical studies	Required to demonstrate safety in animal models	Required to test mRNA stability and safety	Required to ensure safety and efficacy of the vector	Required for safety and efficacy in animals
Clinical trials	Phase 1 (safety), phase 2 (efficacy), and phase 3 (large scale)	Phase 1 (safety), phase 2 (efficacy), and phase 3 (large scale)	Phase 1 (safety), phase 2 (efficacy), and phase 3 (large scale)	Phase 1 (safety), phase 2 (efficacy), and phase 3 (large scale)
Manufacturing requirements	Large-scale virus production and inactivation	Sophisticated facilities for mRNA synthesis and lipid nanoparticle formulation	Genetic engineering and virus production facilities	Protein expression systems and purification processes
Storage and stability	Standard refrigeration temperatures	Ultra-cold storage required for stability	Generally stable at standard temperatures, but varies	Standard refrigeration temperature, varies by formulation
Adjuvants	Often used to enhance immune response	Not typically used; lipid nanoparticles are used	Not always required, but may include stabilizers	Adjuvants may be used to boost immune response
Regulatory considerations	Requires adherence to good manufacturing practices (GMP)	Requires adherence to GMP, and specific conditions for mRNA	Requires GMP, and adherence to vector-specific regulations	Requires GMP and adherence to protein-specific guidelines
Safety monitoring	Extensive historical data available	Newer technology with evolving safety data	Safety data depends on the vector used	Well-established safety profiles, but varies by protein
Examples	Covaxin by Bharat Biotech	No mRNA vaccines approved yet in India	Covishield (AstraZeneca/ Oxford)	Novavax (not yet widely used in India)

response. This involves studying the pathogen's biology, virulence factors, and potential vulnerabilities that can be targeted by a vaccine.

- *Antigen design*: Once a target is identified, scientists design potential antigens (e.g., proteins and peptides) that can stimulate an immune response. This often involves genetic engineering to create these antigens in the laboratory.
- *In vitro studies*: The candidate antigens are tested in vitro (in the laboratory) to evaluate their ability to induce an immune response. These studies might involve assays to test binding affinity to immune cells or the production of antibodies.
- *In vivo studies*: Animal models (e.g., mice, rats, and nonhuman primates) are used to assess the vaccine's safety, immunogenicity (ability to provoke an immune response), and efficacy in preventing disease.

Phase I Clinical Trials

Phase I clinical trials aim to assess the vaccine's safety, dosage range, and immunogenicity in a small group of healthy volunteers (20–100 individuals) and for finding out the maximum tolerable dose (MTD). Typically, phase I trials are open-label or blinded and often involve dose-escalation studies to determine the appropriate dosage. Participants are monitored for adverse effects and immunogenicity.

Phase II Clinical Trials

Phase II clinical trials aim to evaluate the vaccine's immunogenicity, safety, and initial efficacy in a larger group (several hundred participants), often including individuals who are at higher risk for the disease. Phase II trials are usually randomized and controlled, often with a placebo or active comparator group. This phase may include different formulations or delivery methods to optimize the vaccine.

Phase III Clinical Trials

Phase III clinical trials aim to assess the vaccine's efficacy and safety in a much larger population (thousands to tens of thousands of participants), often across multiple countries and diverse populations. Phase III trials are typically randomized, double-blind, and placebo-controlled to provide robust data on the vaccine's ability to prevent the disease. These studies also monitor for rare adverse events that may not have been detected in earlier phases. The main objective is to demonstrate the vaccine's efficacy in preventing the target disease and to gather comprehensive safety data. Successful completion of phase III trials is critical for regulatory approval.

Regulatory Review and Approval

- *Submission of data*: Upon successful completion of phase III trials, the vaccine developer submits a Biologics License Application (BLA) or equivalent to regulatory agencies [e.g., Food and Drug Administration (FDA) and European Medicines Agency (EMA)].
- *Regulatory review*: The regulatory agency reviews the data, including preclinical, clinical, and manufacturing information. This process may include advisory committee meetings and inspections of manufacturing facilities.
- *Approval*: If the data demonstrate that the vaccine is safe, effective, and can be consistently manufactured, the regulatory agency grants approval for the vaccine to be marketed.

Phase IV Clinical Trials and Postmarketing Surveillance

- *Phase IV trials*: Also known as postmarketing studies, these trials continue to monitor the vaccine's safety and effectiveness in the general population. They may involve several thousand participants and focus on specific subgroups or long-term effects.
- *Pharmacovigilance*: Continuous monitoring for adverse events through national and international surveillance systems (e.g., VAERS in the US) is essential. This process helps to identify rare or long-term side effects and assess the vaccine's performance in real-world conditions.
- *Postmarketing commitments*: In some cases, regulatory agencies may require the manufacturer to conduct additional studies to further evaluate safety, efficacy, or specific populations (e.g., pediatric studies).

Manufacturing and Distribution

After approval, the vaccine production is scaled up to meet global demand. This involves ensuring the consistency, quality, and stability of the vaccine across large batches. Each batch of the vaccine undergoes rigorous testing to ensure it meets predefined standards for potency, purity, and sterility. The vaccine is distributed to healthcare providers, often requiring cold chain logistics to maintain efficacy. Healthcare workers are trained to administer the vaccine safely.

MAJOR COMPARISON BETWEEN VACCINE DEVELOPMENT AND DRUG DEVELOPMENT

The development of vaccines and drugs are critical processes in healthcare aimed at preventing and treating diseases, respectively. While both follow a structured pathway from discovery to market approval, there are distinct differences and similarities in their development processes, objectives, regulatory requirements, and challenges **(Table 2)**.

TABLE 2: Differences between vaccine development and drug development.

Aspect	Vaccine development	Drug development
Target identification	• Identifying a pathogen (virus, bacteria) or its components (e.g., proteins and peptides) that can stimulate an immune response • Identifying antigens capable of eliciting protective immunity	• Identifying biological targets (e.g., proteins, enzymes, and receptors) involved in disease pathophysiology • Screening of chemical libraries for molecules that modulate these targets
Molecule/Antigen design	• Antigens are designed to mimic parts of the pathogen, such as surface proteins, to provoke an immune response without causing disease • Can include live-attenuated, inactivated, subunit, or mRNA vaccines	• Molecules are designed or selected based on their ability to interact with the biological target to correct or modulate a pathological process • Can include small molecules, biologics (antibodies and peptides), or gene therapies
Preclinical testing	• Involves testing in vitro (lab-based) and in vivo (animal) models to assess immunogenicity (ability to induce an immune response), safety, and preliminary efficacy • Focuses on identifying the best formulation and delivery method	• Involves in vitro and in vivo testing to assess pharmacodynamics (PD), pharmacokinetics (PK), safety, and preliminary efficacy • Includes metabolism studies and toxicity evaluations (acute, chronic, reproductive, etc.).
Phase I clinical trials	• Conducted in a small group (20–100) of healthy volunteers • Focuses on safety, tolerability, and immunogenicity • Often includes dose-escalation studies to determine the optimal dose	• Conducted in a small group (20–100) of healthy volunteers or patients with the target disease • Focuses on safety, tolerability, and PK/PD • Often includes dose-escalation studies to determine the optimal dose
Phase II clinical trials	• Conducted in several hundred participants, often including higher-risk groups • Focuses on safety, immunogenicity, and initial efficacy • May include different formulations or delivery methods	• Conducted in several hundred patients with the target disease • Focuses on efficacy, safety, and optimal dosing • May include different patient subgroups or dose regimens
Phase III clinical trials	• Conducted in thousands to tens of thousands of participants across diverse populations • Focuses on confirming efficacy, safety, and immunogenicity in preventing disease • Usually involves randomized, double-blind, placebo-controlled trials	• Conducted in thousands of patients across multiple sites and diverse populations • Focuses on confirming efficacy and safety in treating or managing the disease • Usually involves randomized, double-blind, placebo-controlled trials
Regulatory submission	• Submission of a Biologics License Application (BLA) to regulatory authorities (e.g., FDA and EMA) • Includes data on preclinical studies, clinical trials, and manufacturing processes	• Submission of a New Drug Application (NDA) for small molecules or a BLA for biologics • Includes data on preclinical studies, clinical trials, and manufacturing processes
Regulatory review and approval	• Regulatory agencies review the safety, efficacy, and manufacturing data • May involve advisory committees and inspections of manufacturing facilities • Approval leads to vaccine distribution and administration to the public	• Regulatory agencies review the safety, efficacy, and manufacturing data • May involve advisory committees and inspections of manufacturing facilities • Approval leads to the drug being made available for prescription

Continued

Continued

Aspect	Vaccine development	Drug development
Phase IV clinical trials	• Postmarketing studies to monitor long-term safety and effectiveness in the general population • Focuses on specific subgroups (e.g., children and elderly) and rare adverse events • May involve large-scale observational studies or additional randomized trials	• Postmarketing studies to monitor long-term safety, effectiveness, and adverse effects in the general population • Focuses on specific subgroups and rare adverse events • May involve additional randomized trials, observational studies, or registries
Postmarketing surveillance	• Continuous monitoring for adverse events through national and international surveillance systems (e.g., VAERS) • Pharmacovigilance activities ensure ongoing safety and effectiveness • Potential for vaccine updates or recalls based on new data	• Continuous monitoring for adverse events through pharmacovigilance systems (e.g., MedWatch) • Monitoring includes reporting from healthcare providers, patients, and manufacturers • Potential for drug label updates, warnings, or recalls based on new safety data
Manufacturing and distribution	• Involves scaling up production, while maintaining consistency, quality, and stability across large batches • Requires cold chain logistics for distribution to maintain vaccine potency • Training healthcare workers for proper administration is critical	• Involves scaling up production while maintaining consistency, quality, and stability across large batches • Distribution logistics depend on the drug's formulation (e.g., oral and injectable) and stability • May require special training for healthcare providers, especially for complex biologics
Adaptation and updates	• Vaccines may require updates or reformulations in response to new variants of a pathogen or emerging scientific data • Ongoing studies are essential to evaluate the effectiveness of new formulations or booster doses	• Drugs may require label updates, new formulations, or new indications based on emerging data • Ongoing research may lead to new therapeutic uses, dose adjustments, or safety warnings

(EMA: European Medicines Agency; FDA: Food and Drug Administration)

COMPARISON OF THE REGULATORY DIFFERENCES BETWEEN VACCINE DEVELOPMENT AND DRUG DEVELOPMENT PROCESSES ACROSS THE FDA (USA), EUROPEAN MEDICINES AGENCY, AND DCGI CDSCO (DRUGS CONTROLLER GENERAL OF INDIA AND CENTRAL DRUGS STANDARD CONTROL ORGANIZATION) FROM MOLECULE IDENTIFICATION THROUGH PHASE 4 CLINICAL TRIALS AND POSTMARKETING SURVEILLANCE (TABLE 3)[1-14]

While the regulatory frameworks for vaccine and drug development across the FDA, EMA, and DCGI CDSCO are similar in structure, the key differences lie in the scale and focus of trials, especially in the later phases. Vaccines undergo more extensive testing for immunogenicity and are subject to rigorous postmarketing surveillance due to their public health impact. Drug development, while also stringent, is more focused on efficacy in treating specific conditions, with some flexibility in trial designs based on the therapeutic area and population. The timelines and specific requirements may vary across regions, but the core principles of safety, efficacy, and quality are universally maintained.

TABLE 3: Comparison of the regulatory differences.

Aspect	Vaccine development (FDA, USA)	Vaccine development (DCGI CDSCO, India)	Drug development (FDA, USA)	Drug development (EMA, Europe)	Drug development (DCGI CDSCO, India)
Regulatory authority	• Regulated by the Center for Biologics Evaluation and Research (CBER) under the FDA • Oversees all aspects of vaccine development, including preclinical and clinical trials, licensing, and postmarketing surveillance	• Regulated by the Central Drugs Standard Control Organization (CDSCO) under the Ministry of Health and Family Welfare • The office of DCGI oversees the approval and regulation of vaccines in India	• Regulated by the Center for Drug Evaluation and Research (CDER) under the FDA • Handles small molecule drugs, biologics (under CBER), and ensures drug safety and efficacy	Regulated by the EMA's CHMP for centralized approval across EU member states	• Regulated by CDSCO under the office of DCGI • Manages approval, regulation, and postmarketing surveillance of pharmaceuticals
Preclinical requirements	• Extensive requirements for animal studies focusing on safety, immunogenicity, and efficacy • FDA may require studies in multiple animal models to predict human response	• CDSCO mandates preclinical studies in at least two species, including nonhuman primates, especially for new vaccine platforms • Requires local studies even if global data is available	• FDA requires preclinical studies focusing on toxicity, pharmacokinetics/pharmacodynamics (PK/PD), and efficacy • Includes detailed carcinogenicity and reproductive toxicity studies	EMA's preclinical requirements are aligned with ICH guidelines but may allow more flexibility in study design depending on the drug's nature	• CDSCO requires local preclinical studies for novel drugs, with an emphasis on toxicology and PK/PD • Global data can be supplemented with local studies for approval
Clinical trial approval process	• Requires an Investigational New Drug (IND) application for starting clinical trials • IND review includes preclinical data, manufacturing information, and trial protocols	• Requires a Clinical Trial Permission (CTP) from DCGI • Also requires ethics committee approval and registration with the Clinical Trials Registry-India (CTRI)	• IND application required for drug trials • Includes detailed protocols, preclinical data, and manufacturing details	CTA process is similar to vaccines but may vary slightly based on the drug's nature	• Similar to vaccines, a CTP from DCGI and ethics committee approval are required before trials • Registration with CTRI is mandatory
Phase I clinical trials	• Conducted under stringent safety protocols with emphasis on immunogenicity and dosage • Focus on first-in-human safety data and immunogenicity profiles	• CDSCO requires local phase I trials even if global data is available • Trials focus on safety, immunogenicity, and dose selection	• Focus on safety, tolerability, and PK/PD • May include healthy volunteers or patients depending on the drug's indication	• Phase I trials must adhere to EMA's Good Clinical Practice (GCP) guidelines • Focus on safety and PK/PD data	• Local phase I trials are mandatory unless an exemption is granted based on existing global data • Focus on safety and PK/PD in Indian populations

Continued

Continued

Aspect	Vaccine development (FDA, USA)	Vaccine development (DCGI CDSCO, India)	Drug development (FDA, USA)	Drug development (EMA, Europe)	Drug development (DCGI CDSCO, India)
Clinical trial regulations	• Must adhere to the FDA's regulations on Good Clinical Practice (GCP) • Trials must be registered on ClinicalTrials.gov.	• Must comply with Indian GCP guidelines and Schedule Y of the Drugs and Cosmetics Act • Mandatory registration on CTRI	Must follow FDA regulations on GCP and be registered on ClinicalTrials.gov.	• Compliance with CTR and GCP guidelines is mandatory • Trials must be registered on EudraCT	• Must follow Indian GCP guidelines and Schedule Y of the Drugs and Cosmetics Act • Registration on CTRI is mandatory
Vaccine-specific regulatory requirements	• FDA has specific guidelines for vaccine potency, safety, and efficacy, particularly for adjuvanted and live-attenuated vaccines • Requires stability studies to ensure vaccine viability throughout its shelf life	• CDSCO has strict guidelines for vaccine trials, focusing on immunogenicity, population diversity, and safety, especially in the pediatric population • Local clinical trials are often required even if global data is available	• Drug-specific guidelines focus on therapeutic efficacy and safety • FDA has specific pathways for orphan drugs, generics, and biosimilars	EMA has specific guidelines for different drug classes, including biosimilars, generics, and orphan drugs	CDSCO requires adherence to local guidelines for drug approval, including biosimilars and generics, with a focus on local trials
Fast-track and conditional approvals	• Vaccines can receive Fast Track, Breakthrough Therapy, or Emergency Use Authorization (EUA) during public health emergencies • Postmarketing commitments are required under EUA	• DCGI can grant Accelerated Approval or EUA for vaccines, particularly during public health emergencies • Conditional approvals often come with postmarketing study requirements	• Drugs may qualify for Fast Track, Breakthrough Therapy, Priority Review, or Accelerated Approval • Conditional approvals often require additional postmarketing studies	Similar expedited pathways available, including Conditional Marketing Authorization and Accelerated Assessment	Accelerated Approval can be granted for drugs, particularly those addressing unmet medical needs, with mandatory postapproval studies
Postmarketing surveillance	• FDA requires ongoing surveillance via Vaccine Adverse Event Reporting System (VAERS) and additional postmarketing studies (Phase IV) • Periodic Safety Update Reports (PSURs) are mandatory	• CDSCO requires extensive postmarketing surveillance through the Pharmacovigilance Programme of India (PvPI) • Mandatory submission of PSURs and may require additional local phase IV studies	• Ongoing safety monitoring via MedWatch and other pharmaco-vigilance systems • PSURs are required to monitor long-term safety	• EMA requires ongoing pharmaco-vigilance via EudraVigilance and RMPs • PSURs must be submitted regularly	CDSCO mandates postmarketing surveillance through PvPI, including PSUR submissions and may require local postmarketing studies

Continued

Continued

Aspect	Vaccine development (FDA, USA)	Vaccine development (DCGI CDSCO, India)	Drug development (FDA, USA)	Drug development (EMA, Europe)	Drug development (DCGI CDSCO, India)
Ethical review and approval	• Requires IRB review and approval in line with the FDA's regulations on human subject protection • Focuses on informed consent, especially for vulnerable populations like children	• Requires approval from an ethics committee registered with CDSCO • Strict guidelines on informed consent, especially in vulnerable populations • Additional oversight by the Indian Council of Medical Research (ICMR) in some cases	• Requires IRB approval following FDA regulations • Emphasis on informed consent and protection of vulnerable subjects	Ethical approval is mandatory across member states, with a strong focus on informed consent and patient safety	• Ethics committee approval is required, with strict guidelines on informed consent and protection of vulnerable populations • ICMR may provide additional guidelines and oversight
Indigenous vaccine/drug development	The FDA encourages the development of vaccines for specific populations or rare diseases through incentives like the Orphan Drug Designation				

(DCGI CDSCO: Drugs Controller General of India and Central Drugs Standard Control Organization; EMA: European Medicines Agency; FDA: Food and Drug Administration; IRB: Institutional Review Board)

COMPARISON OF THE VACCINE DEVELOPMENT PROCESS BEFORE AND AFTER THE COVID-19 PANDEMIC, HIGHLIGHTING THE CHANGES IN REGULATORY PROCESSES AS PER THE US FDA, EUROPEAN EMA, AND INDIAN DCGI CDSCO

The COVID-19 pandemic led to a paradigm shift in vaccine development, with regulatory processes becoming more flexible, collaborative, and focused on speed without compromising safety. The introduction of emergency use authorizations, rolling reviews, and parallel trial phases allowed for the rapid development and deployment of vaccines globally, a stark contrast to the lengthy and sequential processes seen before the pandemic. Enhanced surveillance systems postapproval further ensured the ongoing safety and efficacy of vaccines in real-world settings **(Tables 4 and 5)**.[1-15]

TABLE 4: Comparison of the vaccine development process before and after the COVID-19 pandemic.

Aspect	Pre-COVID vaccine development (FDA, USA)	Post-COVID vaccine development (FDA, USA)	Pre-COVID vaccine development (EMA, Europe)	Post-COVID vaccine development (EMA, Europe)	Pre-COVID vaccine development (DCGI CDSCO, India)	Post-COVID vaccine development (DCGI CDSCO, India)
Timeline for development	• Typically took 10–15 years from discovery to licensure • Includes preclinical research, several clinical trials phases, and regulatory review	• Condensed timeline: 12–24 months due to emergency measures • Parallel phases and rolling reviews adopted	• Similar 10–15 years for full development • Emphasis on comprehensive clinical data before approval	• Condensed timeline: 12–24 months or even shorter • Rolling reviews and accelerated assessments were key	• Similar 10–15 years, including mandatory local trials • Regulatory and ethical approvals were sequential and often lengthy	• Accelerated timeline of 12–24 months or less • Regulatory reviews were expedited, and trials were conducted in parallel
Regulatory pathways	• Standard pathway via Biologics License Application (BLA) • Emergency Use Authorization (EUA) was rarely used	• EUA became a critical tool for rapid deployment • BLA still required but could be submitted after initial EUA	• Standard Marketing Authorization Application (MAA) process • Conditional Marketing Authorizations (CMA) were used but less frequently	• CMAs and rolling reviews were heavily utilized • EMA developed specific COVID-19 guidance for vaccine approval	• Standard New Drug Application (NDA) or BLA • Emergency authorizations were uncommon	• EUA became central • Expedited review processes and conditional approvals were implemented
Clinical trial phases	• Sequential phases (I, II, and III) with significant gaps between phases • Phase IV conducted postlicensure	• Phases were often overlapped or combined (e.g., phase I/II, II/III) • Post-EUA phase IV commitments were common	• Sequential clinical trials with comprehensive data required before progressing to the next phase • Phase IV as postmarketing	• Parallel phase trials with overlapping phases to accelerate development • Postapproval phase IV studies were mandatory	• Sequential phases with mandatory local trials • Often long intervals between phases due to regulatory and ethical reviews	• Combined and overlapping trial phases • Regulatory and ethical approvals were fast-tracked, with post-EUA phase IV studies being critical
Manufacturing scale-up	• Scale-up typically began after phase III results were positive • Manufacturing was done at risk but was slower	• Manufacturing scale-up began during early clinical trials to ensure rapid deployment postapproval • Risk of early scale-up was high but necessary	• Manufacturing scale-up followed successful phase III trials • Limited at-risk manufacturing unless there was strong evidence of success	• Large-scale manufacturing began in parallel with late-phase trials • Public–private partnerships were key to funding at-risk production	• Scale-up was often slow and began post-phase III • Reliance on established manufacturing facilities, which could delay rollout	• Manufacturing began in parallel with early-phase trials • Government support and private sector involvement were critical in rapid scale-up

Continued

Continued

Aspect	Pre-COVID vaccine development (FDA, USA)	Post-COVID vaccine development (FDA, USA)	Pre-COVID vaccine development (EMA, Europe)	Post-COVID vaccine development (EMA, Europe)	Pre-COVID vaccine development (DCGI CDSCO, India)	Post-COVID vaccine development (DCGI CDSCO, India)
Safety and efficacy data	• Extensive safety and efficacy data were required before licensure • Long-term follow-up was standard	• Short-term data were accepted under EUA, with long-term follow-up required postapproval • Real-world evidence became critical	• Robust safety and efficacy data were mandatory before approval • Long-term data collection was a key requirement	• Acceptance of interim data for emergency approvals with ongoing studies to confirm long-term efficacy and safety • Real-world data collection was essential	• Long-term safety and efficacy data were required before approval • Strict local trial requirements delayed the process	• Short-term data were accepted for emergency approvals, with a requirement for long-term follow-up • Real-world evidence was emphasized postapproval
Regulatory review process	• Standard review timelines were 10–12 months for a BLA • Priority review could shorten this to 6 months	• Rolling submissions allowed for ongoing data review • EUA reviews were conducted in weeks to months, depending on urgency	• Standard review timelines were 210 days for an MAA • Accelerated review available but not commonly used	• Rolling reviews and conditional approvals allowed for much faster decision-making • Reviews were often completed within 3–6 months	• Standard review timelines were often long, with additional delays for local data requirements • Priority reviews were rare	• Rolling reviews and accelerated approval processes were implemented • Reviews could be completed in a few weeks to a few months
Emergency use provisions	• EUA was rarely invoked and typically used only for rare, high-risk situations • Focus was on ensuring long-term safety	• EUA became central to the vaccine rollout strategy • Allowed deployment based on interim data, with ongoing data collection and monitoring	• Conditional approvals were used infrequently, mostly for urgent cases or unmet needs • Extensive preapproval data were still required	• CMA and rolling reviews were widely used • Allowed for rapid deployment while additional data were collected	• Emergency approvals were rare and typically required extensive local data even in emergencies • Local trials were mandatory	• EUA became a primary tool • Conditional approvals were granted with ongoing data collection and real-world evidence requirements
Postmarketing surveillance	• Standard postmarketing surveillance (phase IV) with VAERS and PSURs • Focus on long-term safety and rare adverse events	• Enhanced surveillance with extensive real-world data collection • Active monitoring for adverse events through VAERS, PSURs, and additional real-world evidence	• Standard phase IV surveillance, focusing on safety and efficacy in larger populations • Routine PSUR submissions	• Expanded postmarketing surveillance with a strong focus on rare adverse events and real-world evidence • Enhanced pharmacovigilance systems were employed	• Standard postmarketing surveillance focusing on safety in the local population • Phase IV studies were often required	• Intensive postmarketing surveillance, including additional studies and real-world evidence collection • Enhanced safety monitoring through the Pharmacovigilance Programme of India (PvPI)

Continued

Continued

Aspect	Pre-COVID vaccine development (FDA, USA)	Post-COVID vaccine development (FDA, USA)	Pre-COVID vaccine development (EMA, Europe)	Post-COVID vaccine development (EMA, Europe)	Pre-COVID vaccine development (DCGI CDSCO, India)	Post-COVID vaccine development (DCGI CDSCO, India)
Public–private partnerships	Limited to large-scale government contracts and established global health initiatives (e.g., Gavi, WHO)	• Extensive use of public–private partnerships to fund research, development, and manufacturing • Operation Warp Speed in the US is an example	• Public–private partnerships existed but were less critical in vaccine development • Funding primarily from EU institutions or pharmaceutical companies	• Public–private partnerships were central to the rapid development and distribution of COVID-19 vaccines • EMA facilitated cooperation between industry, academia, and governments	• Public-private partnerships were limited, with most funding coming from government and international bodies • Scale and speed were challenges	• Strong emphasis on public–private partnerships to accelerate development • Government incentives and international collaboration were crucial
Global collaboration	• International collaboration was primarily through WHO, Gavi, and similar organizations • Collaboration was slower and less coordinated	• Unprecedented global collaboration with initiatives such as COVAX, CEPI, and WHO • Regulatory agencies worked together to harmonize guidelines and accelerate approvals	• EMA participated in global initiatives but focused on the European context • Collaboration with WHO and global bodies was important but less central	• EMA played a key role in global collaboration for COVID-19 vaccines • Active participation in COVAX, CEPI, and coordination with WHO	• Limited international collaboration, with a strong focus on local trials and approvals • Participation in global health initiatives but with slower uptake	• Active participation in global initiatives like COVAX • Collaboration with international regulatory bodies to align guidelines and expedite approval
Ethical and regulatory oversight	• Ethical approvals were strict, with a focus on long-term safety and informed consent • Regulatory oversight was sequential and thorough	• Ethical guidelines were adapted for rapid deployment but maintained strict oversight • Informed consent processes were streamlined, with enhanced regulatory oversight	• Standard ethical review processes with an emphasis on patient safety and informed consent • Reviews were conducted in sequence with thorough oversight	• Ethical and regulatory processes were streamlined without compromising safety • Adaptive trial designs and rolling reviews required enhanced ethical oversight	• Standard ethical reviews often caused delays due to mandatory local trials and additional approvals • Strict oversight with a focus on local conditions	• Ethical reviews were expedited, with ongoing oversight to ensure safety and consent • Stremlined process may be implemented

(CEPI: Coalition for Epidemic Preparedness Innovations; DCGI CDSCO: Drugs Controller General of India and Central Drugs Standard Control Organization; EMA: European Medicines Agency; EU: European Union; FDA: Food and Drug Administration; PSURs: Periodic Safety Update Reports; WHO: World Health Organization)

TABLE 5: Various vaccines developed in the USA, Europe, and India over the last one decade.

Vaccine	Country/Region	Disease targeted	Development timeline	Development start	Approval year	Notes
Gardasil 9	USA (Merck)	Human papillomavirus (HPV)	~12 years	Early 2000s	2014	Expanded from original Gardasil to cover 9 HPV types
Cervarix	Europe (GlaxoSmithKline)	HPV	~10 years	Early 2000s	2007	Focused on HPV types 16 and 18
Rotarix	Europe (GlaxoSmithKline)	Rotavirus	~9 years	Late 1990s	2006	Oral vaccine for rotavirus infections
RotaTeq	USA (Merck)	Rotavirus	~15 years	Late 1980s	2006	Another oral vaccine, underwent extensive clinical trials
Prevnar 13	USA (Pfizer)	Pneumococcal disease	~10 years	Late 1990s	2010	Covers 13 strains of *Streptococcus pneumoniae*
MenAfriVac	India (Serum Institute of India)	Meningitis A	~5 years	2004	2010	Developed specifically for use in African meningitis belt, fast-tracked development
Shingrix	USA/Europe (GlaxoSmithKline)	Herpes zoster (Shingles)	~10 years	2005	2017	Adjuvanted recombinant subunit vaccine for shingles
Covaxin	India (Bharat Biotech)	COVID-19	~1 year	Early 2020	2021	Inactivated virus vaccine, developed under emergency conditions
Comirnaty (Pfizer-BioNTech)	USA/Europe (Pfizer-BioNTech)	COVID-19	~1 year	Early 2020	2020	mRNA vaccine, one of the first COVID-19 vaccines to be approved
Vaxzevria (AstraZeneca)	Europe/India (AstraZeneca/ Serum Institute of India)	COVID-19	~1 year	Early 2020	2021 (in India as Covishield)	Viral vector vaccine, widespread global use. Developed in collaboration with Oxford University
Sputnik V	Russia/India (Gamaleya Institute)	COVID-19	~1 year	Early 2020	2021 (in India)	First approved in Russia, later rolled out in other countries including India
BCG revaccination	India (Serum Institute of India)	Tuberculosis (TB)	~8 years	2008	2016	Revaccination program for TB, not a new vaccine but a revised application in TB-endemic areas

DNA VACCINE DEVELOPMENT IN INDIA

DNA vaccine development in India has been an exciting area of progress, especially given the innovative approaches and potential for rapid development and deployment. Here is an overview of DNA vaccine development in India.

ZyCoV-D

- *Developer*: Cadila Healthcare
- *Disease targeted*: COVID-19
- *Technology*: DNA vaccine
- *Details*:
    - *Description*: ZyCoV-D is a needle-free DNA vaccine that uses plasmid DNA to induce an immune response against the SARS-CoV-2 virus. The vaccine's DNA plasmids encode for the spike protein of the virus, prompting the body to generate an immune response.
    - *Administration*: It is delivered using a needle-free device known as the "PharmaJet," which uses a high-pressure stream to inject the vaccine.
    - *Clinical trials*: ZyCoV-D has undergone multiple phases of clinical trials to assess its safety, efficacy, and immunogenicity.

- *Approval*: It received emergency use authorization from the Drugs Controller General of India (DCGI) in August 2021, making it one of the first DNA vaccines to be approved for COVID-19.
- *Impact*: It is noted for its potential for rapid development and scalability, offering a promising tool for vaccination against emerging infectious diseases.

Other DNA Vaccine Research

- *Ongoing research*: Besides ZyCoV-D, there are other ongoing research and development efforts in India focused on DNA vaccines for various diseases, including cancer and other infectious diseases. These efforts are often in preclinical or early clinical stages.
- *Collaborations*: Indian research institutions and companies are collaborating with international partners to explore DNA vaccine technology for a range of applications, leveraging advancements in genomics and biotechnology.

Advantages of DNA Vaccines

- *Rapid development*: DNA vaccines can be developed quickly once the genetic sequence of the pathogen is known, which is beneficial in responding to emerging infectious diseases.
- *Stability*: DNA vaccines are generally more stable than some other types of vaccines, reducing the need for stringent cold chain requirements.
- *Scalability*: They can be produced in large quantities using established plasmid production techniques.

Challenges:

- *Delivery*: Effective delivery of DNA vaccines can be challenging, although needle-free devices like the PharmaJet are addressing this issue.
- *Regulatory approval*: Navigating regulatory pathways for new vaccine technologies can be complex, requiring extensive clinical data and safety evaluations.

UTILIZATION OF ARTIFICIAL INTELLIGENCE AND DIGITAL TECHNOLOGY IN VACCINE DEVELOPMENT AS PER FDA (USA), EMA (EUROPE), AND DCGI CDSCO (INDIA) FROM MOLECULE IDENTIFICATION TO VACCINE AVAILABILITY

The integration of artificial intelligence (AI) and digital technology in vaccine development has transformed the process from molecule identification to postmarketing surveillance. The **FDA (USA), EMA (Europe), and DCGI CDSCO (India)** have all embraced AI to varying degrees, leading to more efficient vaccine development, regulatory review, and distribution. AI has particularly enhanced the speed and accuracy of preclinical testing, clinical trial management, and postmarketing surveillance. While the adoption is more advanced in the US and Europe, India is rapidly incorporating these technologies to improve its vaccine development and regulatory processes **(Table 6)**.[1-16]

TABLE 6: Utilization of artificial intelligence (AI) and digital technology in vaccine development.

Stage	FDA (USA)	EMA (Europe)	DCGI CDSCO (India)
Molecule identification	• *AI in drug discovery*: FDA supports the use of AI/ML in identifying vaccine candidates • *Guidance*: Limited specific guidance, but AI is subject to general drug development regulations	• *AI in discovery*: EMA recognizes AI's role in identifying antigens and molecules • *Guidance*: EMA provides frameworks for AI use in medicinal product development	• *AI in discovery*: DCGI CDSCO acknowledges AI's potential but lacks specific guidelines • *Policy*: Regulatory framework is evolving to include AI in drug and vaccine discovery
Preclinical studies	• *Digital simulations*: FDA encourages the use of digital models for preclinical testing under strict validation standards • *Regulations*: Must comply with GLP (Good Laboratory Practice)	• *Virtual modeling*: EMA supports the use of AI for predictive modeling in preclinical studies • *Compliance*: Models must be validated under EU regulations	• *Preclinical AI*: Limited specific guidance, but AI tools can be used if validated • *Regulatory expectations*: Must follow national preclinical testing regulations

Continued

Continued

Stage	FDA (USA)	EMA (Europe)	DCGI CDSCO (India)
Clinical trial design	• *AI in trial design*: FDA allows AI to optimize trial design, including patient recruitment • *Digital tech*: FDA's Digital Health Innovation Action Plan supports AI in clinical trials	• *AI in design*: EMA supports AI in optimizing trial protocols and predictive analytics for trial outcomes • *Digital innovations*: EMA has issued guidelines on the integration of digital technologies in trials	• *AI and digital tech*: DCGI CDSCO is beginning to incorporate AI in trial designs; however, specific regulations are still under development • *Guidance*: Follows ICH GCP guidelines with AI tools being supplementary
Clinical trial conduct	• *Remote monitoring*: FDA permits digital health tools for remote patient monitoring and data collection • *eSource data*: FDA accepts electronically sourced data if compliant with 21 CFR Part 11	• *Digital tools*: EMA supports digital tools in patient monitoring and data collection, provided they adhere to data integrity and security standards • *Remote trials*: EMA has issued guidance on decentralized trials	• *AI and remote tools*: Growing acceptance of digital tools for remote monitoring; however, specific AI regulations are evolving • *Data integrity*: Requires adherence to local data protection laws and trial guidelines
Data analysis	• *AI in analysis*: FDA supports AI/ML algorithms for analyzing clinical trial data but insists on transparency and explainability • *Validation*: Algorithms must be validated according to regulatory standards	• *AI-driven analytics*: EMA allows the use of AI for data analysis in clinical trials, with strict validation and traceability requirements • *Guidance*: EMA provides detailed guidelines on the validation of AI tools	• *AI in data processing*: DCGI CDSCO recognizes AI in data analysis but requires clear validation and adherence to regulatory standards • *Guidance*: Under development, with an emphasis on validation and transparency
Regulatory submission	• *eSubmissions*: FDA encourages the use of AI tools for preparing regulatory submissions via eCTD (Electronic Common Technical Document) • *Regulatory framework*: AI-generated data must meet existing regulatory submission standards	• *Digital submissions*: EMA accepts eCTD submissions, including AI-generated analysis, if compliant with EU regulations • *Guidance*: EMA requires clear documentation of AI use in regulatory submissions	• *Digital submissions*: DCGI CDSCO is adapting to eCTD submissions, including AI data; however, guidelines are in the process of being fully established • *Regulatory process*: Focus on validation and compliance with local standards
Manufacturing process	• *AI in manufacturing*: FDA supports AI in manufacturing for process optimization and quality control, under cGMP (Current Good Manufacturing Practice) • *Regulations*: Requires AI tools to be validated and integrated into quality systems	• *AI in production*: EMA allows AI in manufacturing processes, especially in real-time monitoring and predictive maintenance • *Regulatory compliance*: Must adhere to EU GMP standards and be validated	• *AI in manufacturing*: DCGI CDSCO is beginning to incorporate AI into manufacturing, with guidelines in development • *Compliance*: AI tools must be validated according to Indian GMP standards
Postmarketing surveillance	• *AI in pharmacovigilance*: FDA encourages the use of AI for signal detection in postmarket surveillance • *Digital monitoring*: FDA supports real-time digital monitoring tools for adverse event reporting	• *AI in vigilance*: EMA supports AI in pharmacovigilance for automating signal detection and adverse event reporting • *Guidance*: Detailed guidelines on AI use in postmarket safety monitoring	• *AI in surveillance*: DCGI CDSCO is exploring AI in pharmacovigilance, focusing on automated signal detection and reporting • *Framework*: Guidelines are evolving, with an emphasis on AI validation and transparency

Continued

Continued

Stage	FDA (USA)	EMA (Europe)	DCGI CDSCO (India)
Vaccine distribution and access	• *Digital supply chains*: FDA supports digital tools and AI in optimizing vaccine distribution, ensuring cold chain integrity, and monitoring distribution • *AI applications*: AI used for predictive analytics in distribution planning	• *AI in logistics*: EMA supports the use of AI and digital tools for vaccine distribution, focusing on supply chain optimization and real-time monitoring • *Regulatory standards*: Requires adherence to EU regulations on cold chain and distribution integrity	• *AI in distribution*: DCGI CDSCO is adopting digital technologies and AI for vaccine distribution, especially for ensuring cold chain integrity • *Implementation*: Guidelines are being developed to integrate AI into national immunization programs

(AI: artificial intelligence; DCGI CDSCO: Drugs Controller General of India and Central Drugs Standard Control Organization; EMA: European Medicines Agency; EU: European Union; FDA: Food and Drug Administration; ML: machine learning)

CONCLUSION

Vaccine development is an important aspect of public health strategy for prevention of diseases. Complete process is expedited during COVID era for drug and vaccine development and same need to be gold standard for future vaccine development. Emergency use authorization of vaccine is the newer provisions under the law being utilized in emergency situations for early roll out of the vaccine for public health. Vaccine development process is as per International and National guidelines and regulations so as to be available all resource-poor as well as resource-rich settings. Newer technology-based mRNA and DNA-based vaccines are being developed. AI will reduce the time period further from molecule identification to animal studies to various phases of vaccine trials.

REFERENCES

1. FDA (United States)

1. U.S. Food and Drug Administration. 21st Century Cures Act. Pub. L. No. 114-255, 130 Stat. 1033. 2016.
2. U.S. Food and Drug Administration. (2020). Emergency Use Authorization for Vaccines to Prevent COVID-19. [online] Available from https://www.fda.gov/media/144673/download [Last accessed March, 2025].
3. U.S. Food and Drug Administration. (2020). Guidance for Industry: Development and Licensure of Vaccines to Prevent COVID-19. [online] Available from https://www.fda.gov/media/139638/download [Last accessed March, 2025].
4. U.S. Food and Drug Administration. Vaccines and Related Biological Products Advisory Committee (VRBPAC) Guidance Updates. [online] Available from https://www.fda.gov/advisory-committees/advisory-committee-calendar [Last accessed March, 2025].

2. EMA (European Medicines Agency)

5. European Medicines Agency. (2004). Regulation (EC) No 726/2004 of the European Parliament and of the Council. [online] Available from: https://eur-lex.europa.eu/legal-content/EN/TXT/?uri=CELEX%3A32004R0726 [Last accessed March, 2025].
6. European Medicines Agency. (2020). Guideline on the Clinical Development of Vaccines Intended to Provide Protection against COVID-19. [online] Available from https://www.ema.europa.eu/en/documents/scientific-guideline/guideline-clinical-development-vaccines-intended-provide-protection-against-covid-19_en.pdf [Last accessed March, 2025].
7. European Medicines Agency. (2020). Good Manufacturing Practice (GMP) for COVID-19 Vaccines. [online] Available from https://www.ema.europa.eu/en/documents/scientific-guideline/gmp-guidance-covid-19-vaccines_en.pdf [Last accessed March, 2025].
8. European Medicines Agency. COVID-19 Vaccine Assessment Reports. [online] Available from https://www.ema.europa.eu/en/medicines/human/EPAR [Last accessed March, 2025].

3. DCGI CDSCO (India)

9. Government of India. Drugs and Cosmetics Act, 1940 & Rules, 1945. [online] Available from http://www.cdsco.gov.in/ [Last accessed March, 2025].
10. Central Drugs Standard Control Organization. Guidelines for Evaluation of COVID-19 Vaccines. 2020 [online] Available from https://cdsco.gov.in/opencms/opencms/en/Guidelines/COVID-19/ [Last accessed March, 2025].
11. Central Drugs Standard Control Organization. (2020). Standard Operating Procedures for COVID-19 Vaccines Approval and Monitoring. [online] Available from https://cdsco.gov.in/opencms/opencms/en/Guidelines/COVID-19/ [Last accessed March, 2025].
12. New Drugs & Clinical Trial Rules, 2019. [online] Available from https://cdsco.gov.in/opencms/opencms/system/modules/CDSCO.WEB/elements/download_file_division.jsp?num_id=OTI4MA== [Last accessed March, 2025].
13. ICMR. (2017). National Ethical Guidelines for Biomedical and Health Research Involving Human Participants. [online] Available

from https://ethics.ncdirindia.org/asset/pdf/ICMR_National_Ethical_Guidelines.pdf [Last accessed march, 2025].

14. ICMR. (2017). National Ethical Guidelines for Biomedical Research Involving Children. [online] Available from https://main.icmr.nic.in/sites/default/files/guidelines/National_Ethical_Guidelines_for_BioMedical_Research_Involving_Children_0.pdf [Last accessed march, 2025].
15. ICMR. (2020). National Guidelines for Ethics Committees Reviewing Biomedical & Health Research During Covid-19 Pandemic. [online] Available from https://ethics.ncdirindia.org//asset/pdf/EC_Guidance_COVID19.pdf [Last accessed march, 2025].
16. ICMR. (2023). Ethical Guidelines for Application of Artificial Intelligence in Biomedical Research and Healthcare. [online] Available from https://ethics.ncdirindia.org//asset/pdf/Ethical_Guidelines_Application_Artificial_Intelligence_Biomed_Rsrch.pdf [Last accessed march, 2025].

Index

Page numbers followed by *f* refer to figure, *fc* refer to flowchart, and *t* refer to table.

U

V

W

Y

Z